Eduardo Anitua • Ramón Cugat
Mikel Sánchez
Editors

Platelet Rich Plasma in Orthopaedics and Sports Medicine

Springer

Editors
Eduardo Anitua
Director of the University Institute
for Regenerative Medicine and Oral
Implantology (UIRMI) from the University
of Basque Country (UPV/EHU)
Vitoria, Spain

Mikel Sánchez
Arthroscopic Surgery Unit
Hospital Vithas San José
Vitoria, Spain

Ramón Cugat
Hospital Quirón
Artroscopia GC
Barcelona, Spain

ISBN 978-3-030-09702-8 ISBN 978-3-319-63730-3 (eBook)
https://doi.org/10.1007/978-3-319-63730-3

Printed on acid-free paper

This Springer imprint is published by the registered company Springer International Publishing AG part of Springer Nature.
The registered company address is: Gewerbestrasse 11, 6330 Cham, Switzerland

EDITORS

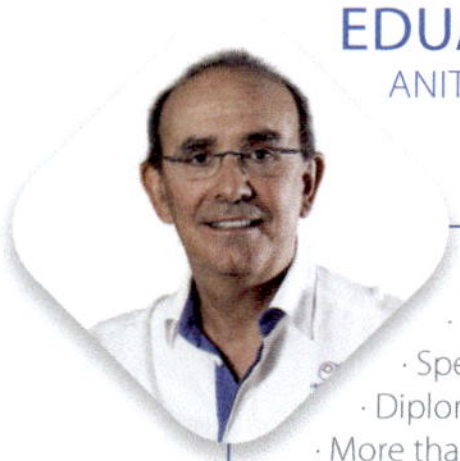

EDUARDO ANITUA

Director of the University Institute for Regenerative Medicine and Oral Implantology (UIRMI) from the University of Basque Country (UPV/EHU).
Director of the Eduardo Anitua Institute for Basic and Clinical Research.
Scientific Director of BTI Biotechnology Institute.
President of the Eduardo Anitua Foundation for biomedical research.

- Degree in General Medicine and Surgery from the University of Salamanca (1979).
- PhD in Medicine from the University of Valencia.
- Specialist in Stomatology from the University of Basque Country (UPV/EHU) (1982).
- Diploma in Prosthodontics and Occlusion from the Pankey Institute (Florida, USA).
- More than 300 papers published in national and international journals.
- Author of 14 books and co-author of 7 books and chapters, being translated languages.
- 46 international patents in the fields of regenerative therapy and implant dentistry.
- Director of the programme "Continuing Education on Oral Implantology and Rehabilitation" given in Spain and various other countries for the last 25 years.
- More than 600 courses and conferences around the world on Tissue Regeneration, Implantology, Prosthodontics and Aesthetic Dentistry.

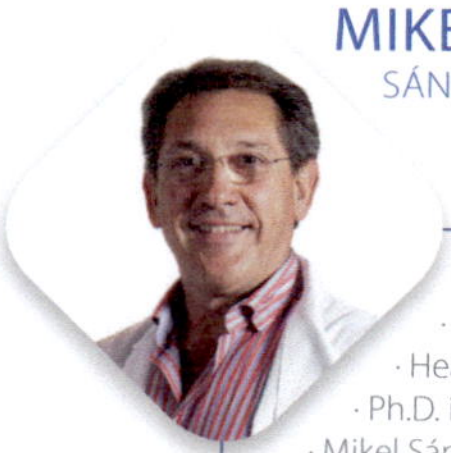

MIKEL SÁNCHEZ

Medical and Scientific Director of the Arthroscopic Surgery Unit (UCA), Hospital Vithas San José.

- Degree in Medicine and Surgery from the University of Bordeaux, France (1978).
- Specialized in Traumatology and Orthopedics at the University of the Basque Country, Spain. (1984).
- Head of the Arthroscopic Surgery Unit (UCA), Vitoria-Gasteiz, Spain (1995)
- Ph.D. in Medicine by the University of the Basque Country,, Spain (2017).
- Mikel Sánchez has been one of the pioneers in the advance of Arthroscopic Surgery in Spain.
- Part of Leeds-Keio teamwork (1986-1997), an Anglo-Japanese collaboration in order to boost developed prototypes of surgical equipment for the anterior and posterior cruciate ligament reconstruction and for the treatment of shoulder chronic instability.
- In 2000, he understood the therapeutic potential of PRP and its applications in traumatology.
- Since 2012 is a precursor in Spain of the use in surgery of 3D printing technology.
- Author of more than 250 national and international lectures, book chapters, international patents and more than 65 international scientific articles.

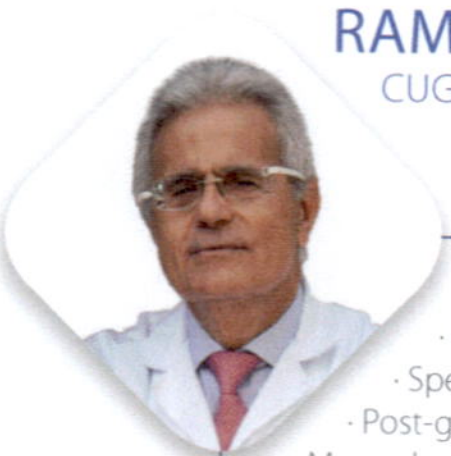

RAMÓN CUGAT

President of the Board of Trustees of the Garcia Cugat Foundation for Biomedical Research.
Director of the Garcia Cugat Foundation Chair at the CEU-Cardenal Herrera University on Regenerative Medicine and Surgery.
President of the medical council of the Catalonian Soccer Federation and member of medical staff of the Spanish Soccer Federation.
Co-Director of the Orthopaedic Surgical Department, Arthroscopia GC; an ISAKOS-Approved Teaching Center.

- Degree in Medicine and Surgery from the University of Barcelona (1975).
- PhD in Medicine from the University of Barcelona (1978).
- Specialist in Orthopaedic and Trauma surgery (1979).
- Post-graduate studies on Arthroscopy and Sports Medicine at Massachusetts General Hospital, Harvard Medical School Massachusetts-U.S.A.
- Associated Professor at the Medical School at Barcelona University and UIC.
- Active member of the Royal European Academy of Doctors.
- Member and honorary member of many national and international societies including ISAKOS, AAOS, AANA, ICRS, SLARD, ESSKA, AGA, SECOT, AEA, FEMEDE, HERODICUS SOCIETY, ASIAM PACIFIC INSTITUTE (Member of BOD) among others.
- Over 150 publications between specialised journal articles and book chapters.
- He has given lectures in congresses and collaborates in Teaching Courses of Arthroscopic Surgical Techniques and Sports Medicine around the world.

AUTHORS

ALAN NURDEN, PAQUITA NURDEN, EDUARDO ANITUA, SABINO PADILLA, FELIPE PROSPER, MIKEL SÁNCHEZ, VICTOR VAQUERIZO, RAMÓN CUGAT, JAMES H-C WANG, MATTHEW J. KRAEUTLER, FERNANDO KIRCHNER, STEVEN SAMPSON, ROBERTO PRADO, IONE PADILLA, BEATRIZ PELACHO, ANA PÉREZ, LAURA PIÑAS, MOHAMMAD HAMDAN ALKHRAISAT, NICOLÁS FIZ, ORLANDO POMPEI, JUAN AZOFRA, DIEGO DELGADO, PEIO SÁNCHEZ, MARÍA DEL MAR RUIZ DE CASTAÑEDA, XAVIER CUSCÓ, ROBERTO SEIJAS, DAVID BARASTEGUI, PEDRO ÁLVAREZ DÍAZ, EDUARD ALENTORN GELI, MARTA RIUS, GILBERT STEINBACHER, ESTHER SALA, JUAN BOFFA, SEBASTIÁN GROSSI, MONTSERRAT GARCÍA BALLETBÓ, SUE-SONIA TIZOL, PATRICIA LAIZ, MIGUEL MARÍN, XAVIER ÁLVAREZ, NIEVES LAMA, YIQIN ZHOU, XAVIER NIRMALA, TIGRAN GARABEKYAN, OMER MEI DAN, ANE GARATE, ANE MIREN BILBAO, BEATRIZ AIZPURUA, JORGE GUADILLA, HUNTER VINCENT, MARY AMBACH.

PROLOGUE

It is not routine to be asked to write the prologue to a book on a topic somewhat removed from one's area of expertise. In trying to justify my acceptance to do this prologue I certainly took into account my long friendship with Eduardo Anitua, but thinking about reasons to do it I thought that having only little more than a layman knowledge about platelet rich plasma would give me a more unbiased view of this controversial subject.

PRP and its relative, stem cells, have been for some years at the forefront of innovative therapies for many medical conditions, especially musculoskeletal affections. And, as it has happened many times before with new techniques or therapeutics, they have been embraced enthusiastically by many, unfortunately including entrepreneurs and even charlatans. This has led to indiscriminate use and even abuse of these therapies before clinical evidence of their value was obtained. And both industry and individuals have benefitted greatly when basically no or minimal information about their real effect was available.

But with the passage of time more information is accumulating on the real importance of these substances and their unquestionable value in the treatment of many conditions. For example, there are now systematic literature reviews of randomized and prospective studies showing that injections of PRP into osteoarthritic knees secure better functional outcomes at 6 months than placebo or hyaluronic acid injections, although no difference in pain or patient satisfaction was shown.

This book represents a compendium of the knowledge available today on Platelet-rich plasma preparations, their formulations, methods of production, mechanism of action, different effects, and their applications to musculoskeletal conditions. It represents an attempt to "drain the swamp" and to provide evidence-based information in a field where that is painfully scarce.

In 16 chapters the authors have provided abundant information on the basic science of Platelet-rich plasma preparations, the already classical applications of these formulations to orthopedic conditions, primarily joints, tendons and muscle injuries, the use in dentistry and oral surgery (so the book extends beyond the realm of sports medicine), but there are also chapters that address other less common applications, such as nerve injuries or low back pain. One may frown at these novel uses of PRP, or at its intraosseous use in knee osteoarthritis. I would reason that background science for their use in these conditions appears sound and it seems reasonable that it should be up to the "developers" to first explore with well-designed studies the limits of these therapies.

The book is attractively produced, nicely illustrated and represents the authors long experience with PRP. It should be read by anybody who intends to use or has been using PRP in clinical settings. It will be therefore a valuable asset for orthopedists, oral surgeons, sport medicine physicians and all those interested in musculoskeletal conditions. The editors and authors deserve congratulations and thanks from all those of us that will benefit from reading this text.

Miguel E Cabanela, MD, MS (Orth Surg)

Emeritus Professor of Orthopedic Surgery | College of Medicine
Consultant, Orthopedic Surgery | Mayo Clinic | Rochester, Minnesota, USA

INDEX

INTRODUCTION

The adventure of the plasma rich in growth factors began in 1995 as a result of questioning ourselves about what were the biological mechanisms involved in the regeneration of the post extraction socket. I was deeply concerned to understand why a patient who underwent a tooth extraction healed in a few days and the process for other patients was instead slow and painful. The key to this question was in the blood clot and so we began to investigate what would be the clot's optimal characteristics in order to make it extendable to all patients and thus achieve an optimal healing.

We began investigating ways of anti-coagulating the blood and how to reverse the coagulation cascade, and as we closed fronts, others were opened. What was the effective concentration of platelets? Would it make sense that the plasma we prepared had white blood cells? At this point, I have to thank the extraordinary collaboration with Drs. Nurden, with whom we at our foundation have been tireless collaborators during all these years. Throughout these 25 years, we have studied many of the biological repair processes using different cellular phenotypes. We have also defined the release kinetics of proteins from the fibrin matrix, a fundamental process to be able to understand the effect of these molecular signals at the injury site. A pioneering work published in 1999 on the use of an autologous PRP from small volumes of blood was the key in the development of this biological system.

Following the path of the evolution of mammals, where the tooth was first and then bone and vertebrae, in 2001 and with the extraordinary collaboration of Dr. Mikel Sánchez, we began to investigate the possibilities of clinical application in the area of Orthopedics and sports medicine.

Everything was uncertain, and in the arduous path of intuition to evidence, a great effort had to be made, both in the laboratory and in the surgical experimental room, performing innumerable surgeries in animals that would eventually derive the gold standard in orthobiology in the clinical protocols that are currently used worldwide.

Thanks to Mikel and all his team, this path has been exciting and so much so that a 2003 article appears as the first work on the application of a PRP in the area of orthopedics and sports medicine in the world literature.

They have been years of hope and passion, where everything was yet to be discovered. There was nothing written on this subject and therefore the canvas was blank, which made the project even more interesting at the same time as challenging.

I believe that we have provided a new biological approach to orthopedic surgery where other teams have contributed to consider PRP as an irreplaceable tool in the therapeutic arsenal of the orthopedic surgeon and sports doctor.

Thanks to the extraordinary collaboration of my good friends, Drs. Mikel Sánchez and Ramón Cugat, as well as of all the authors, we offer the reader the most up-to-date information on the use of plasma rich in growth factors in orthopedics and sports medicine.

I would like to also express my gratitude to Dr. Miguel Cabanela for the preparation of the prologue. I hope that the reader will enjoy and be passionate about this book as much as we all have enjoyed working on it.

Dr. Eduardo Anitua

CHAPTER 1
Platelets at the Interface between Inflammation and Tissue Repair

AUTHORS

Nurden A.T.[1], Nurden P.[1]

[1] Institut de Rhythmologie et de Modélisation Cardiaque, Plateforme Technologique d'Innovation Biomédicale, Hôpital Xavier Arnozan, Pessac, France

SUMMARY

Blood platelets are produced in large numbers from megakaryocytes in the bone marrow. Anucleate, their principal role is to prevent blood loss on vascular injury and to promote tissue repair, and for this they adhere, aggregate and secrete a wide variety of metabolites and biologically active proteins. The latter are stored in organelles that undergo exocytosis when platelets are stimulated. Activated platelets may also become procoagulant, participate in thrombin formation and help constitute a stable fibrin-based clot. They liberate microparticles (MPs) that act as drones participating in hemostatic and pathologic events far from the parent thrombus. Platelets are also major players in angiogenesis, innate and adaptive immunity and participate in inflammation and host defense. For this, they possess membrane glycoproteins that include receptors for leukocytes and store or synthetize a multitude of adhesive proteins, coagulation and fibrinolytic factors, growth factors, chemokines and cytokines, anti-microbial proteins, proteases and protease inhibitors. On secretion, these components are vital in promoting such events as stem cell recruitment, tissue cell migration and maturation, blood vessel development, and DNA-NET formation. At the same time, platelets and MPs intervene in the progression of major illnesses including cardiovascular disease (atherosclerosis and thrombosis), cancer (tumor cell diffusion and metastasis) and inflammatory diseases (e.g. rheumatoid arthritis) and sepsis. Enigmatically, they often secrete proteins that have opposing roles (e.g. pro- and anti-angiogenic proteins). The challenge is to decipher the roles of secreted proteins and to adapt these natural processes for the therapeutic use of platelet-derived therapies in injury and disease.

E. Anitua et al. (eds.), *Platelet Rich Plasma in Orthopaedics and Sports Medicine*,
https://doi.org/10.1007/978-3-319-63730-3_1

1. INTRODUCTION

Platelets are produced in vast numbers from megakaryocytes (MKs), a large multinucleate cell formed from hematopoietic stems cells (HSC) in a multistep process regulated by thrombopoietin (TPO) in the bone marrow. After initial mononuclear cell proliferation, MKs undergo polyploidy: when mature, they migrate to the endothelial barrier of the vascular sinus and extend long processes termed proplatelets into the blood stream (fig. 1)[1]. Platelets either bud off directly or proplatelets are released as large fragments that break up in the circulation, particularly in the lungs. Intermediate steps include the division of dumb-bell shaped preplatelets and even multiplication of platelets themselves[2]. Anucleate discoid platelets circulate in large numbers; the normal range is 150,000-400,000/μL of blood and their life span is 7 to 10 days. Their primary role is to assure hemostasis and to prevent bleeding (fig. 2). For this, they possess a unique range of receptors. For adhesion these include glycoprotein Ib (GPIb) that has matrix-bound von Willebrand factor (VWF) as ligand and GPVI that recognizes collagen, a major subendothelial matrix component. Platelet receptors for soluble agonists mostly belong to the seven transmembrane domain superfamily and include P2Y1 and P2Y12 that bind ADP while proteinase-activated receptor-1 (PAR-1) and PAR-4 coordinate the response to thrombin. A more complete list of surface receptors is found in figure 3. Multiple intracellular signaling pathways

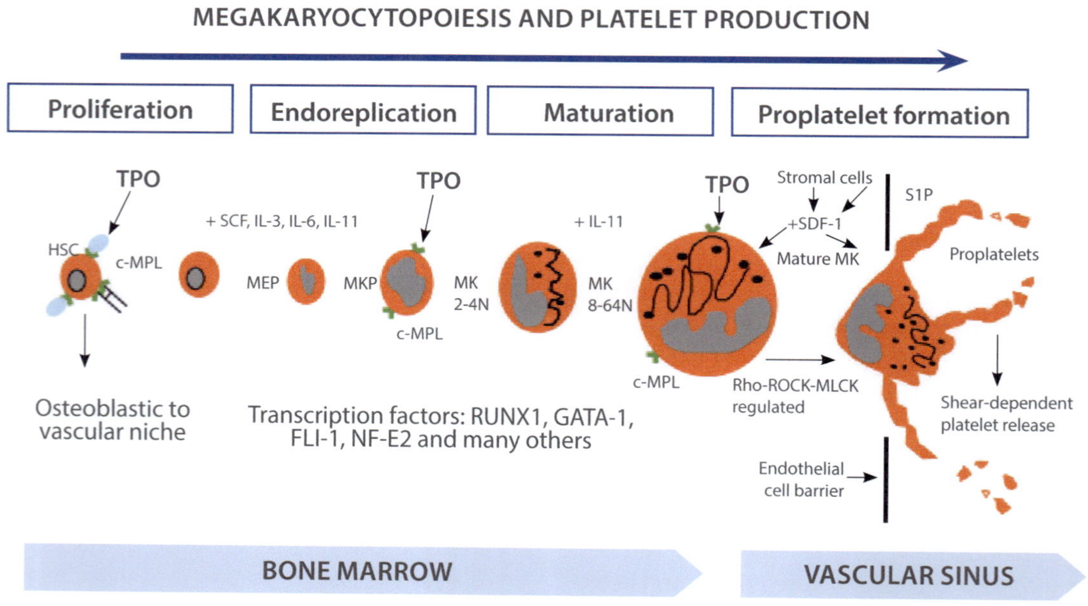

FIG. 1
Schematic representation of the essential steps of megakaryocytopoiesis and platelet production. The process starts with pluripotent hematopoietic stem cells (HSC) that migrate to the vascular niche within the bone marrow and first proliferate before undergoing a series of changes beginning with endoreplication and maturation, a process highly dependent on thrombopoietin (TPO). The chromosome content of mature megakaryocytes (MKs) can be as high as 64 or 128n, a step allowing the formation of the membrane systems and proteins required for platelet production. Many transcription factors are involved in MK maturation with multiple interactions between MKs and their environment (stromal cells, ECM proteins). Finally, mature MKs migrate to the vascular sinus where intracellular signaling pathways favour the formation of long projections termed proplatelets that penetrate across endothelial cell junctions into the blood stream and either bud off platelets directly from their ends or break off as larger structures under the influence of shear and which themselves divide into platelets in the circulation. MEP, MK-erythroid precursors; MKP, MK precursors.

lead to conformational changes in integrin αIIbβ3 enabling it to bind fibrinogen (Fg) or other adhesive proteins that form platelet-to-platelet bridges in the final common step of platelet aggregation. Platelet-to-platelet contacts allow other membrane GPs to interact and to consolidate the aggregate (fig. 3). Endothelial cells form a protective barrier to blood and limit platelet reactivity by secreting nitric oxide (NO) and prostacyclin (PGI2) that dampen down platelet activation; or by expressing enzymes that degrade ADP. But after the loss of ECs or their structural modification (such as during atherosclerosis or inflammation), platelets intervene. Attached and activated platelets spread on exposed extracellular matrix (ECM), particularly collagen, secrete metabolites and release the contents of storage organelles (dense granules, α-granules). These processes promote both flow-dependent thrombus formation and the ensuing tissue repair (fig. 2).

After strong platelet activation, transport of phosphatidylserine (PS) from the inner to the outer leaflet of the phospholipid bilayer makes the platelet membrane procoagulant. Platelets in the central core of the aggregate (or thrombus) are more tightly packed and undergo more extensive changes than those in the outer shell; thereby regulating intra-thrombus solute transport and local thrombin activity, fibrin formation and thrombus stability[3]. Fibrin is essential for blood clotting and wound repair, entrapping other blood cells while platelet aggregates act as hubs within the fibrin network ultimately mediating clot retraction. ADP-related formation of stable platelet aggregates, not fibrin, limits plasma extravasation and promotes tissue repair. In pathology, hyperactive platelets and spontaneous formation or uncontrolled embolization of platelet masses that severely perturb or occlude the circulation are at the origin of arterial thrombosis and stroke[4].

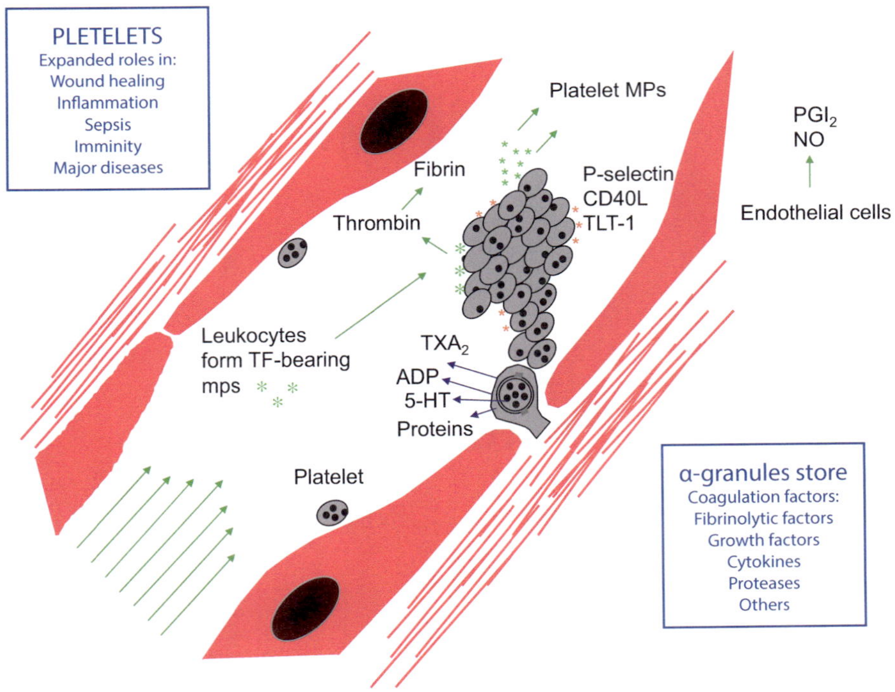

FIG. 2
Cartoon highlighting the biological roles of platelets. Platelets attach when they meet subendothelial elements, become activate and secrete metabolites and granule stores that promote stable aggregate formation at the injured site. Thrombus size is limited by blood flow and regulators secreted from endothelial cells (NO, PGI2). Thrombin generation within the aggregate promotes fibrin formation, consolidation of the hemostatic plug and the release of procoagulant MPs. Also highlighted are the α-granule secreted storage pools of biologically active proteins and the major non-hemostatic roles of platelets.

Platelets are either used up in hemostasis or, when aged undergo glycosylation changes that promote removal from the circulation in the liver, a process that stimulates TPO production in a feedback mechanism that masterminds platelet production[5]. Inherited or acquired defects (induced by certain drugs, chemotherapy, viral or bacterial infections, autoimmune-mediated destruction) that result in a dramatic fall in platelet numbers (i.e. below 30,000/μL) and/or a loss of platelet function favor bleeding. In addition to their essential hemostatic role, platelets also intervene in inflammation and infection, tissue repair, metastasis and tumor growth, and innate immunity[6-9]. This short review will now largely concentrate on describing the role of platelets in non-hemostatic events and to providing the background to their therapeutic use in healing and combatting disease.

2. PLATELETS AS A SOURCE OF BIOLOGICALLY ACTIVE PROTEINS AND METABOLITES

Certain features of the typical discoid anuclear platelet stand out (fig. 3A). These include an outer plasma membrane linked to an extensive intracellular open canalicular membrane system (OCS) that likens the platelet to a sponge. Under the membrane is a microtubular network that interacts with an actin-rich cytoskeleton, while the cytoplasm contains mitochondria and a series of secretory organelles. Platelet activation after adhesion and/or the binding of soluble stimuli results in Ca2+ fluxes and the generation of a plethora of second messengers. Important is the production of lipid metabolites such as thromboxane A2 (TXA2) that act in feedback mechanisms promoting platelet aggregation, a process

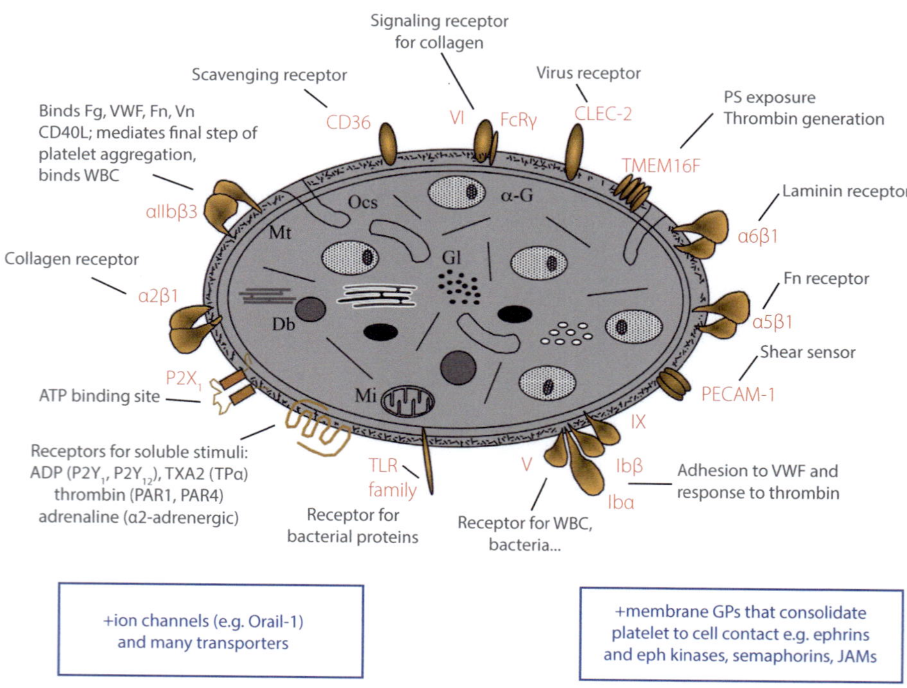

FIG. 3
Schema highlighting the surface structure of resting platelets showing many of the essential membrane GPs that mediate platelet adhesion and aggregation responses in hemostasis. By far the most abundant receptor is αIIbβ3 present at over 100,000 copies per platelet thereby reflecting its importance in platelet function. JAMs: junction adhesion molecules; α-G, α-granule; Db, dense body; Mio, mitochondria; Gl, glycogen store, Mt, microtubule ring; Ocs, open surface canalicular system.

inhibited by aspirin. Sphingosine 1-phosphate, a metabolite able to stimulate mitogenesis and cell proliferation, is released from platelets during clotting and favors fibronectin (Fn) matrix assembly, endothelial barrier integrity, and tissue factor (TF) expression in the vasculature[6]. Lysophosphatidic acid and platelet activating factor (PAF) are other released metabolites. A major early response of the platelet, and a primary subject of this review, is the release of the storage pools of biologically active agents from granules.

(i) Dense granules

These small lysosome-related organelles (3 to 8 per platelet) contain serotonin (actively taken up and stored by circulating platelets), ADP, ATP, polyphosphosphate, Ca2+ (itself a potential central regulator of wound healing) as well as small amounts of other amines such as histamine and dopamine. The dense granule membrane contains molecules associated with the uptake and storage of their contents such as two-pore channel 2 (for Ca2+ uptake), vesicular monoamine transporter 2 (serotonin) as well as membrane glycoproteins such as P-selectin that are shared with other organelles. Dense granule release from platelets requires a complex secretory mechanism involving SNARE (soluble N-ethylmaleimide sensitive factor attachment protein receptor) proteins and a series of proteins involved in vesicular trafficking and the late membrane fusion events required for exocytosis[10]. ADP has a universal role in assuring stable platelet aggregation by other agonists[3]. Highly charged polyphosphate promotes coagulation and enhances fibrin clot structure; in so doing, it provides an early link between platelets, coagulation and inflammation[11]. Released serotonin induces vasoconstriction while increasing vascular permeability. Although the subject of debate, release from dense granules is thought to occur faster than from α-granules.

(ii) α-Granules

These are the principal storage organelles of biologically active proteins (fig. 4, Table I). They are formed from intermediate multivesicular bodies (MVB) originating from the trans-Golgi network in maturing MKs and are numerous with 50-80 α-granules per platelet[10, 12]. Some MVB and α-granules may contain smaller vesicular struc-

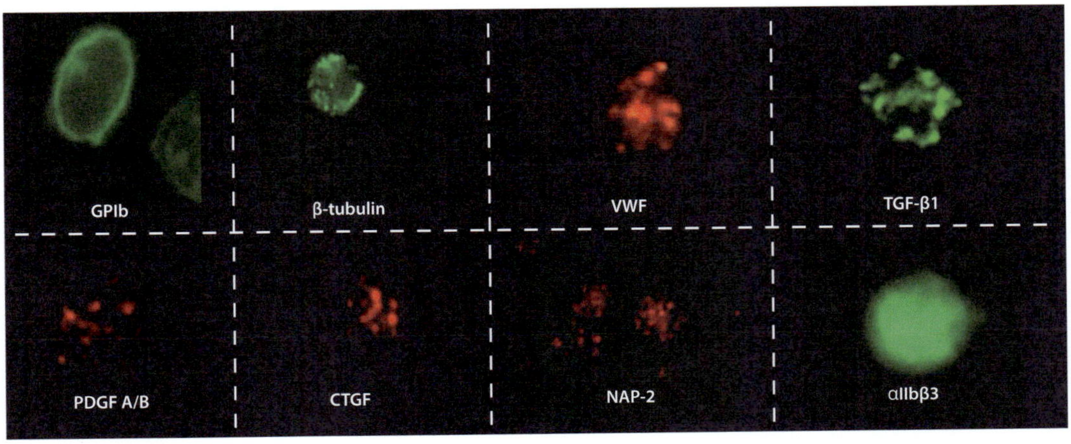

FIG. 4
Fluorescent detection of selected proteins in platelets. Parafarmaldehyde fixed and permeabilized resting human platelets were sequentially incubated with monospecific primary antibodies and fluorochrome-labeled anti-IgG subtype antibodies prior to visualization of bound antibodies by fluorescence microscopy [see 16 for Methods]. Note the presence of the adhesion receptor, GPIb, as primarily a plasma membrane component whereas the aggregation mediator, αIIbβ3, is abundantly distributed throughout the different membrane systems of the platelet. The microtubule component, β-tubulin, is revealed with a sub-membranous distribution whereas selected α-granule components, VWF, TGF-β1, PDGF A/B, CTGF and NAP-2 are localized to discrete organelles within the platelet ready to be released on platelet activation.

tures called exosomes that are enriched in CD63 and secreted intact; their significance is largely unknown. Proteomics show just how wide and diverse is the platelet protein content and several hundred secreted proteins have been identified[13]. Table I highlights a selection of the more prominent proteins that are somewhat arbitrarily grouped into functional categories. For the most part, stored proteins are synthesized in MKs and traffic in endosomes to developing granules; however, some are captured by MKs or platelets from their environment by endocytosis (e.g. Fg, factor V (FV), albumin, immunoglobulin G (IgG))[12]. Ca2+ and Mg2+ are enriched in α-granules that also contain acidic glycosaminoglycans (mainly chondroitin-4-sulphate) localized to distinct domains

Adhesive proteins	VWF + pro-peptide, Fg, Fn, Vn, TSP-1, TSP-2, laminin-8, osteonectin	Cell contact interactions, platelet function and clotting, wound healing, bone metabolism, inflammation
Clotting factors and their inhibitors	FV (+ multimerin), FXI, FXIII, TF*, prothrombin, HMWK, protein S, protease nexin-2 (amyloid β/A4 protein precursor (APP) (also see membrane glycoproteins)), C1 inhibitor, TFP1, protein C inhibitor, gas6**	Thrombin production and clotting, wound healing, inflammation
Fibrinolytic factors and their inhibitors	Plasminogen/plasmin, urokinase-PA, PAI-I, α2-antiplasmin, histidine-rich glycoprotein, thrombin-activatable fibrinolysis inhibitor (TAFI)	Plasmin production and fibrinolysis. Vascular modelling
Other proteases and anti-proteases	Metalloprotease (MMP)-1-4, -9, -14, ADAMTS-13, ADAM-10 (α-secretase), ADAM-17, TIMPs 1-4, α1-antitrypsin, α2-antitrypsin, α2-macroglobulin, granzyme B	Platelet function, angiogenesis, vascular modelling, regulation of coagulation, inflammation
Growth and mitogenic factors	PDGF (A, B and C), EGF, FGF, HGF, IGF, VEGF (A-D), bone morphogenetic proteins, IGFBP3, CTGF, connective tissue activating peptides	Chemotaxis, cell proliferation and growth, angiogenesis, wound healing, bone metabolism, cancer
Cytokines, chemokines and related compounds	TGF-β1, IL-1β⊠⊠⊠, IL-1α, Il-2, IL-4, TNF-α, CCL2 (MCP-1), CCL3 (MIP-1α), CCL4 (MIP-1β), CCL5 (RANTES), CCL7 (MCP-3), CCL14, CCL15 (MIP-5), CCL17, CCL19 (MIP-3b), CCL20 (MIP-3a), CXCL1 (GROα), CXCL2 (MIP-2α), CXCL3 (MIP-2β), CXCL4 (PF4), CXCL4L1 (PF4alt), CXCL4L (PFAalt)CXCL5 (ENA-78), CXCL7 (β-thromboglobulin, platelet basic protein or CTAP-III), CXCL8 (IL-8), CXCL12 (SDF-1α), TPO*, angiopoietin-1	Regulation of angiogenesis, cellular proliferation and differentiation, chemotaxis, vascular modelling, cellular interactions, immunity, bone metabolism, immune-regulatory and inflammatory processes, cancer
Anti-microbial proteins	Several chemokines and truncated derivatives often grouped globally as thrombocidins (from CTAP-III or NAP-2) and kinocidins (from the PF4 family)****, human β-defensin-1, -2, -3*****, thymosin-β4, fibrinopeptides A/B	Bactericidal and fungicidal properties, chemoattractants, inflammation, infections (sepsis)
Others	Serglycin (secretory granule proteoglycan core), chondroitin 4-sulfate, albumin, IgG, IgA and IgM, C3 and C4 precursor, properdin factor D, Factor H, bile salt-dependent lipase, autotaxin, lysophospholipase-2, clusterin, (+ APP), PDI******, HMGB1*, dickkopf-1, osteoprotegerin (OPG), substance P, brain-derived neurotrophic factor (BDNF)*, endostatin (proteolytic fragment of collagen), angiostatin (proteolytic fragment of plasminogen), angiogenin	Various functions including tissue remodelling, inflammation, immunity and disease states including cancer
Membrane glycoproteins	αIIbβ3, αvβ3, GPIb, PECAM-1, ICAM-2, semaphorin 3A, semaphorin 4D, PLEXIN-B1, CD147, TLR-1-7, -9, Siglec-7, receptors for primary agonists, P-selectin, TLT-1, JAM-1, JAM-3, claudin-5, PSGL, CD40L, Glut-3, TRAIL (Apo2-L), TWEAK (Apo3-L (TNF), APP (amyloid beta (A4) precursor), gC1qR, Fas ligand (CD95), beta-2-microglobulin, hyaluronidase-2	Platelet aggregation and adhesion, endocytosis of proteins, thrombin generation, platelet-leukocyte and platelet-vascular cell interactions, inflammation, wound healing, immune modulation, disease states

TABLE 1

(or cores) where they concentrate basic proteins such as platelet factor 4 (PF4, chemokine CXC motif ligand 4 (CXCL4)). The granule membrane contains intrinsic GPs (e.g. P-selectin, Trem-like transcript-1 (TLT-1) and CD40L) as well as many of the plasma membrane receptors and the abundant presence of αIIbβ3. Their surface expression confers new properties to the activated platelet promoting platelet-leukocyte tethering or platelet interactions with other cells as well as consolidating platelet interactions within the thrombus.

Adhesive proteins are abundant in the α-granule storage pool (Table I); secreted VWF, Fg, Fn and vitronectin (Vn) all participate in platelet-to-platelet interactions even if Fg plays the major role. Fibrillar cellular Fn in the vessel wall is an excellent substrate for thrombus formation. Special mention should be made of thrombospondin-1 (TSP-1), one of the most abundant α-granule proteins; TSP-1 plays an important role in thrombus stability and clot retraction. Adhesive proteins may also act directly as mitogens or they may promote mitogen activity of growth factors. The α-granules are also a source of coagulation and fibrinolytic factors. However, they also contain inhibitors of coagulation (e.g. tissue factor pathway inhibitor (TFPI), protease nexin-2) and of fibrinolysis (plasminogen activator inhibitor type I, PAI-1). This illustrates the fundamental enigma of platelet α-granules that store proteins with contrasting effects and also of the corresponding roles of platelet as compared to plasma pools.

Questions were raised on how stimulators and inhibitors of angiogenesis were stored. Italiano et al[14] localized pro- (e.g. vascular endothelial growth factor (VEGF), basic fibroblast growth factor (bFGF)) and anti-angiogenic proteins (e.g. endostatin, TSP-1) to distinct granule sub-populations in platelets and in MKs; they also backed up earlier work that these cargos were released with different kinetics. Nevertheless, high-resolution and scanning transmission electron microscopy (STEM) suggested another explanation; that granule cargos are compartmentalized zonally but within the same organelle while three-dimensional images obtained by cryo-electron tomography showed α-granules with microvesicular and tubular internal structures consistent with structural heterogeneity[10, 15]. Tissue inhibitors of metalloproteases (TIMPs) were clearly stored separately from VWF as platelets from a donor with an inherited disorder of α-granule production failed to label for VWF while normally containing TIMPs that were organized in individual compartments[16]. Another granule cargo stored in specific granules (termed T-granules by some) is protein disulfide isomerase (PDI), a secreted protein that co-localizes with toll-like receptor-9 (TLR9) and which on secretion stabilizes a fibrin clot together with the cross-linking protein, FXIII[17]. The presence of TLR9 suggests a link with innate and adaptive immune responses as well as infectious inflammation.

Platelet release of α-granule constituents requires docking of the granule membrane with either the plasma membrane or the OCS followed by membrane fusion. Similarly to dense granules, exocytosis resolves around vesicle- and plasma membrane-bound SNARE proteins and their chaperones[10, 18]. STEM tomography further revealed how α-granules can liberate their contents through tubular extensions reacting directly with the plasma membrane while OCS membranes join independently with the plasma membrane thereby increasing platelet surface area[15]. Differential sorting of α-granules has also been shown, with granules labeling for VAMP-7 sorting to a more peripheral localization during platelet spreading as compared to those expressing VAMP-3 or VAMP-8[18]. Differentially packaged and segregated proteins may have different diffusion rates to the exterior while the spatial localization of the granules, determined by VAMP isoforms, and the size of the fusion pores may also influence secretion kinetics, as will the strength and nature of the stimulus initiating secretion.

(iii) Lysosomes

These contain enzymes such as cathepsins D and E, elastase, β-glucuronidase and acid phosphatase; while their membranes resemble dense granules in expressing CD63 and lysosome-associated membrane protein-2. Platelets also contain a constitutively active autophagy pathway[19].

3. OTHER PLATELET CHANGES ON ACTIVATION

PS expression on platelets allows the binding of coagulation factors (e.g. FVIII) and the rapid formation of an activated FXa/Va complex. The latter transforms prothrombin into thrombin in a Ca2+-dependent process. Thrombin itself is a powerful mitogen. However, its main immediate role is in the formation of the fibrin clot. PS expression is also essential for the release of membrane-bound MPs by platelets; these bud off from the platelet surface following calcium-dependent uncoupling of the underlying cytoskeleton from the plasma membrane. Procoagulant in nature, MPs intervene in thrombotic disease and inflammation being, for example, active mediators of rheumatoid arthritis[20]. MPs express P-selectin and 12-lipoxygenase and the release of 12(S)-hydroxyeicosatetranoic acid promotes their internalization by neutrophils. Quite surprisingly, platelets can also release mitochondria, both within MPs and as free organelles[21]. Degradation of the mitochondrial membrane by soluble phospholipase A2 leads to the release of inflammatory mediators while mitochondria themselves can bind to neutrophils.

4. PLATELETS AND WOUND HEALING

Platelets intervene at many stages of wound healing including restoring the integrity of blood vessels after injury or after atherosclerotic plaque rupture. Collagens, proteoglycans and adhesive proteins such as Fn are major constituents of the ECM; providing a molecular scaffold for incoming platelets and migrating cells such as fibroblasts[22]. Thrombus growth at the injured site concentrates platelets to participate in tissue remodeling by secreting a variety of growth factors, cytokines, chemokines and other factors (Table I). For example, VEGF, platelet-derived growth factor (PDGFa/b and c), fibroblast growth factor (FGF), hepatocyte growth factor (HGF), epidermal growth factor (EGF), connective tissue growth factor (CTGF) and insulin-like growth factor (IGF) form chemotactic gradients through binding to matrix components or to newly generated fibrin. Transforming growth factor-β1 (TGF-β1) recruits inflammatory cells into the wound area and stimulates fibroblasts to produce connective tissue and the ECM; Fg itself can enhance wound closure by increasing cell proliferation and migration while it forms matrix fibrils with Fn, a substrate for αvβ3 on fibroblasts[22]. PDGF particularly stimulates fibroblast migration. Fibrin is very important for wound healing, providing an additional meshwork for cells; but it is the platelet mass that limits plasma loss[3]. Fibrin degradation products also attract leukocytes and aid the transition between inflammation and tissue repair.

Platelets favor angiogenesis by recruitment, proliferation and differentiation of endothelial and other vascular cells. Growth factors such as VEGF, bFGF and PDGF, also enhance late events such as endothelial tube formation and sprouting of new vessels[23]. Yet we underline the apparent paradox that platelets also store and release anti-angiogenic factors such as endostatin, PF4, TSP1 and the TIMPs that may counterbalance the effect of the pro-angiogenic mediators[14]. PF4 is perhaps the best studied of these. It binds with high affinity to heparin and to heparin-like molecules on the endothelial cell surface and is a negative regulator of angiogenesis by inhibiting VEGF and FGF as well as blocking the cell cycle making it a molecule with anti-cancer properties[24]. Stromal cell derived factor 1 (SDF-1) is an α-granule stored chemokine that through binding to CXCR4 and CXCR7 on progenitor or mesenchymal stem cells enhances their recruitment to the site of vascular lesions[25]. Platelets also are capable of modulating the balance between cell survival and apoptosis. SDF-1 acts with serotonin, ADP and sphingosine-1 phosphate to favor cell survival. In contrast, a number of tumor necrosis factor-α (TNF-α) related apoptosis regulators secreted from platelets (e.g. CD40L, soluble Fas Ligand, TNF-related apoptosis-inducing ligand (TRAIL)) can induce inflammatory responses in fibroblasts, smooth muscle cells, neutrophils, monocytes and other cells as well as promoting apoptosis[23]. Not only biologically active proteins participate in wound healing. Serotonin plays an active role in liver regeneration[26].

Defining how platelets control the balance between cell proliferation and cell elimination at the wound site will be a key feature of future research. Tissue factor (TF) is the initiator of the extrinsic pathway of coagulation; it also plays a key role in angiogenesis and wound healing. Whether circulating platelets intrinsically possess TF is unclear; however, they can (i) take it up by transfer from monocytes and their MPs by a P-selectin dependent mechanism and (ii) on activation, can synthetize it from preformed mRNA via their spliceosome. Platelets are a rich source of metalloproteases (MMPs) possessing MMP1-4, -9, -14, ADAMTS-13 (a disintegrin and metalloprotease with thrombospondin type I repeats-13), ADAM-10 and -17 among others. MMPs have many biological roles that include tissue remodeling[27].

5. PLATELETS AND INFLAMMATION

A) Inflammatory proteins

Inflammation involves close interplay between platelets, leukocytes and cells of the immune system. It is critically linked with thrombosis in many major acquired diseases. Some secreted platelet metabolites are pro-inflammatory including TXA2 and PAF while dense granules are sources of serotonin and histamine[28]. Platelet α-granules contain many proteins able to influence inflammation[12, 28]. Activated platelets within the growing thrombus recruit and bind immune cells by secreting chemoattractants and expressing granule-derived P-selectin and other targets for leukocyte GPs. Monocytes, neutrophils and lymphocytes are all recruited and once present become activated as part of their inflammatory response[9]. Secreted chemokines and cytokines such as CXCL4, CXCL7 and CCL5 (chemokine C-C motif ligand 5 (regulated upon activation normally T-expressed and secreted (RANTES)) favor immune cell recruitment and activation; specifically, neutrophil-activating peptide-2 (NAP-2, a proteolytic derivative of CXCL7) induces immune cells to traverse the thrombus and enter the vessel wall[29]. Other chemokines of interest are interleukin-8 (IL-8), macrophage migration inhibitory factor (MIF), growth-regulated oncogene-α (Gro-α), epithelial activating protein-78 (ENA-78) and monocyte chemoattractant protein-3 (MCP-3) (Table I)[29]. Platelet expression of adhesive proteins, membrane GPs and the surface exposure of P-selectin helps stabilize the interaction between platelets and endothelial or immune cells via interplay between surface receptor pairs. Significantly, many of these mechanisms are involved in atherosclerotic plaque formation[22]. The importance of platelets is confirmed by the increased bleeding in inflammatory states when the platelet count is low[30]. The role of platelets extends well beyond the vascular system. For example, regardless of the blood-brain barrier, platelets influence central nervous system repair through leukocyte recruitment to inflammatory sites and by promoting regenerative processes in the nervous system including the incoming of stem/progenitor cells[31].

B) Antimicrobial proteins

A special and increasingly recognized function of platelets is in host defense both in the circulation and at sites of vascular lesions such as in infectious endocarditis[12, 32]. Bacteria can bind to platelets indirectly via adhesive proteins such as Fg or VWF that recognize receptors on platelets and the bacterial surface or they may even bind αIIbβ3 or GPIb directly. Platelets also contain FcγRIIA that recognizes IgG bound to bacteria and a host of specific receptors for bacterial proteins including TLR1-7; 9, whose occupancy leads to platelet release of microbicidal proteins and cytokines with recruitment of circulating inflammatory cells and bacterial destruction[33]. Bacteria can be internalized by platelets and they can promote apoptosis; platelet interactions with bacteria can modify platelet function with release of immunomodulators leading to falls in platelet count or even thrombosis. Taking a specific example, inflammation drives thrombosis in the liver after Salmonella infection and does so in a TLR4-dependent cascade via ligation of C-type lectin-like receptor-2 (CLEC-2) on platelets by the membrane glycoprotein, podoplanin, on monocytes and kupffer cells[34]. As well as bacteria, platelets can directly bind and internalize many types of virus including human immunodeficiency virus; capture involves multiple platelet receptors including CLEC-2[35]. Some cytokines released from platelets have direct microbicidal activities (Table I) including CXCL4, CXCL7, thymosin-β4 and RANTES. Of particular importance are NAP-2 and thrombocidins (TC-1 and -2), small C-terminal proteolytic derivatives of CXCL7. Platelets also store and secrete from α-granules elements of the complement (C) cascade (C3, C4 precursor) as well as proteins that regulate complement activity. The ability of platelets to bind complement is another element in the interaction of activated platelets with bacteria[32].

C) Sepsis

An extreme condition combining infection, an uncontrolled immune response and inflammation, sepsis is associated with a high degree of mortality. Platelet accumulation in inflamed tissues accelerates immune cell recruitment and the excessive response can promote organ dysfunction. The onset of disseminated intravascular coagulation can lead to a fall in platelet count and increased vascular permeability (aided by platelet VEGF and serotonin release) with edema, shock and organ failure. Sepsis is a progressive systemic inflammatory condition and the kallikrein/kinin systems, elements of which can be secreted from platelets (Table I), can have a prominent role[36]. As discussed earlier, as well as secreting their granule contents, anucleate platelets entrapped in a clot can synthesize proteins such as Il-1β and TF from preformed mRNA. Il-1β can bind to fibrin where it retains its activity while TF favors thrombosis. Significantly, as well as producing inflammatory molecules, a major role for secreted ADP either from platelets and/or tissue cells, in systemic inflammation and sepsis, has been confirmed through the use of anti-platelet P2Y12 drugs in man[37]. In inflammatory states, hepatic TPO production is upregulated by IL-6 leading to an overproduction of platelets; at the same time, platelet clearance in the liver may be part of the acute phase response and help increase the chance of survival in sepsis[5]. Also, a highly inflammatory state can lead to an upregulation of platelet production by caspase-dependent direct fragmentation of MKs, a process promoted by IL-1α/IL-1 type I receptor signaling[38].

Wnt/β-catenin signaling has a major influence in lung repair and activated platelets are sequestered in pulmonary vascular beds. Modulation of Wnt/β-catenin signaling by platelet-derived Dickopf-1 (Dkk1) is a major factor in promoting neutrophil trafficking and the inflammatory response in the lungs; Dkk1 is another example of a relatively unknown α-granule protein[39].

6. INNATE AND ADAPTIVE IMMUNITY

Platelets are now known to act as sentinel innate immune cells[40, 41]. This role will now be illustrated with reference to three platelet α-granule proteins.

A) CD40L

A much-studied platelet cytokine is CD40 ligand (CD40L, CD154), first identified on activated helper T cells and a member of the tumour necrosis factor (TNF) family[41]. It binds to CD40 on antigen-presenting cells; other receptors include αMβ2, α5β1 and αIIbβ3 on platelets thereby also linking it to thrombosis. In the immune system, the CD40L/CD40 interaction drives B-cell proliferation and antibody production; it plays a primary role in immunoglobulin (Ig) class switching and it has been implicated in autoimmune disorders. Platelets constitute the major reservoir for CD40L in blood; present in the α-granule membrane, it is transported to the platelet surface on platelet activation. Here, it is available to bind vascular and immune cells and participate in inflammation, in stimulating interleukin and cytokine production and in the release of reactive oxygen species. Surface-expressed platelet CD40L is a substrate for MMP activity with release of the smaller but still biologically active soluble CD40L (sCD40L) that has become a plasma marker for inflammation.

B) TREM-like transcript-1

The triggering receptors expressed on myeloid cells (TREMs) contain a single V-set Ig domain, and are involved in cell activation within the innate immune system with a key role in sepsis. A GP with significant homology to the TREMs, TLT-1, is exclusive to the mouse and human megakaryocyte

(MK) lineages where it co-localizes with P-selectin in the α-granule membrane. It is translocated to the platelet surface when platelet activation leads to secretion and supports platelet aggregation thereby protecting against bleeding during inflammation. Like CD40L (and P-selectin), TLT-1 can be the object of cleavage by MMPs with liberation of a soluble form that has a regulatory role in sepsis by modulating platelet-neutrophil crosstalk[42].

C) High mobility group box 1 (HMGB1) protein
HMGB1, principally known as a nuclear protein, is also secreted by immune cells when it acts as a cytokine-mediator of inflammation. It was recently recognized to be stored in platelet α-granules from which it is translocated both to the platelet surface and secreted on platelet activation in multiple inflammatory diseases[43]. As repeatedly stated by us, thrombosis and inflammation are inseparably linked and in this context HMGB1 appears as a critical player in both processes. Mice specifically lacking HMGB1 in their platelets have increased bleeding risk, reduced thrombus formation and platelet aggregation, and reduced inflammation and organ damage during experimental trauma/hemorrhagic shock[43]. HMGB1 offers yet another excellent example of a previously unrecognized platelet protein with multiple functions in health and disease. Activated platelets commit neutrophils to form neutrophil extracellular DNA traps (NETs) with released HMGB1 playing a key role by binding to neutrophils and through the induction of autophagy[44]. Platelets play a key role in NET formation. NETs are important for the host response to infection and inflammation but can have harmful effects such as promoting microvascular and deep vein thrombosis).

7. CONCLUDING REMARKS

Space restrictions have necessitated that we make our review highly selective. Platelets participate in many major illnesses. For example, circulating tumor cells may bind platelets and even aggregate them; an interaction that can protect tumor cells from the immune system and also help deposit them within the vasculature by way of platelet adhesive receptors (e.g. GPIb, integrins, P-selectin)[8]. Release of ADP and ATP, the expression of P-selectin after platelet activation and the generation of thrombin on the now procoagulant platelet surface may all favor metastasis within the vessel wall and help tumor stability. The release of α-granule proteins may promote angiogenesis and vascularization of the tumor; a novel enzyme secreted from platelets that liberates lysophosphatidylcholine and stimulates tumor cell mobility is autotaxin[45].

By acting as a major source of secretable pools of amyloid-β precursor, a substrate for α-secretase (ADAM10), and by being activated by amyloid-β in the walls of cerebral vessels leading to thrombus formation and granule release, platelets participate actively in the progression of Alzheimer's disease, an age-related neurodegenerative disorder[46, 47]. Amyloid-β binds directly to αIIbβ3 integrin and stimulates release of ADP and the chaperone protein clusterin from platelets. The latter promotes the formation of fibrillar amyloid-β aggregates while ADP further promotes αIIbβ3 activation and clusterin release in a feedback mechanism. The pro-inflammatory potential of platelets and MPs lead to roles in acute lung injury, asthma, inflammatory bowel disease (with elevated levels of RANTES) and migraine (through IL-1 and β-thromboglobulin) among many examples[9].

Yet in this context, studies using platelet-rich plasma derivatives therapeutically confirm many in vitro studies showing how platelets stimulate the growth of many types of cell including osteogenic cells, brain and nerve cells and various cellular constituents of muscles and tendons [see chapters 4 and 14 in this book]. It will be exciting to see how these therapies advance and how the active players are identified. It will also be interesting to see the progression of alternative approaches such as using genetically modified progenitor cells or MKs so that platelets are produced with α-granules containing proteins of therapeutic benefit such as FVIII as a treatment for hemophilia; an approach that may also ultimately be of benefit in cardiovascular disease, cancer and Alzheimer's disease[48].

1. *Machus KR, Italiano JE, Jr. The incredible journey: From megakaryocyte development to platelet formation. J Cell Biol 2013; 201:785-96.*

2. *Schwertz H, Köster S, Kahr WH, Michetti N, Kraemer BF, Weitz DA, Blaylock RC, Kraiss LW, Greinacher A, Zimmerman GA, Weyrich A. Anucleate platelets generate progeny. Blood 2010; 115:3801-9.*

3. *Welsh JD, Muthard RW, Stalker TJ, Taliaferro JO, Diamond SL, Brass LF. A systems approach to hemostasis: 4. How hemostatic thrombi limit the loss of plasma-borne molecules from the microvasculature. Blood 2016; 127:1598-605.*

4. *Jackson SP. Arterial thrombosis-insiduous, unpredictable and deadly. Nat Med 2011; 17:1423-36.*

5. *Grozovsky R, Begonja AJ, Liu K, Visner G, Hartwig JH, Falet H, Hoffmeister KM. The Ashwell-Morell receptor regulates hepatic thrombopoietin production via JAK2-STAT3 signaling. Nat Med 2015; 21:47-54.*

6. *Nurden AT, Nurden P, Sanchez M, Andia I, Anitua E. Platelets and wound healing. Front Biosci 2008; 13:3532-48.*

7. *Rondina MT, Weyrich AS, Zimmerman GA. Platelets as cellular effectors of inflammation in vascular diseases. Circ Res 2013; 112:1506-19.*

8. *Franco AT, Corken A, Ware J. Platelets at the interface of thrombosis, inflammation, and cancer. Blood 2015; 126:582-8.*

9. *Golebiewska EM, Poole AW. Platelet secretion: From hemostasis to wound healing and beyond. Blood Rev 2015; 29:153-62.*

10. *Heijnen H, van der Sluijs P. Platelet secretory behavior: as diverse as the granules…or not? J Thromb Haemost 2015; 13:2141-51.*

11. *Morrissey JH, Choi SH, Smith SA. Polyphosphate: an ancient molecule that links platelets, coagulation, and inflammation. Blood 2012; 119:5972-9.*

12. *Blair P, Flaumenhaft R. Platelet α-granules: Basic biology and clinical correlates. Blood Rev 2009; 23:177-89.*

13. *Burkhart JM, Vaudel M, Gambaryan S, Radau S, Walter U, Martens L, Geiger J, Sickmann A, Zahedi RP. The first comprehensive and quantitative analysis of human platelet protein composition allows the comparative analysis of structural and functional pathways. Blood. 2012;120:e73-82.*

14. *Italiano JE Jr, Richardson AL, Patel-Hyatt S, Battinelli E, Zaslavsky A, Short S, Ryeom S, Folkman J, Klement GL. Angiogenesis is regulated by a novel mechanism: pro- and antiangiogenic proteins are organized into separate platelet α-granules and differentially released. Blood 2008; 111:1227-33.*

15. *Pokrovskaya ID, Aronova MA, Kamykowski JA, Prince AA, Hoyne JD, Calco GN, Kuo BC, He Q, Leapman RD, Storrie B. STEM tomography reveals that the canalicular system and α-granules remain separate compartments during early secretion stages in blood platelets. J Thromb Haemost 2015; 13:1-13.*

16. *Villeneuve J, Block A, Le Bousse-Kerdilès M-C, Lepreux S, Nurden P, Ripoche J, Nurden AT. Tissue inhibitors of matrix metalloproteinases in platelets and megakaryocytes: a novel organization for these secreted proteins. Exp Hematol 2009; 37:849-56.*

17. *Thon JN, Peters CG, Macchlus KR, Aslam R, Rowley J, Macleod H, Devine MT, Fuchs TA, Weyrich AS, Semple JW, Flaumenhaft R, Italiano JE Jr. T granules in human platelets function in TLR9 organization and signaling. J Cell Biol 2012; 198:561-74.*

18. Peters GC, Michelson AD, Flaumenhaft R. Granule exocytosis is required for platelet spreading: differential sorting of α-granules expressing VAMP-7. Blood 2012; 120:199-206.

19. Ouseph MM, Huang Y, Banerjee M, Joshi S, MacDonald L, Zhong Y, Li X, Xiang B, Zhang G, Komatsu M, Yue Z, Li Z, Storrie B, Whiteheart SW, Wang QI. Autophagy is induced upon platelet activation and is essential for hemostasis and thrombosis. Blood 2015; 126:1224-33.

20. Boilard E, Nigrovic PA, Larabee K, Watts GF, Coblyn JS, Weinblatt ME, Massarotti ME, Remold-O'Donnell E, Farndale RW, Ware J, Lee DM. Platelets amplify inflammation in arthritis via collagen-dependent microparticle production. Science 2010; 237:580-3.

21. Boudreau LH, Duchez AC, Cloutier N, Soulet D, Martin N, Bollinger J, Paré A, Rousseau M, Naika GS, Lévesque T, Laflamme C, Marcoux G, Lambeau G, Farndale RW, Pouliot M, Hamzeh-Cognasse H, Cognasse F, Garraud O, Nigrovic PA, Guderley H, Lacroix S, Thibault L, Semple JW, Gelb MH, Boilard E. Platelets release mitochondria serving as substrate for bactericidal group IIA-secreted phospholipase A2 to promote inflammation. Blood. 2014; 124:2173-83.

22. Nurden AT. Platelets, inflammation and tissue regeneration. Thromb Haemost 2011; 105 Suppl 1: S13-33.

23. Gawaz M, Vogel S. Platelets in tissue repair: control of apoptosis and interactions with regenerative cells. Blood 2013; 122:2550-4.

24. Wang Z, Huang H. Platelet factor 4 (CXCL4/PF-4): an angiostatic chemokine for cancer therapy. Cancer Lett 2013; 33:147-53.

25. Massberg S, Konrad I, Schürzinger K, Lorenz M, Schneider S, Zohlnhoefer D, Hoppe K, Schiemann M, Kennerknecht E, Sauer S, Schulz C, Kerstan S, Rudelius M, Seidl S, Sorge F, Langer H, Peluso M, Goyal P, Vestweber D, Emambokus NR, Busch DH, Frampton J, Gawaz M. Platelets secrete stromal cell-derived factor 1alpha and recruit bone marrow-derived progenitor cells to arterial thrombi in vivo. J Exp Med 2006; 203:1221-33.

26. Lesurtel M, Graf R, Aleil B, Walther DJ, Tian Y, Jochum W, Gachet C, Bader M, Clavien PA. Platelet-derived serotonin mediates liver regeneration. Science 2006; 312:104-7.

27. Selzer P, May AE. Platelets and metalloproteases. Thromb Haemost 2013; 110:903-9.

28. Semple JW, Italiano JE, Freedman J. Platelets and the immune continuum. Nat Rev Immunol 2011; 11:264-74.

29. Karshovska E, Weber C, von Hundelshausen P. Platelet chemokines in health and disease. Thromb Haemost 2013; 110:894-902.

30. Goerge T, Ho-Tin-Noe B, Carbo C, Benarafe C, Remold-O'Donnell E, Zhao BQ, Cifuni SM, Wagner DD. Inflammation induces hemorrhage in thrombocytopenia. Blood 2008; 111:4958-64.

31. Rivera FJ, Kazanis I, Ghevaert C, Aigner L. Beyond clotting: A role of platelets in CNS repair. Front Cell Neurosci 2016; Feb 4;10:20. doi: 10.3389/fncel.2016.00020.

32. Hamzeh-Cognasse H, Damien P, Chabert A, Pozzedtto B, Cognesse F, Garraud O. Platelets and infections – complex interactions with bacteria. Front Immunol 2015; Feb 26;6:82. Doi: 103389/fimmu.2015.00083.ecollection 2015. Review. PMID: 25767472.

33. Kapur R, Zufferey A, Boilard E, Semple JW. Nouvelle cuisine: platelets served with inflammation. J Immunol 2015; 194:5579-87.

34. Hitchcock JR, Cook CN, Bobat S, Ross EA, Flores-Langarica A, Lowe KL, Khan M, Dominguez-Medina CC, Lax S, Carvalho-Gaspar M, Hubscher S, Rainger GE, Cobbold M, Buckley CD, Mitchell TJ, Mitchell A, Jones ND, Van Rooijen N, Kirchhofer D, Henderson IR, Adams DH, Watson SP, Cunningham AF. Inflammation drives thrombosis after Salmonella infection via CLEC-2 on platelets. J Clin Invest 2015; 125:4429-46.

35. Yeaman MR. Platelets: At the nexus of antimicrobial defence. Nat Rev Microbiol 2014; 12:426-37.

36. Schmaier AH. The contact activation and kallikrein/kinin systems: pathophysiologic and physiologic activities. J Thromb Haemost 2016; 14:28-39.

37. Thomas MR, Outteridge SN, Ajjan RA, Phoenix F, Sangha GK, Faulkner RE, Ecob R, Judge HM, Khan H, West LE, Dockrell DH, Sabroe I, Storey RF. Platelet P2Y12 inhibitors reduce systemic inflammation and its prothrombotic effects in an experimental human model. Arterioscler Thromb Vasc Biol 2015; 35:2562-70.

38. Nishimura S, Nagasaki M, Kunishima S, Sawaguchi A, Sakata A, Sakaguchi H, Ohmori T, Manabe I, Italiano JE Jr, Ryu T, Takayama N, Komuro I, Kodowaki T, Eto K, Nagai R. Il-1a induces thrombopoiesis through megakaryocyte rupture in response to acute platelet needs. J Cell Biol 2015; 209:453-66.

39. Guo Y, Mishra A, Howland E, Zhao C, Shukla D, Weng T, Liu L. Platelet-derived Wnt antagonist Dickkopf-1 is implicated in ICAM-1/VCAM-1-mediated neutrophilic acute lung inflammation. Blood 2015; 126:2220-9.

40. Morrell CN, Aggrey AA, Chapman LM, Modjeski KL. Emerging roles for platelets as immune and inflammatory cells. Blood 2014; 123:2759-67.

41. Dewitte A, Tanga A, Villeneuve J, Lepreux S, Quattara A, Desmoulière A, Combe C, Ripoche J. New frontiers for platelet CD154. Exp Hematol Oncol 2015; March 1;4 :6. Doi: 10.1.1186/s40164-015-0001-6.

42. Derive M, Bouazza Y, Sennoun N, Marchionni S, Quigley L, Washington V, Massin F, Max JP, Ford J, Alauzet C, Levy B, McVicar DW, Gibot S. Soluble TREM-like transcript-1 regulates leukocyte activation and controls microbial sepsis. J Immunol. 2012; 188:5585-92.

43. Vogel S, Bodenstein R, Chen Q, Feil S, Feil R, Rheinlaender J, Schäffer TE, Bohn E, Frick JS, Borst O, Münzer P, Walker B, Markel J, Csanyi G, Pagano PJ, Loughran P, Jessup ME, Watkins SC, Bullock GC, Sperry JL, Zuckerbraun BS, Billiar TR, Lotze MT, Gawaz M, Neal MD. Platelet-derived HMGB1 is a critical mediator of thrombosis. J Clin Invest 2015; 125:4638-54.

44. Maugeri N, Campana L, Gavina M, Covino C, De Metrio M, Panciroli C, Maiuri L, Maseri A, D'Angelo A, Bianchi ME, Rovere-Querini P, Manfredi AA. Activated platelets present high mobility group box 1 to neutrophils, inducing autophagy and promoting the extrusion of neutrophil extracellular traps. J Thromb Haemost 2014; 12:2074-88.

45. Leblanc R, Peyruchaud O. Platelet-derived autotaxin with tumor integrin αvβ3 controls metastasis of breast cancer cells to bone. Blood 2016; May 6. pii: blood-2016-01-636399. [Epub ahead of print].

46. Canobbio I, Guidetti GF, Oliviero B, Manganaro D, Vara D, Torti M, Pula G. Amyloid β-peptide-dependent activation of human platelets : essential role for Ca2+ and ADP in aggregation and thrombus formation. Biochem J. 2014; 462:513-23.

47. Donner L, Fälker K, Gremer L, Klinker S, Pagani G, Ljungberg LU, Lothmann K, Rizzi F, Schaller M, Gohlke H, Willbold D, Grenegard M, Elvers M. Platelets contribute to amyloid-β aggregation in cerebral vessels through integrin αIIbβ3-induced outside-in signaling and clusterin release. Sci Signal. 2016; 9(429):ra52. doi: 10.1126/scisignal.aaf6240.

48. Du LM, Nurden P, Nurden AT, Nichols T, Bellinger DA, Jensen ES, Haberichter SL, Merricks E, Raymer RA, Fang J, Koukouritaki SB, Jacobi PM, Hawkins TB, Cornetta K, Shi Q, Wilcox DA. Platelet-targetted gene therapy with human factor VIII establishes hemostasis in dogs with haemophilia A. Nat Commun 2013; 4:2773.doi: 10.1038/ncomms3773.

CHAPTER 2

Characterization of Plasma Rich in Growth Factors (PRGF): Components and Formulations

AUTHORS

Anitua E.[1,2,3], Prado R.[2], Nurden A.T.[4], Nurden P.[4]

[1] Eduardo Anitua Fundation. Vitoria-Gasteiz, Spain
[2] BTI-Biotechnology Institute, Vitoria-Gasteiz, Spain
[3] University Institute for Regenerative Medicine and Oral Implantology (UIRMI) from the University of Basque Country (UPV/EHU)
[4] Institut de Rhythmologie et de Modélisation Cardiaque, Plateforme Technologique d'Innovation Biomédicale, Hôpital Xavier Arnozan, Pessac, France

SUMMARY

Platelet-rich Plasma (PRP) is a set of autologous platelet products used to reduce pain and speed up recovery from injury while maintaining the tissue function. Its basic rationale is to mimic yet enhance the natural processes of healing by bringing to the injury site a set of molecules that will accelerate functional recovery, and even regenerate the tissue. In the array of PRP-products, Plasma Rich in Growth Factors (PRGF)-Endoret is a pioneering autologous regenerative technology with multiple therapeutic potentials. It can be produced in at least four different formulations, depending on coagulation and degree and type of activation. PRGF-Endoret technology is safe and versatile, and has a wide range of applications.

E. Anitua et al. (eds.), *Platelet Rich Plasma in Orthopaedics and Sports Medicine*,
https://doi.org/10.1007/978-3-319-63730-3_2

1. POTENTIAL OF PLASMA RICH IN GROWTH FACTORS (PRGF-ENDORET): MIMICKING THE NATURAL HEALING PROCESS

The increasing number of musculoskeletal injuries has produced a concurrent stimulus in both the number and the effectiveness of different treatments of these lesions, especially in the search for minimally invasive procedures or adjuvants[1-3]. One of these cutting-edge technologies is Plasma Rich in Growth Factors (PRGF-Endoret)1. This biological treatment mimics the natural pathways of wound healing[4] by driving to the injury site the whole protein array of PRGF that is involved in the repair of damaged tissues. In this way, all the bioactive molecules (including growth factors and other proteins) necessary for tissue repair are efficiently and locally released.

The tissue repair process occurs naturally in a staged fashion[5] and includes removal of dead cells, proliferation, migration of cells to the injury site, production of new vascular structures, and other events. The organization of all these elements influences healing in a given injury, preventing fibrotic elements that cause loss of functional capacity in that tissue[6,7] i Growth factors play an important role coordinating the whole process in an orchestrated fashion in all tissues of the musculoskeletal system, including muscle[8], tendon[9], bone[10,11], and cartilage[12]. Growth factors act on other tissues as well, including skin[13], oral soft tissue[14,15], and cornea[16] among others.

PRGF-Endoret technology mimics the natural healing mechanisms, but with two special features: avoiding loss of functionality (fibrous tissue) and shortening healing times. This is achieved in part by adjusting the PRGF-Endoret formulation and dosage to the type of tissue and injury.

PRGF-Endoret therapy accelerates and improves tissue healing by local delivery of autologous bioactive molecules and hence, contributing a first line provisional scaffold[1]. This autologous therapeutic toolbox consists of platelets as both reservoir and vehicle of a large repertoire of proteins[17,18.] Recently, a proteomic dissection of PRGF scaffold was performed[19]. In this research, the authors studied those proteins that remained most closely bound to the fibrin network and that were therefore retained by the mesh itself, rather than being released into the supernatant. The high-throughput proteomic techniques used in this characterization allowed us to produce a catalogue of these proteins and subsequently to classify them into families on the basis of their function and gene ontology. The results of this process showed that the fibrin network is enriched in proteins specifically involved in tissue regeneration and wound healing. Interestingly, there was found to be an enrichment in certain lipoproteins, which are involved in regenerative processes, particularly by delaying degradation (fibrinolysis) of the fibrin network, thereby extending the controlled release of other molecules. Similarly, an important family of proteins involved in the acute phase reaction was found to be present. These proteins form the first line of defence in the immune system[19].

In the last decade, several systems have been developed to produce a biologically active product, both commercially and in-house, but they differ in the presence of white blood cells, growth factors concentration, and architecture of fibrin scaffold[20-24]. The different PRP commercial systems can be certified for various medical applications, but the therapeutic outcome will depend on the type of platelet-rich plasma used and the dosage employed. Establishing a proper classification of PRPs and identifying the biological differences among them is absolutely necessary to understand some of the controversial results obtained with these types of technologies so far[25].

One of the most relevant and controversial issues is the presence of leukocytes in the platelet-rich plasma. In order to distinctly define the PRGF technology, and thus be able to compare other PRPs, PRGF can be categorized according to three of the most cited classifications that have been proposed for PRPs. The first and most widely used[26] classifies PRGF as pure-PRP (P-PRP) since it does not contain WBC. The PRGF is classified as type 4-B (Minimal WBCs, activated with $CaCl_2$, and platelet concentration below 5x) as has been proposed[27] for sports medicine classification. Finally, PRGF would fit in the P2-x-Bβ category (platelet count greater than baseline levels to 750,000 platelets/μL, exogenous activation with $CaCl_2$, with WBC -and specifically neutrophils- below to baseline levels) according to the PAW (platelets, activation and WBC) classification[28].

2. UNDERSTANDING THE PROPERTIES OF PLATELET-RICH PLASMA PRODUCTS

Several key biological mediators are present in a PRP. The more studied growth factors contained in platelet-rich plasma that are important during tissue repair include IGF-I (Insulin-like Growth Factor type I), TGF-β1 (Transforming Growth Factor β type 1), PDGF (Platelet Derived Growth Factor), HGF (Hepatocyte Growth Factor), VEGF (Vascular Endothelial Growth Factor), EGF (Epithelial Growth Factor) and bFGF (basic Fibroblastic Growth Factor) among others (Table 1)[29,30]. Some of them (IGF-I and HGF) are plasmatic proteins, and their concentration does not depend on the platelet enrichment. However, most of the growth factors are indeed platelet proteins, both synthesized and adsorbed, and thus their quantity does depend on the platelet concentration. To understand the properties of platelet-rich plasma products, it is necessary to detail the different roles of molecules that it contains:

- IGF-I: This protein circulates in plasma as a complex with binding proteins (IGFBP). This determines the bioavailability and regulates the interaction between this IGF-I and its receptor[31,32]. IGF-I is involved in keratinocyte migration and wound healing[33,34], stimulates bone matrix formation and maintenance[35] by promoting pre-osteoblast proliferation[36,37], and also is involved in striated muscle myogenesis[38]. Furthermore, knockout mice for IGF-IR in muscle exhibited impaired muscle regeneration and deficient myoblast differentiation[39]. Recently, It has been observed that IGF-1 promotes tissue repair of skeletal muscle without scar tissue formation by increasing fibre size and muscle size hypertrophy[40]. Also, and related to this, IGF-1 is considered a potent enhancer of tissue regeneration, and its overexpression in muscle injury leads to hastened resolution of the inflammatory phase[41].

- TGF-β1: The role of TGF- β family proteins in wound healing has been recently reviewed[42]. TGF-β has different effects, depending on the tissue and the cell type[6]. The release and posterior bioactivation of latent TGF-β contributes to the early cellular reparative responses, such as migration of cells and neovascularization and angiogenesis[43] into the wound area. In bone, TGF-β1 induces osteogenic differentiation of mesenchymal cells of the bone marrow, upregulating osteoblast differentiation markers[44]. TGF- β plays a crucial role in maintaining homoeostasis of both articular cartilage and subchondral bone[45].

- PDGF: This growth factor is a mitogen and chemotactic factor for all cells of mesenchymal origin[46]. It is important in the repair of joint tissue, including cartilage and meniscus[47,48]. Bone is also a target of PDGF, influencing its metabolism and acting in repair mechanisms[49,50], including the recruitment of pericytes to stabilize new blood vessels[51].

- HGF: Also called scatter factor, it regulates cell growth, migration and morphogenesis[52] and plays an important role in wound-healing through an epithelial-mesenchymal interaction[53]. HGF modulates central inflammatory and immune events that are common to many diseases and organ systems[54]. The antifibrotic effect of HGF has been shown in various tissues[55,56], through induction of Smad[7], and thus regulates the myofibroblast phenotype, allowing the initial contraction of the wound, but gradually making the myofibroblast disappear[57].

- VEGF: This growth factor is a key mediator in wound healing[58] and the main inducer of angiogenesis since it stimulates chemotaxis and proliferation of endothelial cells[59]. This protein is crucial in the sprouting of new capillaries from preexisting vasculature, mainly initiated by hypoxia in ischemic tissue[60]. Also, VEGF is involved in the regulation of many organ homeostases, such as brain, heart, kidney, and liver[61], and its role may be crucial in cell-mediated tissue regeneration[62].

- EGF: This protein promotes chemotaxis and mitogenesis in epithelial and mesenchymal cells[63,64] by acting on the regeneration of multiple tissues. It has an important role in skin, cornea, gastrointestinal tract and nervous system[65-69].

- bFGF: This factor, also called FGF-2, is a potent inductor of cell proliferation, angiogenesis and differentiation[70,71]. Its role in the repair process has been observed in several tissues[72], including bone[73-75], tendon[76,77], and periodontal tissue[78-80].

Classification	Protein	Biological effects
Adhesive proteins	Von Willebrand factor (vWF) propeptide, Fibrinogen, Fibronectin, Vitronectin, Thrombospondin 1 (TSP-1), laminin-8 (alpha4- and alpha5- laminin subunits), signal peptide-CUB-EGF domain containing protein 1 (SCUBE 1)	Cell contact interactions, homeostasis and clotting, and extracellular matrix composition
Clotting factors and associated proteins	FactorV/Va, FactorXI-like protein, multimerin, protein S, high-molecular weight kininogen, antithrombin III, tissue factor pathway inhibitor (TFPI)1	Thrombin production and its regulation
Fibrinolytic factors and associated proteins	Plasminogen, Plasminogen activator inhibitor-1 (PAI-1), urokinase plasminogen activator (uPA), alpha2-antiplasmin, histidine-rich glycoprotein, thrombin activatable fibrinolysis inhibitor (TAFI), alpha2-macroglobulin (α2M)	Plasmin production and vascular modelling
Proteases and anti-proteases	Tissue inhibitor of metalloprotease 1–4 (TIMPs 1–4), metalloprotease-1, -2, -4, -9, A disintegrin and metalloproteinase with a thrombospondin type 1 motif, member 13 (ADAMTS13), tumor necrosis factor-alpha-converting enzyme (TACE), protease nexin-2, C1 inhibitor, serpin proteinase inhibitor 8, alpha1-antitrypsin	Angiogenesis, vascular modelling, regulation of coagulation, and regulation of cellular behaviour
Growth factors	PDGF, TGF-beta1 and -beta2, EGF, IGF-1, VEGF (A and C), bFGF (FGF-2), HGF, Bone morphogenetic protein (BMP)-2, -4, -6, connective tissue growth factor (CTGF)	Chemotaxis, cell proliferation and differentiation, and angiogenesis
Chemokines, cytokines and others	Regulated upon Activation - Normal T-cell Expressed, and Secreted (RANTES), Interleukin-8 (IL-8), Macrophage inflammatory protein-1 (MIP-1) alpha, Epithelial Neutrophil-Activating Peptide 78 (ENA-78), Monocyte chemotactic protein-3 (MCP-3), Growth regulated oncogene- alpha (GRO-alpha), angiopoietin-1, IGF-1 binding protein 3 (IGF-BP3), interleukin-6 soluble receptor (IL-6sR), Platelet factor 4 (PF4), beta-thromboglobulin (bTG), platelet basic protein, neutrophil-activating protein-2 (NAP-2), connective tissue-activating peptide III, high-mobility group protein 1 (HMGB1), Fas ligand (FasL), Homologous to lymphotoxins, exhibits inducible expression, and competes with herpes simplex virus (HSV) glycoprotein D for herpes virus entry mediator, a receptor expressed by T lymphocytes (LIGHT), Tumor necrosis factors (TNF)-related apoptosis-inducing ligand (TRAIL), Stromal cell-derived factor-1 (SDF-1) alpha, endostatin-I, osteonectin-1, bone sialoprotein	Regulation of angiogenesis, vascular modelling, cellular interactions, and bone formation
Anti-microbial proteins	Thrombocidins, defensins	Bactericidal and fungicidal properties
Others	Chondroitin 4-sulfate, albumin, immunoglobulins, disabled-2, semaphorin 3A, Prion protein (PrPC)	
Human adipose-derived stromal cells	PRP releseate after thrombin activation	Increased cell proliferation, ALP activity and mineralization

TABLE 1
Platelet protein classification and their biological role. A set of proteins present in platelets and its physiological role in the regeneration of tissues is shown. Reproduced with permission [126]

Growth factors classically promote several important functions in the regenerative milieu: they are able to stimulate cell proliferation (mitosis), cellular migration (chemotaxis), differentiation (morphogenic effect), angiogenesis, and the combination of several of these effects. These peptides exert the above-mentioned functions in the local environment, close to the site of the application.

However, it is difficult to dissect the contribution of each molecule contained in platelet-rich plasma and examine its effect separately, since many have multiple effects, some of which overlap with others. Also, many molecules are activated in the presence of others, such as TGF-β, which is in a latent state[81] and becomes functional after proteolytic activation or in the presence of other molecules, such as thrombospondin-1[82] or various integrins.

The idea that platelet-rich plasma contains only factors that stimulate angiogenesis and proliferation would be a little simplistic. In fact, another important property of the PRP is the bacteriostatic effect[83]. These antibacterial effects were observed against Staphylococcus aureus and Escherichia coli[84]. Classically, these properties have been shown in leukocyte-enriched platelet-rich plasma. However, recently these antimicrobial properties have been evidenced in PRGF-Endoret[85], which by definition has no white cells. Specifically, PRGF-Endoret has bacteriostatic effect against Staphylococcal strains. Moreover, the addition of leukocytes to the PRGF-Endoret preparation did not yield greater bacteriostatic potential than it already had. This data raise questions about the role that leukocytes may play in a platelet-rich plasma preparation, since they do not improve the bacteriostatic properties but, on the contrary, they might significantly increase the presence of pro-inflammatory molecules.

Platelet-rich products also act as anti-inflammatory mediators by blocking monocyte chemotactic protein-1 (MCP-1), released from monocytes, and lipoxin A4 production[86]. HGF in PRP inhibits NF-kB, a key nuclear factor implicated in inflammatory responses, by activation of its inhibitor (ikBα). In this same study, it was also observed that PRP reduced the chemotaxis of the monocytic line U937[87]. In addition, serotonin, a neurotransmitter and hormone present in platelets, has been reported to directly mediate liver regeneration[88].

3. PRGF-ENDORET: A PIONEERING TECHNOLOGY

For almost two decades our research group has characterized this technology and has studied its therapeutic potential in tissue repair and wound healing[1]. PRGF-Endoret contains a moderated platelet concentration, a two-third fold increase compared to peripheral blood, a dosage shown to induce optimal biological benefit[89]. In fact, lower platelet concentrations can lead to suboptimal effects, whereas higher concentrations might have an inhibitory effect[90]. PRGF-Endoret does not contain leukocytes, and activation is performed only with $CaCl_2$.

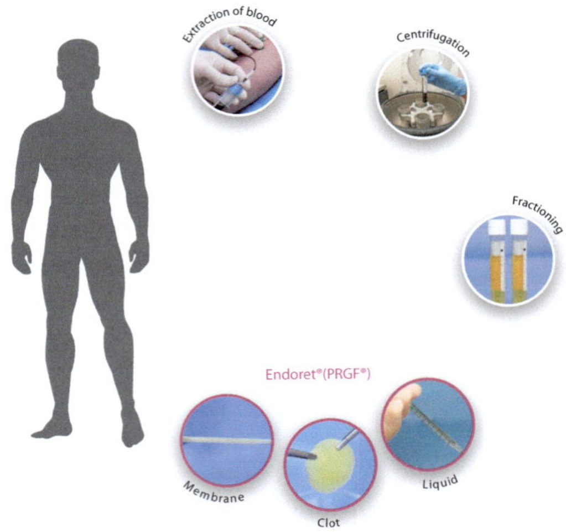

FIG. 1
PRGF-Endoret technology overview. PRGF-Endoret aids in the preparation of different autologous therapeutic formulations from patient's own blood.

The process to produce PRGF-Endoret is easy, fast and reproducible (fig. 1). Blood collection is performed in tubes containing sodium citrate as anticoagulant. Thus, platelets are well preserved. Subsequently, centrifugation is achieved in a specifically designed centrifuge (PRGF System V). The centrifuge has specific parameters to maximize the production of platelets and keep the plasma leukocyte-free. Three typical layers are obtained after centrifugation: (i) a yellowish top layer, the plasma, which contains a gradient of platelets, with maximum concentration of those platelets above the buffy coat; (ii) the leukocyte layer, or buffy coat, is located below the plasma layer; and (iii) the bottom layer, that is the layer containing the red cells. Regarding the plasma volume, it is possible to empirically differentiate between two different fractions, depending on the respective concentration of platelets. The upper fraction will contain a similar number of platelets as peripheral blood whereas the lower fraction will contain 2 to 3-fold the concentration of platelets compared with blood. However, depending on the application, as in the case of PRGF eye drops, it is possible to collect the entire PRGF column without performing two fractions[91]. The basic characteristics of PRGF (whole plasma column) are shown in Table 2.

N=30	Whole blood	PRGF
Leukocytes (x 103/μL)	6.1 ± 1.4	0.3 ± 0.2
Erythrocytes (x 106/μL)	4.78 ± 0.41	0.01 ± 0.01
Platelets (x 103/μL)	235 ± 41	517 ± 107
Leukocyte concentration factor (LCF)	-	0.05 ± 0.03
Platelet concentration factor (PCF)	-	2.2 ± 0.2
Platelet yield (%)	-	66 ± 7

TABLE 2
Summary of the characterization of whole blood and PRGF samples from thirty donors. The values for PRGF correspond to the whole plasma column. Leukocyte, platelet and erythrocyte concentration was measured in whole blood and PRGF. Leukocyte and platelet concentration factor (enrichment as fold increase) relative to the level of peripheral blood (LCF and PCF) and platelet yield (%) are also indicated. Data are expressed as mean ± SD. Reproduced with permission [95].

With the aim of collecting these plasma fractions from PRGF-Endoret technology, we have recently developed an optimized device, the plasma transfer device (PTD2) (fig. 2). The PTD2 is a disposable and sterile aspiration system that allows separating the different fractions obtained after centrifugation. In contrast to the traditional pipetting system, the PTD2 system is faster, avoiding intermediate pipetting steps. In addition, the plasma transfer device does not require maintenance of the pipetting system. Depending on clinical needs, the fractionation can be made in one or two fractions, achieving higher volume - lower concentration of platelets (a single fraction), or lower volume - higher concentration of platelets (two fractions, F1 and F2). After fractionation, PRGF-Endoret can be activated in a controlled way by the addition of $CaCl_2$, providing a clot that mimics its natural structure. Moreover, the coagu-

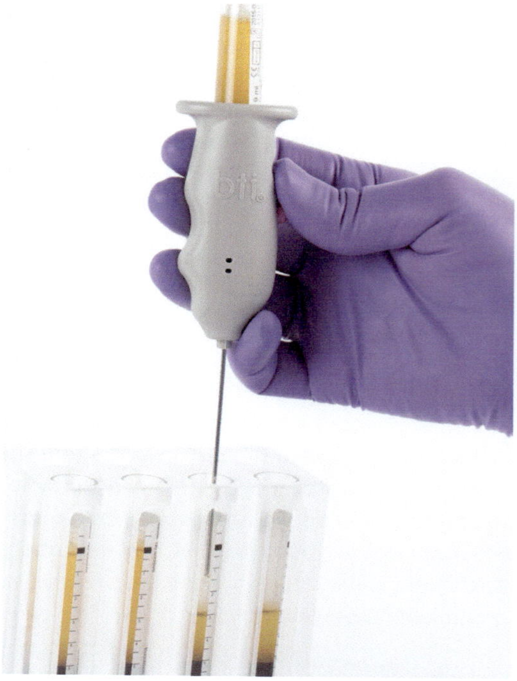

FIG. 2
The plasma transfer device 2 (PTD2) is a disposable and sterile aspiration system that allows the fractionation of PRGF. The device contains an ergonomic button that allows fine control of the suction flow. The suction is performed by the vacuum contained in the fractionation tube (TF9). The aspiration needle is a blunt needle to prevent accidental stab injuries. In this way, PRGF-Endoret is obtained directly in a fractionation tube, where it can be directly activated with calcium chloride. It is possible to perform the whole procedure without opening the extraction tubes, using an adapter needle.

lation is conducted at a speed that allows control of the whole process. Activation with $CaCl_2$ avoids the use of exogenous bovine thrombin, a source of possible immunological reactions[92-94]. Recently, the PRGF obtaining protocol has been improved[95] in order to reduce both the amount of anticoagulant and activator: the new blood extraction tubes (TB9) contain 400 µL of trisodium citrate as anticoagulant, and the new ratio of PRGF Activator would be 20 µL of calcium chloride / mL PRGF.

Another important feature of the PRGF-Endoret technology, when compared with other platelet-rich plasma systems, is the absence of leukocytes, which categorizes it as a safe and homogeneous, because the values of leukocytes are highly variable between donors[96], and within the same donor are highly dependent on small perturbations of the body homeostasis. In addition, polymorphonuclear neutrophils (PMN) contain molecules designed to kill microorganisms, but can seriously damage the body tissues. For example, PMNs are important producers of matrix metalloproteinases (MMP), mainly MMP-8 and MMP-9, which can hamper the regeneration of damaged tissue. PMNs also produce free radicals, reactive oxygen species and nitrogen, which can destroy not only microorganisms but surrounding cells[97]. Of special concern would be to avoid leukocytes if muscle regeneration is required, as in vivo PMNs increase muscle damage[98] and do not provide extra functionality. Therefore, it is recommended to use leukocyte-free platelet-rich plasma in infiltrations of damaged muscle[99].

4. PRGF-ENDORET TECHNOLOGY: A VERSATILE TOOLBOX WITH MULTIPLE FORMULATIONS

A key point that distinguishes the PRGF-Endoret technology from other platelet-rich plasma products is its versatility. Four different formulations (fig. 3) with therapeutic potential are obtained from the patient's blood, depending on the coagulation and activation degree of the samples. These formulations may be used for different therapeutic purposes:

PRGF-Endoret scaffold. This three-dimensional matrix encloses autologous growth factors, both plasma and platelet proteins. This scaffold can be used in various applications, such as the treatment of ulcers[100,101], wound closure and tissue engineering[102]. The three-dimensional structure of the fibrin mesh (fig. 4) allows cell proliferation, since, as mentioned, it contains factors necessary for growth and migration of cells. In addition, this formulation can be combined with other materials[103], such as autologous bone, demineralized freeze-dried bovine bone, and collagen, among others, fine-tuning the resulting characteristics of the scaffold[102].

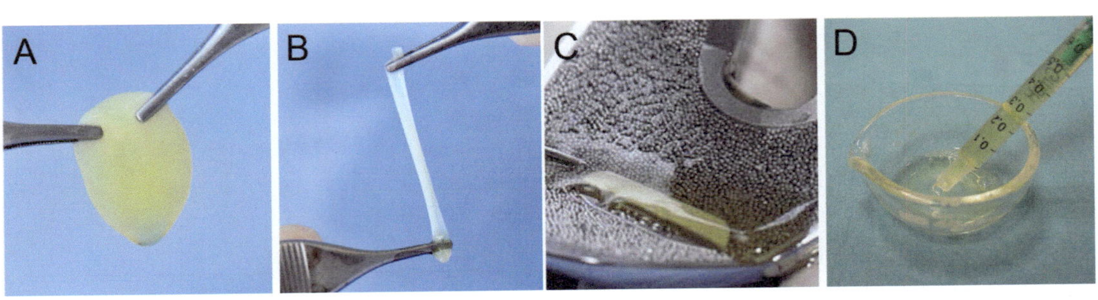

FIG. 3
PRGF-Endoret technology formulations: (A) three-dimensional clot or scaffold, (B) elastic and dense autologous fibrin membrane. (C) liquid formulation activated at the moment and deposited on the implant surface, and (D) the PRGF supernatant, ideal as eye drops or cell culture supplement.

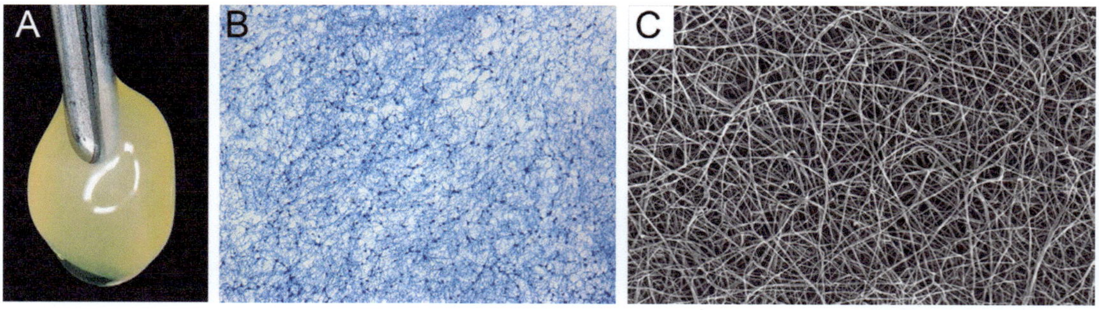

FIG. 4
Three-dimensional structure of PRGF-Endoret clot or scaffold. (A) PRGF scaffold observed with the naked eye. (B) Optical microscopy reveals a 3D network of fibrin with platelet aggregates scattered throughout the network (May-Grunwald-Giemsa staining, original magnification x 400). (C) Closer inspection reveals regular and interconnected intact fibrin strands in a leukocyte-free plasma rich in growth factors (PRGF)-Endoret scaffold (original magnification x 3500). Adapted, with permission,[102].

1. Liquid PRGF-Endoret, activated at the time of use, is used in intra-articular[104-106] and intraosseous[107-109] injections, surgery[110-112], treatment of skin disorders[100,101,113], and implant surface bioactivation by producing a biologically active layer on the titanium surfaces[114,115].

2. The PRGF-Endoret supernatant contains plasma proteins and platelet releasate and can be used as eye drops treatment for dry eye disease[116] and other corneal defects[117,118]. Both in basic research studies and applied areas, this formulation can be used to supplement the cell culture medium[102,119].

3. Autologous fibrin membrane. At the end of the process of coagulation, fibrin scaffold retracts[120]. At that stage, the fibrin membrane can be shaped with tweezers or similar instruments to obtain an elastic, dense and suturable membrane. It is an excellent tool to seal the post-extraction tooth sockets[121-123] and to promote the full epithelialization of other soft tissues[124].

The autologous platelet products have a high therapeutic potential and can be used in various formulations and in various fields of medicine and tissue engineering. At present, there are over forty of these products with different characteristics, in terms of enrichment of platelets, presence of leukocytes, activator type, and final volume among others. This great variability makes it difficult to standardize protocols and compare results. Furthermore, this large variability can engender confusion among clinicians and researchers[125]. It is, therefore, necessary to reach a consensus and better definition of each product. Our research team has spent more than 20 years developing this technology, which makes PRGF-Endoret one of the best characterized autologous platelet-rich plasma, with multiple and growing therapeutic applications, as result of a continuous research translation to the clinical setting.

1. Padilla S, Sanchez M, Orive G, Anitua E. Human-Based Biological and Biomimetic Autologous Therapies for Musculoskeletal Tissue Regeneration. Trends Biotechnol. 2017;35:192-202.

2. Sánchez M, Garate A, Delgado D, Padilla S. Platelet-rich plasma, an adjuvant biological therapy to assist peripheral nerve repair. Neural Regeneration Research. 2017;12:47-52.

3. O'Cearbhaill ED, Ng KS, Karp JM. Emerging medical devices for minimally invasive cell therapy. Mayo Clinic proceedings. 2014;89:259-73.

4. Eming SA, Martin P, Tomic-Canic M. Wound repair and regeneration: mechanisms, signaling, and translation. Science translational medicine. 2014;6:265sr6.

5. Singer AJ, Clark RAF. Cutaneous wound healing. New England Journal of Medicine. 1999;341:738-46.

6. Beanes SR, Dang C, Soo C, Ting K. Skin repair and scar formation: The central role of TGF-β. Expert Reviews in Molecular Medicine. 2003;5.

7. Satish L, Kathju S. Cellular and molecular characteristics of scarless versus fibrotic wound healing. Dermatology Research and Practice. 2010;2010.

8. Karalaki M, Fili S, Philippou A, Koutsilieris M. Muscle regeneration: Cellular and molecular events. In Vivo. 2009;23:779-96.

9. Muller SA, Todorov A, Heisterbach PE, Martin I, Majewski M. Tendon healing: an overview of physiology, biology, and pathology of tendon healing and systematic review of state of the art in tendon bioengineering. Knee Surg Sports Traumatol Arthrosc. 2015;23:2097-105.

10. Soucacos PN, Johnson EO, Babis G. An update on recent advances in bone regeneration. Injury. 2008;39.

11. Deschaseaux F, Sensébé L, Heymann D. Mechanisms of bone repair and regeneration. Trends in Molecular Medicine. 2009;15:417-29.

12. Fortier LA, Barker JU, Strauss EJ, McCarrel TM, Cole BJ. The role of growth factors in cartilage repair. Clinical Orthopaedics and Related Research. 2011;469:2706-15.

13. Barrientos S, Stojadinovic O, Golinko MS, Brem H, Tomic-Canic M. Growth factors and cytokines in wound healing. Wound Repair and Regeneration. 2008;16:585-601.

14. Dereka XE, Markopoulou CE, Vrotsos IA. Role of growth factors on periodontal repair. Growth Factors. 2006;24:260-67.

15. Smith PC, Martinez C, Caceres M, Martinez J. Research on growth factors in periodontology. Periodontol 2000. 2015;67:234-50.

16. Klenkler B, Sheardown H, Jones L. Growth factors in the tear film: role in tissue maintenance, wound healing, and ocular pathology. The ocular surface. 2007;5:228-39.

17. Nurden AT, Nurden P, Sanchez M, Andia I, Anitua E. Platelets and wound healing. Frontiers in Bioscience. 2008;13:3532-48.

18. Blair P, Flaumenhaft R. Platelet α-granules: Basic biology and clinical correlates. Blood Reviews. 2009;23:177-89.

19. Anitua E, Prado R, Azkargorta M, et al. High-throughput proteomic characterization of plasma rich in growth factors (PRGF-Endoret)-derived fibrin clot interactome. J Tissue Eng Regen Med. 2015;9:E1-E12.

20. Sundman EA, Cole BJ, Fortier LA. Growth factor and catabolic cytokine concentrations are influenced by the cellular composition of platelet-rich plasma. American Journal of Sports Medicine. 2011;39:2135-40.

21. Nishiyama K, Okudera T, Watanabe T, et al. Basic characteristics of plasma rich in growth factors (PRGF): blood cell components and biological effects. Clinical and Experimental Dental Research. 2016;2:96-103.

22. Pifer MA, Maerz T, Baker KC, Anderson K. Matrix Metalloproteinase Content and Activity in Low-Platelet, Low-Leukocyte and High-Platelet, High-Leukocyte Platelet Rich Plasma (PRP) and the Biologic Response to PRP by Human Ligament Fibroblasts. Am J Sports Med. 2014.

23. Osterman C, McCarthy MB, Cote MP, et al. Platelet-Rich Plasma Increases Anti-inflammatory Markers in a Human Coculture Model for Osteoarthritis. Am J Sports Med. 2015;43:1474-84.

24. Braun HJ, Kim HJ, Chu CR, Dragoo JL. The effect of platelet-rich plasma formulations and blood products on human synoviocytes: implications for intra-articular injury and therapy. Am J Sports Med. 2014;42:1204-10.

25. Castillo TN, Pouliot MA, Hyeon Joo K, Dragoo JL. Comparison of growth factor and platelet concentration from commercial platelet-rich plasma separation systems. American Journal of Sports Medicine. 2011;39:266-71.

26. Dohan Ehrenfest DM, Rasmusson L, Albrektsson T. Classification of platelet concentrates: from pure platelet-rich plasma (P-PRP) to leucocyte- and platelet-rich fibrin (L-PRF). Trends Biotechnol. 2009;27:158-67.

27. Mishra A, Harmon K, Woodall J. Sports medicine applications of platelet rich plasma. Curr Pharm Biotechnol. 2011.

28. DeLong JM, Russell RP, Mazzocca AD. Platelet-rich plasma: the PAW classification system. Arthroscopy : the journal of arthroscopic & related surgery : official publication of the Arthroscopy Association of North America and the International Arthroscopy Association. 2012;28:998-1009.

29. Alsousou J, Thompson M, Hulley P, Noble A, Willett K. The biology of platelet-rich plasma and its application in trauma and orthopaedic surgery: A review of the literature. Journal of Bone and Joint Surgery - Series B. 2009;91:987-96.

30. Mazzucco L, Borzini P, Gope R. Platelet-derived factors involved in tissue repair-from signal to function. Transfusion Medicine Reviews. 2010;24:218-34.

31. Clemmons DR. Structural and functional analysis of insulin-like growth factors. British Medical Bulletin. 1989;45:465-80.

32. Yakar S, Courtland HW, Clemmons D. IGF-1 and bone: New discoveries from mouse models. Journal of Bone and Mineral Research. 2010;25:2267-76.

33. Ando Y, Jensen PJ. Epidermal growth factor and insulin-like growth factor I enhance keratinocyte migration. Journal of Investigative Dermatology. 1993;100:633-39.

34. Haase I, Evans R, Pofahl R, Watt FM. Regulation of keratinocyte shape, migration and wound epithelialization by IGF-1 and EGF-dependent signalling pathways. Journal of Cell Science. 2003;116:3227-38.

35. Govoni GE. Insulin-like growth factor-I molecular pathways in osteoblasts: Potential targets for pharmacological manipulation. Curr Mol Pharmacol. 2011.

36. Bikle DD, Harris J, Halloran BP, Roberts CT, Leroith D, Morey-Holton E. Expression of the genes for insulin-like growth factors and their receptors in bone during skeletal growth. American Journal of Physiology - Endocrinology and Metabolism. 1994;267.

37. Meinel L, Zoidis E, Zapf J, et al. Localized insulin-like growth factor I delivery to enhance new bone formation. Bone. 2003;33:660-72.

38. Florini JR, Ewton DZ, Coolican SA. Growth hormone and the insulin-like growth factor system in myogenesis. Endocrine Reviews. 1996;17:481-517.

39. Heron-Milhavet L, Mamaeva D, Leroith D, Lamb NJ, Fernandez A. Impaired muscle regeneration and myoblast differentiation in mice with a muscle-specific KO of IGF-IR. Journal of Cellular Physiology. 2010;225:1-6.

40. Gallego-Colon E, Villalba M, Tonkin J, et al. Intravenous delivery of adeno-associated virus 9-encoded IGF-1Ea propeptide improves post-infarct cardiac remodelling. Npj Regenerative Medicine. 2016;1:16001.

41. Tonkin J, Temmerman L, Sampson RD, et al. Monocyte/Macrophage-derived IGF-1 Orchestrates Murine Skeletal Muscle Regeneration and Modulates Autocrine Polarization. Molecular therapy : the journal of the American Society of Gene Therapy. 2015;23:1189-200.

42. Douglas HE. TGF-ß in wound healing: A review. Journal of Wound Care. 2010;19:403-06.

43. Yang EY, Moses HL. Transforming growth factor β1-induced changes in cell migration, proliferation, and angiogenesis in the chicken chorioallantoic membrane. Journal of Cell Biology. 1990;111:731-41.

44. Zhao L, Jiang S, Hantash BM. Transforming growth factor β1 induces osteogenic differentiation of murine bone marrow stromal cells. Tissue Engineering - Part A. 2010;16:725-33.

45. Zhen G, Cao X. Targeting TGFbeta signaling in subchondral bone and articular cartilage homeostasis. Trends in pharmacological sciences. 2014;35:227-36.

46. Chen PH, Chen X, He X. Platelet-derived growth factors and their receptors: Structural and functional perspectives. Biochimica et biophysica acta. 2013;1834:2176-86.

47. Schmidt MB, Chen EH, Lynch SE. A review of the effects of insulin-like growth factor and platelet derived growth factor on in vivo cartilage healing and repair. Osteoarthritis and Cartilage. 2006;14:403-12.

48. Tumia NS, Johnstone AJ. Platelet derived growth factor-AB enhances knee meniscal cell activity in vitro. Knee. 2009;16:73-76.

49. Canalis E, Varghese S, McCarthy TL, Centrella M. Role of platelet derived growth factor in bone cell function. Growth regulation. 1992;2:151-55.

50. Hock JM, Canalis E. Platelet-derived growth factor enhances bone cell replication, but not differentiated function of osteoblasts. Endocrinology. 1994;134:1423-28.

51. Caplan AI, Correa D. PDGF in bone formation and regeneration: New insights into a novel mechanism involving MSCs. Journal of Orthopaedic Research. 2011;29:1795-803.

52. Nakamura T. Structure and function of hepatocyte growth factor. Progress in Growth Factor Research. 1991;3:67-85.

53. Matsumoto K, Nakamura T. Hepatocyte growth factor (HGF) as a tissue organizer for organogenesis and regeneration. Biochemical and Biophysical Research Communications. 1997;239:639-44.

54. Molnarfi N, Benkhoucha M, Funakoshi H, Nakamura T, Lalive PH. Hepatocyte growth factor: A regulator of inflammation and autoimmunity. Autoimmun Rev. 2015;14:293-303.

55. Mizuno S, Kurosawa T, Matsumoto K, Mizuno-Horikawa Y, Okamoto M, Nakamura T. Hepatocyte growth factor prevents renal fibrosis and dysfunction in a mouse model of chronic renal disease. Journal of Clinical Investigation. 1998;101:1827-34.

56. Shang J, Deguchi K, Ohta Y, et al. Strong neurogenesis, angiogenesis, synaptogenesis, and antifibrosis of hepatocyte growth factor in rats brain after transient middle cerebral artery occlusion. Journal of Neuroscience Research. 2011;89:86-95.

57. Shukla MN, Rose JL, Ray R, Lathrop KL, Ray A, Ray P. Hepatocyte growth factor inhibits epithelial to myofibroblast transition in lung cells via Smad7. American Journal of Respiratory Cell and Molecular Biology. 2009;40:643-53.

58. Bao P, Kodra A, Tomic-Canic M, Golinko MS, Ehrlich HP, Brem H. The Role of Vascular Endothelial Growth Factor in Wound Healing. Journal of Surgical Research. 2009;153:347-58.

59. Ferrara N, Gerber HP. The role of vascular endothelial growth factor in angiogenesis. Acta Haematologica. 2001;106:148-56.

60. Jazwa A, Florczyk U, Grochot-Przeczek A, et al. Limb ischemia and vessel regeneration: Is there a role for VEGF? Vascular pharmacology. 2016;86:18-30.

61. Luo J, Xiong Y, Han X, Lu Y. VEGF non-angiogenic functions in adult organ homeostasis: Therapeutic implications. Journal of Molecular Medicine. 2011;89:635-45.

62. Song SY, Chung HM, Sung JH. The pivotal role of VEGF in adipose-derived-stem-cell-mediated regeneration. Expert Opinion on Biological Therapy. 2010;10:1529-37.

63. Carpenter G, Cohen S. Epidermal growth factor. Journal of Biological Chemistry. 1990;265:7709-12.

64. Kurten RC, Chowdhury P, Sanders Jr RC, et al. Coordinating epidermal growth factor-induced motility promotes efficient wound closure. American Journal of Physiology - Cell Physiology. 2005;288.

65. Schultz G, Clark W, Rotatori DS. EGF and TGF-a in wound healing and repair. Journal of Cellular Biochemistry. 1991;45:346-52.

66. Schultz G, Chegini N, Grant M, Khaw P, MacKay S. EFFECTS OF GROWTH FACTORS ON CORNEAL WOUND HEALING. Acta Ophthalmologica. 1992;70:60-66.

67. Wong RWC, Guillaud L. The role of epidermal growth factor and its receptors in mammalian CNS. Cytokine and Growth Factor Reviews. 2004;15:147-56.

68. Xian CJ, Zhou XF. EGF family of growth factors: Essential roles and functional redundancy in the nerve system. Frontiers in Bioscience. 2004;9:85-92.

69. Berlanga-Acosta J, Gavilondo-Cowley J, López-Saura P, et al. Epidermal growth factor in clinical practice - A review of its biological actions, clinical indications and safety implications. International Wound Journal. 2009;6:331-46.

70. Klagsbrun M. The fibroblast growth factor family: Structural and biological properties. Progress in Growth Factor Research. 1989;1:207-35.

71. Yun YR, Won JE, Jeon E, et al. Fibroblast growth factors: Biology, function, and application for tissue regeneration. J Tissue Eng. 2010;2010.

72. Beenken A, Mohammadi M. The FGF family: biology, pathophysiology and therapy. Nat Rev Drug Discov. 2009;8:235-53.

73. Tabata Y, Yamada K, Hong L, Miyamoto S, Hashimoto N, Ikada Y. Skull bone regeneration in primates in response to basic fibroblast growth factor. Journal of Neurosurgery. 1999;91:851-56.

74. Song K, Rao NJ, Chen ML, Huang ZJ, Cao YG. Enhanced bone regeneration with sequential delivery of basic fibroblast growth factor and sonic hedgehog. Injury. 2011;42:796-802.

75. Kempen DHR, Creemers LB, Alblas J, et al. Growth Factor interactions in bone regeneration. Tissue Engineering - Part B: Reviews. 2010;16:551-66.

76. Chang J, Most D, Thunder R, Mehrara B, Longaker MT, Lineaweaver WC. Molecular studies in flexor tendon wound healing: The role of basic fibroblast growth factor gene expression. Journal of Hand Surgery. 1998;23:1052-58.

77. Thomopoulos S, Das R, Sakiyama-Elbert S, Silva MJ, Charlton N, Gelberman RH. BFGF and PDGF-BB for tendon repair: Controlled release and biologic activity by tendon fibroblasts in vitro. Annals of Biomedical Engineering. 2010;38:225-34.

78. Shimabukuro Y, Ichikawa T, Terashima Y, et al. Basic fibroblast growth factor regulates expression of heparan sulfate in human periodontal ligament cells. Matrix Biology. 2008;27:232-41.

79. Shirakata Y, Taniyama K, Yoshimoto T, et al. Regenerative effect of basic fibroblast growth factor on periodontal healing in two-wall intrabony defects in dogs. Journal of Clinical Periodontology. 2010;37:374-81.

80. Murakami S. Periodontal tissue regeneration by signaling molecule(s): What role does basic fibroblast growth factor (FGF-2) have in periodontal therapy? Periodontology 2000. 2011;56:188-208.

81. Annes JP, Munger JS, Rifkin DB. Making sense of latent TGFβ activation. Journal of Cell Science. 2003;116:217-24.

82. Belotti D, Capelli C, Resovi A, Introna M, Taraboletti G. Thrombospondin-1 promotes mesenchymal stromal cell functions via TGFbeta and in cooperation with PDGF. Matrix Biol. 2016.

83. Mariani E, Filardo G, Canella V, et al. Platelet-rich plasma affects bacterial growth in vitro. Cytotherapy. 2014;16:1294-304.

84. Bielecki TM, Gazdzik TS, Arendt J, Szczepanski T, Król W, Wielkoszynski T. Antibacterial effect of autologous platelet gel enriched with growth factors and other active substances: An in vitro study. Journal of Bone and Joint Surgery - Series B. 2007;89:417-20.

85. Anitua E, Alonso R, Girbau C, Aguirre JJ, Muruzabal F, Orive G. Antibacterial effect of plasma rich in growth factors (PRGF(R)-Endoret(R)) against Staphylococcus aureus and Staphylococcus epidermidis strains. Clin Exp Dermatol. 2012;37:652-7.

86. El-Sharkawy H, Kantarci A, Deady J, et al. Platelet-rich plasma: Growth factors and pro- and anti-inflammatory properties. Journal of Periodontology. 2007;78:661-69.

87. Bendinelli P, Matteucci E, Dogliotti G, et al. Molecular basis of anti-inflammatory action of platelet-rich plasma on human chondrocytes: Mechanisms of NF-κB inhibition via HGF. Journal of Cellular Physiology. 2010;225:757-66.

88. Lesurtel M, Graf R, Aleil B, et al. Platelet-derived serotonin mediates liver regeneration. Science. 2006;312:104-07.

89. Anitua E, Sánchez M, Zalduendo MM, et al. Fibroblastic response to treatment with different preparations rich in growth factors. Cell Proliferation. 2009;42:162-70.

90. Weibrich G, Hansen T, Kleis W, Buch R, Hitzler WE. Effect of platelet concentration in platelet-rich plasma on peri-implant bone regeneration. Bone. 2004;34:665-71.

91. Anitua E, Muruzabal F, de la Fuente M, Merayo J, Duran J, Orive G. Plasma Rich in Growth Factors for the Treatment of Ocular Surface Diseases. Current eye research. 2016;41:875-82.

92. Zehnder JL, Leung LLK. Development of antibodies to thrombin and factor V with recurrent bleeding in a patient exposed to topical bovine thrombin. Blood. 1990;76:2011-16.

93. Landesberg R, Moses M, Karpatkin M. Risks of using platelet rich plasma gel [2]. Journal of Oral and Maxillofacial Surgery. 1998;56:1116-17.

94. Diesen DL, Lawson JH. Bovine thrombin: History, use, and risk in the surgical patient. Vascular. 2008;16.

95. Anitua E, Prado R, Troya M, et al. Implementation of a more physiological plasma rich in growth factor (PRGF) protocol: Anticoagulant removal and reduction in activator concentration. Platelets. 2016;27:459-66.

96. Weibrich G, Kleis WKG, Hitzler WE, Hafner G. Comparison of the platelet concentrate collection system with the plasma-rich-in-growth-factors kit to produce platelet-rich plasma: A technical report. International Journal of Oral and Maxillofacial Implants. 2005;20:118-23.

97. Scott A, Khan KM, Roberts CR, Cook JL, Duronio V. What do we mean by the term "inflammation"? A contemporary basic science update for sports medicine. British Journal of Sports Medicine. 2004;38:372-80.

98. Tidball JG. Inflammatory processes in muscle injury and repair. American Journal of Physiology - Regulatory Integrative and Comparative Physiology. 2005;288.

99. Harmon KG. Muscle injuries and PRP: What does the science say? British Journal of Sports Medicine. 2010;44:616-17.

100. Orcajo B, Muruzabal F, Isasmendi MC, et al. The use of plasma rich in growth factors (PRGF-Endoret) in the treatment of a severe mal perforant ulcer in the foot of a person with diabetes. Diabetes Research and Clinical Practice. 2011;93.

101. Anitua E, Aguirre JJ, Algorta J, et al. Effectiveness of autologous preparation rich in growth factors for the treatment of chronic cutaneous ulcers. Journal of Biomedical Materials Research - Part B Applied Biomaterials. 2008;84:415-21.

102. Anitua E, Prado R, Orive G. Endogenous morphogens and fibrin bioscaffolds for stem cell therapeutics. Trends Biotechnol. 2013;31:364-74.

103. Anitua E, Prado R, Orive G. A lateral approach for sinus elevation using PRGF technology. Clinical Implant Dentistry and Related Research. 2009;11.

104. Anitua E, Sanchez M, Aguirre JJ, Prado R, Padilla S, Orive G. Efficacy and safety of plasma rich in growth factors intra-articular infiltrations in the treatment of knee osteoarthritis. Arthroscopy : the journal of arthroscopic & related surgery : official publication of the Arthroscopy Association of North America and the International Arthroscopy Association. 2014;30:1006-17.

105. Vaquerizo V, Plasencia MA, Arribas I, et al. Comparison of Intra-Articular Injections of Plasma Rich in Growth Factors (PRGF-Endoret) Versus Durolane Hyaluronic Acid in the Treatment of Patients With Symptomatic Osteoarthritis: A Randomized Controlled Trial. Arthroscopy : the journal of arthroscopic & related surgery : official publication of the Arthroscopy Association of North America and the International Arthroscopy Association. 2013;29:1635-43.

106. Sanchez M, Fiz N, Azofra J, et al. A randomized clinical trial evaluating plasma rich in growth factors (PRGF-Endoret) versus hyaluronic acid in the short-term treatment of symptomatic knee osteoarthritis. Arthroscopy : the journal of arthroscopic & related surgery : official publication of the Arthroscopy Association of North America and the International Arthroscopy Association. 2012;28:1070-8.

107. Sanchez M, Fiz N, Guadilla J, et al. Intraosseous infiltration of platelet-rich plasma for severe knee osteoarthritis. Arthrosc Tech. 2014;3:e713-7.

108. Sanchez M, Anitua E, Delgado D, et al. A new strategy to tackle severe knee osteoarthritis: Combination of intra-articular and intraosseous injections of Platelet Rich Plasma. Expert Opin Biol Ther. 2016;16:627–43.

109. Sanchez M, Delgado D, Sanchez P, et al. Combination of Intra-Articular and Intraosseous Injections of Platelet Rich Plasma for Severe Knee Osteoarthritis: A Pilot Study. Biomed Res Int. 2016;2016:4868613.

110. Sanchez M, Anitua E, Cugat R, et al. Nonunions treated with autologous preparation rich in growth factors. Journal of Orthopaedic Trauma. 2009;23:52-59.

111. Seijas R, Santana-Suárez RY, García-Balletbó M, Cuscó X, Ares O, Cugat R. Delayed union of the clavicle treated with plasma rich in growth factors. Acta Orthopaedica Belgica. 2010;76:689-93.

112. Sanchez M, Delgado D, Sanchez P, et al. Platelet rich plasma and knee surgery. Biomed Res Int. 2014;2014:890630.

113. Aguirre J, Anitua E, Francisco S, Cabezas A, Orive G, Algorta J. Efficacy and safety of plasma rich in growth factors in the treatment of venous ulcers: a randomized clinical trial controlled with conventional treatment. Clinical Dermatology. 2015;3:13-20.

114. Anitua E, Tejero R, Alkhraisat MH, Orive G. Platelet-rich plasma to improve the bio-functionality of biomaterials. BioDrugs. 2013;27:97-111.

115. Tejero R, Anitua E, Orive G. Toward the biomimetic implant surface: Biopolymers on titanium-based implants for bone regeneration. Progress in Polymer Science. 2014;39:1406-47.

116. Merayo-Lloves J, Sanchez-Avila RM, Riestra AC, et al. Safety and Efficacy of Autologous Plasma Rich in Growth Factors Eye Drops for the Treatment of Evaporative Dry Eye. Ophthalmic research. 2016;56:68-73.

117. Merayo-Lloves J, Sanchez RM, Riestra AC, et al. Autologous Plasma Rich in Growth Factors Eyedrops in Refractory Cases of Ocular Surface Disorders. Ophthalmic research. 2015;55:53-61.

118. López-Plandolit S, Morales MC, Freire V, Etxebarría J, Durán JA. Plasma rich in growth factors as a therapeutic agent for persistent corneal epithelial defects. Cornea. 2010;29:843-48.

119. Burnouf T, Strunk D, Koh MB, Schallmoser K. Human platelet lysate: Replacing fetal bovine serum as a gold standard for human cell propagation? Biomaterials. 2016;76:371-87.

120. Heemskerk JW, Mattheij NJ, Cosemans JM. Platelet-based coagulation: different populations, different functions. J Thromb Haemost. 2013;11:2-16.

121. Rosano G, Taschieri S, Del Fabbro M. Immediate postextraction implant placement using plasma rich in growth factors technology in maxillary premolar region: a new strategy for soft tissue management. J Oral Implantol. 2013;39:98-102.

122. Taschieri S, Lolato A, Ofer M, Testori T, Francetti L, Del Fabbro M. Immediate post-extraction implants with or without pure platelet-rich plasma: a 5-year follow-up study. Oral and maxillofacial surgery. 2017;DOI: 10.1007/s10006-017-0609-2.

123. Mozzati M, Gallesio G, Gassino G, Palomba A, Bergamasco L. Can plasma rich in growth factors improve healing in patients who underwent

radiotherapy for head and neck cancer? A split-mouth study. The Journal of craniofacial surgery. 2014;25:938-43.

124. *Sánchez M, Anitua E, Cole A, Da Silva A, Azofra J, Andia I. Management of post-surgical Achilles tendon complications with a preparation rich in growth factors: A study of two-cases. Injury Extra. 2009;40:11-15.*

125. *Anitua E, Sánchez M, Prado R, Orive G. The P makes the difference in plasma rich in growth factors (PRGF) technology. Platelets. 2011;22:473-74.*

126. *Anitua E, Prado R, Sánchez M, Orive G. Platelet-Rich Plasma: Preparation and Formulation. Operative Techniques in Orthopaedics. 2012;22:25-32.*

CHAPTER 3

Repair and Regeneration: Connecting the Dots Among Coagulation, Immune System, the Sensory Nervous System and Fibrogenesis

AUTHORS

Padilla S.[1,2,4], Sánchez M.[3], Padilla I.[1], Anitua E.[1,2,4]

[1] Eduardo Anitua Fundation. Vitoria-Gasteiz, Spain
[2] BTI Biotechnology Institute. Vitoria-Gasteiz, Spain
[3] Arthroscopic Surgery Unit Research, Hospital Vithas San José, Vitoria-Gasteiz, Spain
[4] University Institute for Regenerative Medicine and Oral Implantology (UIRMI) from the University of Basque Country (UPV/EHU)

SUMMARY

Two conditions have challenged the survival of living beings with a closed circulatory system, namely trauma and infection. These conditions account for the primary life-threatening emergencies, namely, bleeding and microbial invasion. Through natural selection and conservation, evolution has shaped the biological defence system of vertebrates to cope with bleeding and microbial invasion by systems consisting of several interlinked modules such as coagulation, the innate immune system, and fibrogenesis. In humans, pivotal players in the biological defence system modules are platelets, leukocytes and fibrinogen, located within a connective tissue, namely, the blood, which acts as an incessantly dynamic and renewing kind of container in mammals. Drawing on the regenerative potential of platelets, plasma biomolecules and fibrin matrix, several systems of producing autologous platelets-and plasma derived products (APPDPs) have been developed and aimed at enhancing the natural in vivo tissue regenerative capacity of damaged tissues. However, in spite of skill and care in the elaboration and application of these blood products by medical staff, consistency in the surgical application of platelet rich plasma remains illusive due to a nonuniform approach in both the composition of these products and the modalities of their application. As a consequence, there is both light and shadow in the outcomes of this treatment.

E. Anitua et al. (eds.), *Platelet Rich Plasma in Orthopaedics and Sports Medicine*,
https://doi.org/10.1007/978-3-319-63730-3_3

1. INTRODUCTION

Through natural selection and conservation, evolution has shaped the biological defence system of vertebrates (figure 1) to cope with bleeding and microbial invasion, two conditions, which have challenged the survival of animals with a closed circulatory system[1]. The biological defence system of vertebrates consists of 3 interlinked modules namely, coagulation, the innate immune system, and fibrogenesis[1, 2]. Once tissue damage and/or pathogen invasion is detected, organisms mount both a systemic and a local host defence response[2, 3]. In humans, the systemic response stems mainly from the influence of locally produced prostaglandin E2 (PGE2) and other inflammatory mediators[4] on the central nervous system, producing the response known as sickness behaviour (chiefly fever, anorexia, fatigue, and sleepiness) which appear to have only one purpose: survival[3, 5, 6]. Despite the pivotal role of systemic response in the survival function, this response is not in the scope of this chapter. The local response encompasses procoagulant and proinflammatory mechanisms which, together with the activation of platelets, endothelial cells, tissue-resident macrophages, recruitment of circulant monocytes and neutrophils, release inflammatory mediators in a quick autocrine and paracrine reaction (seconds to a few hours)[6-8]. While platelets manage to halt the bleeding process through platelet aggregation, thrombin generation, and fibrin clot formation[9], neutrophils and monocytes prevent the assault of microbial germ lines by killing them, thereby sterilizing the damaged area[8, 10]. Both processes of hemostasis and inflammation are triggered by the aforementioned disruptor, either trauma and/or infection.

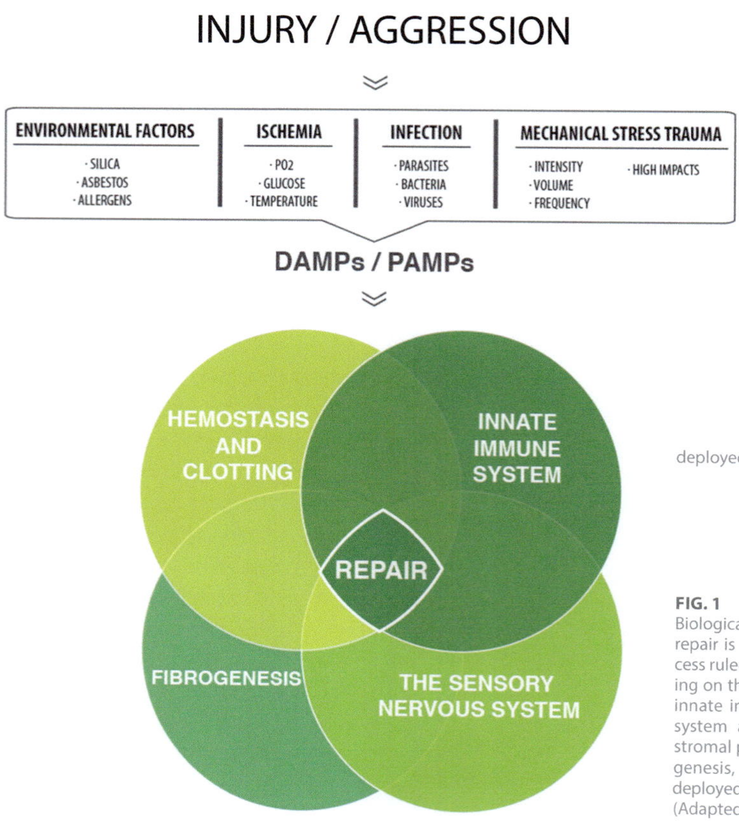

deployed in different ar-

FIG. 1
Biological defense system of mammals. Tissue repair is an open and condition-sensitive process ruled by microenvironment cues. Depending on the balance of hemostasis and clotting, innate immune system, the sensory nervous system and fibrogenesis, parenchymal and stromal processes such as myogenesis, osteogenesis, angiogenesis, and neurogenesis will deployed in different arrays.[1, 2, 15, 53]
(Adapted with permission from Padilla et al.[110])

Immediately after this cascade module, where the pivotal players are platelets, leukocytes and fibrinogen, a dramatic switch from killing to healing occurs in the damaged area known as the resolution of inflammation[6, 11, 12]. As a continuum process, the biological defence program will later address reconstruction of the damaged area, which will require not only resolution of the inflammatory stage, but also the coordinated incorporation and action of other cell effectors such as macrophages, lymphocytes, fibroblasts, EPCs and structural biomolecules aimed at promoting angiogenesis, parenchymal and stromal cell proliferation and differentiation, and extracellular matrix (ECM) synthesis[7, 8, 10], where the new formed fibrin clot acts as a transient scaffold. (Figure 2)[13, 14].

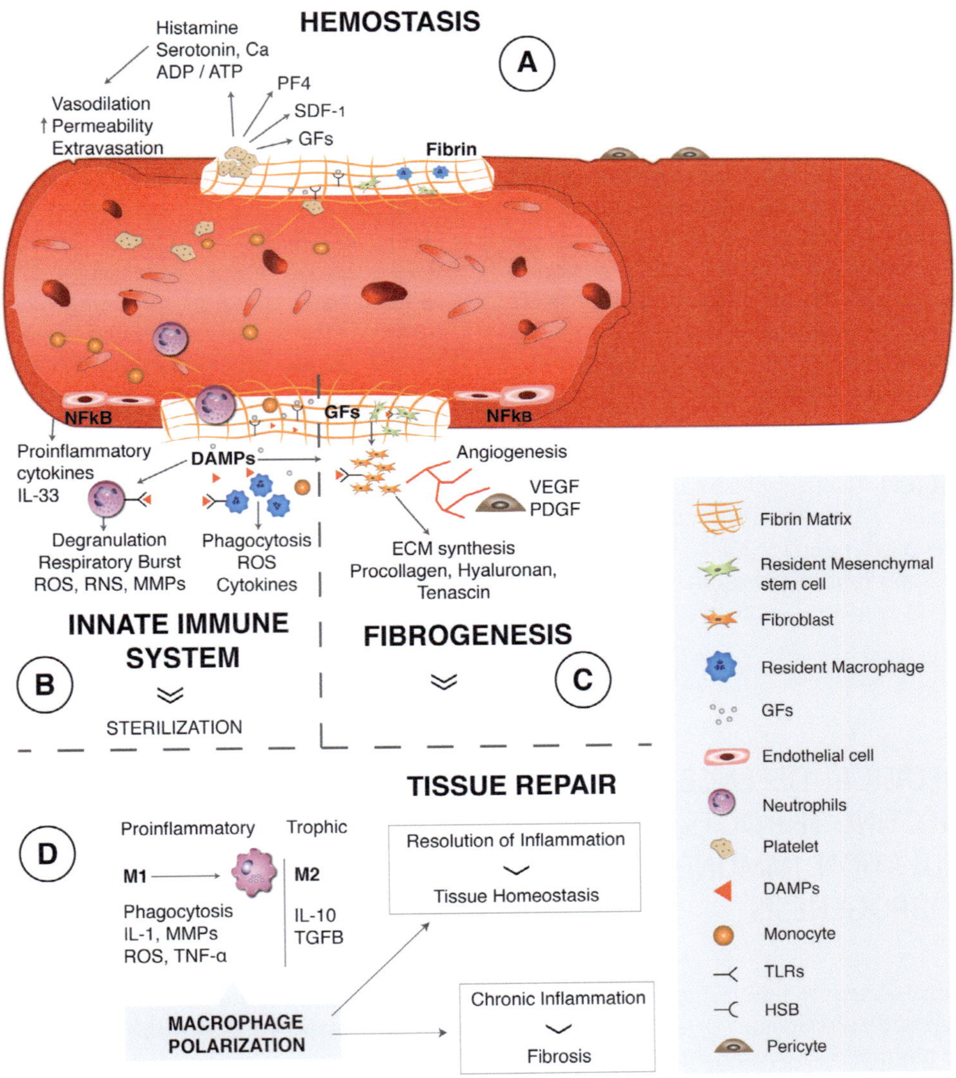

FIG. 2
Connecting the dots among the different modules of the biological defense system. Tissue reconstruction might be considered a byproduct of the mechanisms underlying the biological defense system.[1,2,15,30,37]
(Adapted with permission from Padilla et al.[110])

Drawing on the regenerative potential of platelets, plasma biomolecules and fibrin matrix[13, 15-17], several systems that produce autologous platelets- and plasma-derived products (APPDPs) have been developed, aimed at triggering and enhancing both the natural in vivo tissue morphogenesis and the regenerative capacity of damaged tissues. Platelet-rich plasma (PRPs) are platelet concentrates within a plasma suspension whose composition is determined by the method used to obtain it. PRGF includes plasma and twofold-or-more increases in platelet concentrations above baseline levels, and different collection methods mean the concentration of leukocytes and erythrocytes varies widely, from a complete absence to a high concentration of them[18]. The therapeutic potential of PRPs[19-21] and plasma rich in growth factors (PRGF) for in situ regenerative medicine has yielded extremely promising clinical and surgical outcomes in musculoskeletal system pathologies such as osteoarthritis and cartilage repair[17, 21-27], in oral and maxillofacial surgery[17, 19], as well as in the treatment of diabetic ulcers[19].

In an effort to connect the dots, this chapter is aimed at both clarifying the interactions among coagulation, immune system, and fibrogenesis that may play important roles in tissue healing, and shedding light on some pitfalls in the application of PRPs products as enhancers of tissue repair.

2. BIOLOGICAL DEFENCE SYSTEM: CONNECTING THE DOTS AMONG COAGULATION, IMMUNE SYSTEM, AND FIBROGENESIS

In mammals, the first step in tissue repair is the detection of tissue damage signals such as damage-and pathogen-associated molecular patterns (DAMPs or PAMPs) released as a result of necrotic and apoptotic cell death and damaged microbial and (ECM) host products. These products act as inducers of a complex cascade consisting of hemostasis and clotting, the innate immune system, and fibrogenesis, which are triggered in a sequential and intertwined spatiotemporal manner (figure 2)[10, 28, 29]. DAMPs and PAMPs are damage signals which are recognized by transmembrane toll-like receptors (TLRs) expressed by several tissue cells that act as sensor elements including platelets, mast cells, macrophages, epithelial and endothelial cells, and neutrophils (figure 3)[30-33]. The interaction of DAMPs and PAMPs with TLRs brings about, in these sentinel cells, the activation of a highly conserved intracellular signalling pathway known as NFkB. Its activation will end up inducing the gene expression of growth factors and cytokines, a phenomenon known as inflammatory response (figure 3)[6, 34]. The acute storm of pro-inflammatory cytokines including but not limited to interleukin 1beta (IL-1B), interleukin 6 (IL-6), tumor necrosis factor alpha (TNF-a), interferon gama (IFN-j), transforming growth factor beta (TGFB), platelet derived growth factor (PDGF), vascular endothelial growth factor (VEGF), and connective tissue growth factor (CTGF), mainly coming from activated platelets, endothelial cells, pro-inflammatory macrophages, fibroblasts and mast cells, will attract, recruit, and activate circulating cells such as platelets, neutrophils and monocytes into the injury site[6]. From the beginning, platelets adhere to exposed collagen and tissue factor from damaged ECM, aggregate and facilitate blood clot and thrombin formation and polymerization of fibrinogen to fibrin, thereby halting the bleeding process[9, 13]. In addition to activating platelets and inducing pro-inflammatory cytokines from immune and endothelial cells[1, 35], thrombin performs other important roles as a potent endothelial permeability enhancer, chemoattractant of monocytes and neutrophils, inducer of expression of adhesive molecules and promoter of the degranulation of platelets, as well as influencing the cell cycle of several phenotypes[1, 15, 36]. Simultaneously neutrophils generate a cytotoxic microenvironment[8] as a result of both degranulation of anti-microbial molecules, proteases and metalloproteinases (MMPs), highly reactive oxygen and nitrogen species (ROS and RNS), and by respiratory burst, induce microbial death and sterilize the damaged area (figure 2)[8, 10]. Neutrophils also attract circulating monocytes to the injured site, and activate dendritic cells and macrophages. These resident and migratory mononucleated cells take on a pro-inflammatory phenotype (M1) releasing nitric oxide (NO) and citrulline, ROS, MMPs and a tissue inhibitor of metalloproteinases (TIMPs). Moreover, macrophages express IL-1, IL-6, IL-12, and TNFa, induce Th1 cell infiltration and activation, and phagocytose apoptotic/necrotic cells and other ECM breakdown products, contributing together with the lipoxins (eicosanoids and platelet-activating factors)[7] to tissue repair[6, 28, 37, 38]. This first cell-and bacterial-killing, and matrix destroying microenvironment stems from both the initial noxious agents and the collateral damage inflicted by the inflammatory effectors of the innate immune system which can wreak havoc if the inflammatory process is too intense or too persistent[6, 12]. In addition, platelets release Stromal cell-derived factor (SDF-1), CTGF, TGFB, Platelet factor 4 (PF4) and VEGF, which together with fibrin adhesion cell receptors may well contribute to the resolution of inflammation by recruiting endothelial progenitor cells (EPCs)[39], preventing monocyte apoptosis, promoting trophic macrophages (M2)[40] and activating resident mesenchymal fibroblasts precursor cells[41, 42]. In doing so, these growth factors favour fibrogenesis[30] and generate both a trophic microenvironment, and tissue angiogenesis in a context dependent manner[43]. The formed transient fibrin matrix traps several growth factors and cytokines, promotes adhesion of immune cells, and is chemotactic for phagocytic leukocytes. This natural fibrin scaffold mediates cellular attachment through P-selectin and integrins binding on platelets, monocytes, macrophages, neutrophils, adult stem and hematopoietic progenitor cell antigen (CD34) progenitor cells [1, 13, 14, 43-45], and provides mechanical support and plastic-elastic stiffness all of which have a drastic impact on the fates of diverse cell types such as muscle stem cells[46, 47]. The resolution of inflammation is mainly driven by, but not limited to, the plasticity and polarization of macrophages from phagocytic and pro-inflammatory phenotype (M1) to anti-fibrotic and anti-inflammatory ones (M2)[2, 6, 11, 12], and by the production of lipoxins[7]. In an uninterrupted process, the biological defence system will intensify and address the already ongoing reconstruction of the damaged area, which will require not only resolution of the inflammatory stage, but also the coordinated action of other cell effectors such as trophic macrophages (M2), lymphocytes, activated fibroblasts, EPCs and structural biomolecules aimed at promoting angiogenesis, parenchymal and stromal cell proliferation and differentiation, and ECM synthesis, (figure 2)[10, 28, 48].

As a result of local activation of the tissue plasminogen activator/plasminogen system, fibrinolysis will release the growth factors and cytokines previously trapped in the fibrin network through the cell surface heparan sulphate-binding domains[45, 49] such as SDF-1, PDGF, VEGF, hepatocyte growth factor (HGF), Brain-derived neurotrophic factor (BDNF), Fibroblast growth factor (FGF) among other previously released growth factors by platelets, macrophages, endothelial cells, and newly activated fibroblasts, which will be freed up in the ECM[13, 14, 43-45]. The gradual and sustained release of growth factors[45] from fibrin controls morphogen gradients at the repair scenario[50] and facilitates vascular, epithelial and mesenchymal reconstruction (figure 5)[13, 14, 45]. After the phagocytosis of apoptotic neutrophils, lymphocytes or inflamed parenchymal and stromal cells, inflammatory macrophages (M1) will turn into an anti-inflammatory phenotype and express pro-inflammatory cytokines, including TGF B1, IL-4, IL-10, and PGE2[12]. These cytokines are involved in immunoregulatory functions as well as in the resolution or progression of fibrogenesis[28, 37] which, along with PDGF, and TGFB1, are released from fibrin matrix[14, 45], and lead the switch in the injured area from tissue breakdown to tissue reconstruction[12, 30, 38]. These cytokines allow circulating fibrocytes, perivascular pericytes, and resident mesenchymal cells to differentiate first into fibroblasts and later into alfa-smooth muscle actin myofibroblasts (αSMA) (figure 2)[31, 37, 41, 45]. Fibroblasts and myofibroblasts are highly synthetic and secretory cells that will partially address the loss of tissue in the injured area by synthesizing fibrillar ECM components such as collagen, elastin, fibronectin, tenascin-C, and hyaluronan. They will as well release mitogenic and motogenic cytokines which, together with IL-33 released from the dying cells[51] modulate cells involved in mesenchymal and parenchymal healing response, and which are known as part of the Th2 response[30, 51, 52]. In fibrogenesis (fig. 2), besides the chemical signalling pathways coming chiefly from profibrotic macrophages, the biomechanichal signalling will strongly influence the myofibroblast activity and fate, mainly through the presence of CTGF[10, 41].

These robust and flexible modules will be deployed in many different arrays, and depending on their balance the structural outcome of the repair process will not resolve with a unitary outcome[53]. Therefore, the repair process might be considered as a byproduct, or epiphenomenon of the mechanisms underlying the biological defence system[15, 54] and simply be the way inflammation and fibrogenesis are resolved[28, 55]. Therefore as a secondary outcome of the biological defence system[55], the newly formed tissue often presents several structural and patterning differences from the original one, the fibrotic scarring being the most unsuccessful and nonfunctional secondary outcome (figure 1 and 2)[10, 31, 56]. The resolution of the trophic or reparative period will be followed by the remodelling stage provided that the apoptotic clearance of myofibroblasts by regulatory macrophages is carried out, thereby eliminating the stimuli inducing TGF- ß1 and other profibrotic factors which otherwise would lead to a persistent fibrotic microenvironment[10, 57].

3. HARNESSING THE MORPHOGENETIC POTENTIAL OF AUTOLOGOUS PLATELETS – AND PLASMA DERIVED PRODUCTS (APPDPS)

In mammals, pivotal players in the biological defence system modules are platelets, leukocytes and fibrinogen, located within a connective tissue, namely, the blood, which acts as an incessantly dynamic and renewing kind of container. In addition to the biological defence function, the blood plays a central role in other physiological processes such as the transport of gases by erythrocytes, caloric energy transport and body temperature regulation by water, communication of body systems by hormones, and transport of waste products, among other functions[58]. Therefore, we no longer think of blood as an indivisible tissue-body whose functions reside in the blood as a whole, but rather as a tissue with cellular and acellular elements that carry out a myriad of interactions and specific functions[58, 59].

Platelets are circulating monitors, trackers and surveyors of the integrity of the vascular system and of the internal milieu as well as carriers of cytokines, chemokines and growth factors, taking part in the coordination of coagulation and inflammation as the core of the biological defence system[36, 60] (fig. 2)(see chapter 1). Platelets appear to be crucial in post-embryonic morphogenesis, and their activation in a biological context is carried out by factors such as thrombin, serotonin, or other tissue constituents such as DAMPs[1] (fig. 3). These molecules activate the platelets thereby releasing, by degranulation, growth factors and cytokines which, along with the formation of thrombin, trigger cell migration and proliferation, regulating angiogenesis, chemoattracting circulating progenitor cells, and guiding tissue remodelling and restoration of function[9, 15, 36, 61].

In addition to many bioactive mediators, (α-granules: TGF-®, platelet-derived growth factor (PDGF), vascular endothelial growth factor (VEGF), fibroblast growth factor (FGF), epidermal growth factor (EGF), insulin-like growth factor (IGF-1), hepatocyte growth factor (HGF), bone morphogenic proteins (BMPs), brain-derived neurotrophic factor (BDNF) and the dense granules: Histamine, Serotonin, Calcium (Ca) and ATP/ADP), there are other constituents in the plasma of APPDPs, namely IGF-1, HGF, prothrombin, fibrinogen, fibronectin and other proteins which, together with adhesive proteins expressed by activated platelets, play a central role in the cell signalling pathways which are involved in both tissue injury recognition and in repair of damaged tissues[9, 61].

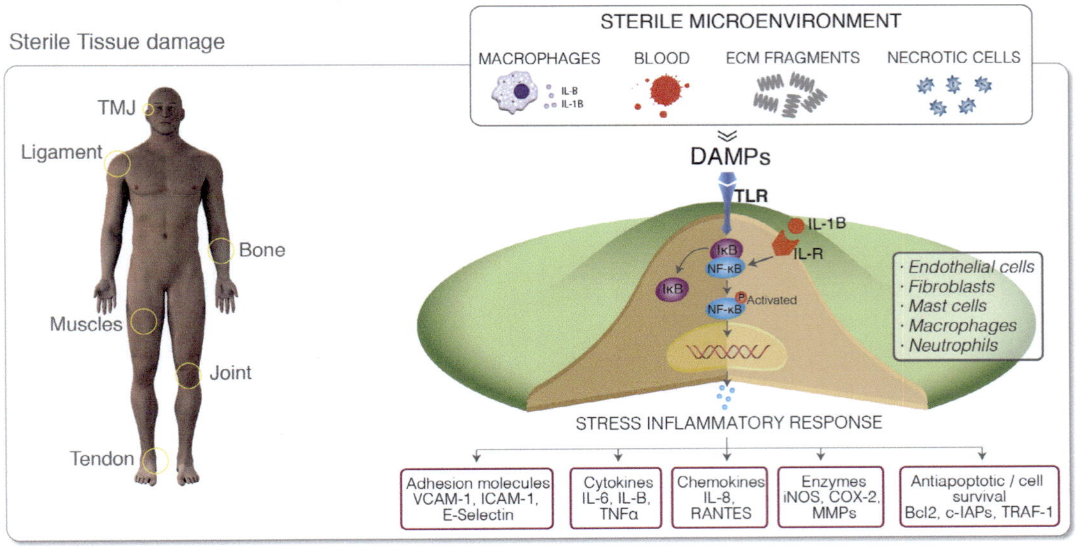

FIG. 3
Tissue repair in sterile conditions. Different types of signals reporting injury such as damage-associated molecular patterns (DAMPs) as well as toxins, minerals, crystals, chemical and antigens can trigger sterile inflammation. [29,33,34,80]
(Adapted with permission from Padilla et al.[110])

For instance, several studies have reported an important HGF-mediated anti-inflammatory effect of platelet-rich plasma on tenocytes, macrophages and chondrocytes[62-64] by attenuating the transactivating activity of NF-kB[62] a highly conserved intracellular signalling pathway whose activation induces tissue inflammation[34]. HGF, a plasmatic key growth factor within APPDPs, has been shown to have a remarkable anti-inflammatory and antifibrotic effect on different tissues[65-67].

PRGF (Plasma rich in growth factors) which is included in APPDPs, conveys growth factors, cytokines, and morphogens contained in the platelets, as well as fibrinogen and other plasmatic proteins in a biologically balanced aggregate, managed and delivered in a pharmacological manner[18, 21] which might account for two special features: the resolution of inflammation and avoidance of fibrosis[68]. In addition, the three-dimensional fibrin network, formed either in vitro as a clot or in situ as an extracellular matrix, contains binding sites for cell adhesion as well as proteins such as thrombospondin-1 (TSP-1), α-1-antitrypsin fibronectin, acute phase proteins or proteins related to lipid metabolism[14, 16, 69]. This fibrin-scaffold formed as a provisional EC serves as a highway for mechanical energy to transit from the environment to the cell, bridges cell-to-cell tissue transition, promotes multi-cellular assembly, provides mechanical support and plastic-elastic stiffness which has a drastic impact on the fates of diverse cell types such as muscle stem cells[46, 47, 70], and endows tissues with a suitable microenvironment for biological restoration[9]. In addition, fibrin matrix, by heparin-binding domains, may sequester growth factors such as PDGF, FGF, HGF, BBNF, and VEGF[14, 45, 71] to gradually release them later.

4. SOME CLARITY IN THE APPLICATION OF PLATELET RICH PLASMA

It is important to shed some light on inconsistent therapeutic application, and bring into focus some common pitfalls regarding the composition of autologous plasma-and platelet derived products (APPDPs) since the biological effects rely quite essentially on their composition and directly depend on particular blood-spinning protocols, as well as on the modalities of their application. They can all deeply influence the success of tissue repair— a process which is already unpredictable — in the abscene of a unitary mechanism (fig. 4)[53].

A. Neutrophils as Engines of Destruction Although Life- Saving cells

A first concern regarding the APPDPs, easily understandable though controversial, is leukocyte concentration. In a repair scenario, leukocytes may aggravate tissue damage and promote a pro-inflammatory microenvironment by releasing TNF-α, IL-6, IFN-γ cytokines which induce the over-expression of MMPs, elastase and cathepsin G among others, thereby breaking down the ECM[8, 72, 73]. The release of reactive oxygen species (ROS) by neutrophils facilitates the removal of necrotic tissue in the repair stage but may exacerbate the initial lesion[74, 75]. In vitro, neutrophils injure cultured myotubes, and, in addition, can cause further muscle injury and disrupt some of the processes involved in skeletal muscle healing[76]. For instance, due primarily to a continual presence of offending elements in the damaged area, leukocyte infiltration may give rise to a nonresolving inflammation[28]. These secretory cells may persist over time, leading to an excessive accumulation of ECM, ultimately producing a pathological and nonfunctional scar tissue (fig. 2)[31, 77]. Anitua et al[78] reported that the inclusion of leukocytes in a fibrin scaffold obtained from APPDPs, both peaked the amount of two molecules involved in inflammation, IL-1 and IL-16, and produced a de-structured and heterogeneous aspect of the fibrin mesh[78]. In the same work and as a way of mimicking pathological conditions in a fibroblast culture exposed to pro-inflammatory cytokines, the addition of leukocytes to an autologous platelet- and plasma derived supernatant triggered over-expression of TGF-β1 and down-regulation of VEGF, an imbalance which may favour the formation of fibrosis. This phenomenon is not observed with an autologous platelet- and plasma-derived product supernatant which is leukocyte-free[78]. The presence of leukocytes in autologous platelet- and plasma-derived product formulations tips the balance of matrix synthesis towards catabolism[79] which may very well lead to a nonresolving inflammation[28]. Filardo and colleagues[22] compared the efficacy and safety of intra-articular injections of a leukocyte-free APPDP with a leukocyte-APPDP in the management of osteoarthritis. Patients treated with the former had fewer side effects than those treated with Leukocyte-APPDP, who presented more pain and more swelling. Tissue injury and microbial infection appear to represent distinct stresses to the host and much of the collateral damage inflicted by neutrophils and macrophages during the hemostatic-inflammatory period might be unnecessary to repair sterile injuries[80] such as musculoskeletal injuries (fig. 3).

Although a less common element in PRPs, erythrocytes too might be detrimental to the repair process, since their phagocytosis by macrophages may induce inflammation, oxidative stress, and promote the persistence of myofibroblasts, thereby leading to fibrosis[57].

B. Fibrogenesis: a double-edged sword

The concern about generating fibrosis has been present since the beginning of the therapeutic application of PRPs, mainly because of the TGF-β1 content in PRP. The TGF-β1 family has been implicated in the development of fibrosis in various tissues[10, 81, 82]. Several studies were conducted both in vitro[83-86] and in vivo[85, 87, 88] to try to tease out the influence of leukocyte-free APPDP on fibrosis. These studies confirmed that, although the TGF-β1family drives fibrogenesis, collagen synthesis and deposition, and it potentially might stimulate the formation of scar tissue[30, 48, 52], the concurrent presence of TGF-β1, VEGF, and HGF in the same local environment makes leukocyte-free APPDP an antifibrotic autologous system. In the molecular network of leukocyte-free APPDP, the fibrotic effect of TGF-β1 would be either modulated, counterbalanced, or even hindered by the presence and local production of HGF, a remarkable antifibrotic regulator[89] and the VEGF, as shown by our work on cells cultured on fibrin matrices[83-86] thus suggesting the pleiotropic behaviour of TGF-β[6]. For instance, in sheep[86] four intratendinous injections of a pre-clotted preparation of leukocyte-free PRGF into the Achilles tendon fascicles triggered a healing response which stemmed from an increase of cellularity, cell organization and angiogenesis. No signs of fibrosis were observed in the histological examination of the sheep Achilles tendons infiltrated with leukocyte-free APPDP[86, 88]. Likewise, the application of leukocyte-free PRGF fibrin matrices on the surgically repaired Achilles tendon tears on 6 athletes showed no wound complication and significantly shortened by 35% the functional recovery time, compared with the group that underwent the same surgical procedure without leukocyte-free PRGF application[90]. In addition, the cross-sectional area of the repaired Achilles tendon, assessed a few years later by ultrasonography, was significantly greater, while minor complications including 1 superficial infection and 2 keloids occurred in the non-treated group[90]. In another study[87], a comparison was made of the overall arthroscopic appearance and the gross morphology and histology of tendon grafts and of the joints of patients treated with leukocyte-free PRGF infiltration with those not treated during anterior cruciate ligament (ACL) surgery[87]. During the remodelling period (6-24 months) the treated group showed more signs of remodelling, maturation, and a synthesis of new connective tissue which wrapped the infiltrated tendon graft with more and better-oriented cells, more akin to the native ACL than in the non-treated one[87].

Recently two other studies assessed the biological effect of leukocyte-free PRGF on other cell lineages such as keratocytes, conjunctival fibroblasts[91] and gingival fibroblasts[92] and synoviocytes[93]. Leukocyte-free APPDP formulations promote the fibroblast phenotype and revert the myofibroblast phenotype to its original fate by protecting and inhibiting TGF-β1-induced myofibroblast differentiation. In conjunctival fibroblasts, leukocyte-free APPDP inhibits and reverses TGF-β1-induced α-SMA expression of fibroblasts as an expression of myofibroblast differentiation[94], thereby preventing the generation of scar tissue. The outcomes of these two studies suggest that leukocyte-free APPDP modulates the fate of myofibroblasts in a way that might be determinant in resolving both inflammation and fibrogenesis, and driving the repair events towards mimicking original tissue, rather than to a tissue-fibrotic outcome[10, 81].

C. APPDPs are not magic products

A third issue related to APPDPs efficacy in healing is the way they are applied in different fields. It has become commonplace to infiltrate APPDPs in the treatment of musculoskeletal injuries as a kind of scatter shot instead of adopting a well thought out and executed biological approach. For instance the application of APPDP to rotator cuff tears is intended to provide the damaged structure with growth factors and cytokines as signalling molecules, one of the three elements involved in the repair process (the two others are cells and 3-dimensional scaffolds). However, as in the case of some studies, it is not enough to add a storm of growth factors to a tendon which for years has been undergoing a degenerative process, and, as a consequence, may have exhausted its healing capacity[95]. There should also be a systematic infiltration of the healthy peripheral tissue surrounding the injury, with the aim of recruiting, activating and mobilizing mesenchymal resident cells to contribute to tissue reparation processes and cell signalling pathways as well as activating endothelial cells and macrophages. A procedure has been developed for the arthroscopic repair of rotator cuff tears assisted by leukocyte-free APPDP which involves 5 infiltration sites, and ultrasound evaluations performed at the third and sixth week after the intervention, during which a subsequent ultrasound-guided infiltration of leukocyte-free PRGF is administered into the repaired tendon[96].

Moreover, we illustrate two examples of the treatment of chronic Achilles tendinopathy[97] in which the authors applied either a single injection of APPDP, following a local anesthetic injection, or two unguided peritendinous injections of autologous whole blood, which showed a negligible clinical effect[98]. In the wake of these two poor clinical results and making inferences about other autologous platelet rich plasma products, some researchers have suggested that all these blood derived products are ineffective in the treatment of mid-portion Achilles tendinopathy. However, a recently published study[99] by Charousset et al. showed clinical and radiological improvement of athletes with chronic Patellar tendinopathy who had been treated using three ultrasound-guided leukocyte-free APPDP infiltrations without any sedation or local injected anesthesia[99].

5. PLEIOTROPY AND ROBUSTNESS OF MECHANISMS UNDERLYING PRP THERAPIES

Wound healing or tissue reconstruction might be considered a byproduct of the mechanisms underlying the biological defence program that entails a set of overlapping complex phenomena encompassing both the recruitment of competent cells to undergo spatiotemporal phenotype commitment and the patterning of cell gene-products to generate ECM and thereby, new tissues (fig. 1)[15, 54]. There is a high degree of self-organization in the regeneration-repair process which may be seen as an open conditon-sensitve process where the environmental cues, both biomechanical and physico-chemical, play a crucial role in influencing and modulating cell phenotypes, in the gene expression, and in patterning the new tissue to mimic the one to be replaced[16, 37, 100, 101].

As is the case in TGF- β1, VEGF and HGF, most of the growth factors and cytokines in PRPs act on a variety of tissues just as they do in any biological system. These proteins exert their regulatory and pleiotropic-biological functions as members of a molecular network linking different modules or systems. Indeed, the results shown in this analysis suggest that applications concerning APPDPs are aptly framed within Nesse and Dawkins' proposal that it is a mistake to seek single, uni-directional causal agents in biological processes; single specific biological factors do not exist for each function[5]. There are simply biological constituents which, in a particular tissue-cell environment, may act together as inhibitions/activations in so-called "genetic switch activities," and induce the expression of cell phenotypes with various behaviours to promote tissue regeneration[5]. This concept, which has been discussed by Huang[102], may account for biological findings that would otherwise appear contradictory, such as the fact that the same molecule, for instance TGF-β1 or a given cell type, such as macrophages, may exert diametrically opposed biological functions [6, 103] or that the same adult stem cell may express different cell phenotypes in different microenvironments or tissue niches[104].

Much scientific evidence, together with the foundations of engineering biology, namely, standardization, decoupling and abstraction[105], has paved the way for several groups to use the blood as a raw material from which to obtain APPDPs as endogenous regenerative technology[19, 106, 107] instead of using the whole blood which conveys a multiplicity of cells and biomolecules whose role in the repair process is negligible or even detrimental (see chapter 4)[57, 75, 76]. At the same time, there are several crucial differences between autologous whole blood and autologous platelet- and plasma derived products (APPDPs), and therefore it is quite inaccurate to infer clinical results from one product as applicable to the other, or to lump all these blood-derived products together[18, 98, 108, 109].

6. CONCLUSIONS

A biological approach to the application of APP-DPs is crucial to obtaining optimum functional repair outcomes in addition to avoiding poor clinical results and drawing misleading inferences. Attempting to optimize the degree of functionality by producing a repaired tissue that is intended to be structurally identical to the damaged tissue might be considered an "artificial" goal imposed by human purposes. In other words, we are creating new goals and placing new demands on cell-based biological programs (to regenerate rather than repair in quiescent and non-dividing tissues) which were selected and conserved over millions of years in different species with a single goal: survival.[1, 36]

Several unanswered questions remain, some regarding molecular mechanisms that give rise to the clinical benefits, and others encompassing dosage aspects such as how many injections would be ideal in a first approach, the interval between them, and whether combining PRPs with stem cells might enhance the healing power of PRPs.

The time has come when we should no longer compare the biological and therapeutic efficacy of very distinct products in musculoskeletal orthopaedic surgery by lumping all autologous platelet-and plasma-derived products together.

1. Delvaeye, M.; Conway, E.M. Coagulation and innate immune responses: can we view them separately? Blood, 2009, 114: 2367-74.

2. Allen, J.E.; Wynn, T.A. Evolution of Th2 immunity: a rapid repair response to tissue destructive pathogens. PLoS Pathog, 2011, 7: e1002003.

3. Medzhitov, R. Inflammation 2010: new adventures of an old flame. Cell, 2010, 140: 771-6.

4. Kumar, V.; Abbas, A.K.; Fausto, N.; Mitchell, R. Robbins basic pathology. Elsevier Health Sciences 2012.

5. Nesse, R.M., Dawkins R. Evolution: Medicine´s most basic science. Oxford University Press 2010.

6. Nathan, C. Points of control in inflammation. Nature, 2002, 420: 846-52.

7. Medzhitov, R. Origin and physiological roles of inflammation. Nature, 2008, 454: 428-35.

8. Nathan, C. Neutrophils and immunity: challenges and opportunities. Nat Rev Immunol, 2006, 6: 173-82.

9. Nurden, A.T.; Nurden, P.; Sanchez, M.; Andia, I.; Anitua, E. Platelets and wound healing. Front Biosci, 2008, 13: 3532-48.

10. Duffield, J.S.; Lupher, M.; Thannickal, V.J.; Wynn, T.A. Host responses in tissue repair and fibrosis. Annu Rev Pathol, 2013, 8: 241-76.

11. Sica, A.; Mantovani, A. Macrophage plasticity and polarization: in vivo veritas. J Clin Invest, 2012, 122: 787-95.

12. Duffield, J.S. The inflammatory macrophage: a story of Jekyll and Hyde. Clin Sci (Lond), 2003, 104: 27-38.

13. Stellos, K.; Kopf, S.; Paul, A.; Marquardt, J.U.; Gawaz, M.; Huard, J.; Langer, H.F. Platelets in regeneration. Semin Thromb Hemost, 2010, 36: 175-84.

14. Anitua, E.; Orive, G. Endogenous regenerative technology using plasma- and platelet-derived growth factors. J Control Release, 2012, 157: 317-20.

15. Brockes, J.P.; Kumar, A. Comparative aspects of animal regeneration. Annu Rev Cell Dev Biol, 2008, 24: 525-49.

16. Nurden, A.T. Platelets, inflammation and tissue regeneration. Thromb Haemost, 2011, 105 Suppl 1: S13-33.

17. Anitua, E.; Alkhraisat, M.H.; Orive, G. Perspectives and challenges in regenerative medicine using plasma rich in growth factors. J Control Release, 2012, 157: 29-38.

18. Dohan Ehrenfest, D.M.; Rasmusson, L.; Albrektsson, T. Classification of platelet concentrates: from pure platelet-rich plasma (P-PRP) to leucocyte- and platelet-rich fibrin (L-PRF). Trends Biotechnol, 2009, 27: 158-67.

19. Burnouf, T.; Goubran, H.A.; Chen, T.M.; Ou, K.L.; El-Ekiaby, M.; Radosevic, M. Blood-derived biomaterials and platelet growth factors in regenerative medicine. Blood Rev, 2013, 27: 77-89.

20. Andia, I.; Abate, M. Platelet-rich plasma: underlying biology and clinical correlates. Regen Med, 2013, 8: 645-58.

21. Anitua, E.; Sanchez, M.; Orive, G. Potential of endogenous regenerative technology for in situ regenerative medicine. Adv Drug Deliv Rev, 2010, 62: 741-52.

22. Filardo, G.; Kon, E.; Pereira Ruiz, M.T.; Vaccaro, F.; Guitaldi, R.; Di Martino, A.; Cenacchi, A.; Fornasari, P.M.; Marcacci, M. Platelet-rich plasma intra-articular injections for cartilage degeneration and osteoarthritis: single- versus double-spinning approach. Knee Surg Sports Traumatol Arthrosc, 2012, 20: 2082-91.

23. Mei-Dan, O.; Carmont, M.R. The role of platelet-rich plasma in rotator cuff repair. Sports Med Arthrosc, 2011, 19: 244-50.

24. Mei-Dan, O.; Carmont, M.R.; Laver, L.; Mann, G.; Maffulli, N.; Nyska, M. Platelet-rich plasma or hyaluronate in the management of osteochondral lesions of the talus. Am J Sports Med, 2012, 40: 534-41.

25. Sanchez, M.; Anitua, E.; Orive, G.; Mujika, I.; Andia, I. Platelet-rich therapies in the treatment of orthopaedic sport injuries. Sports Med, 2009, 39: 345-54.

26. Wang-Saegusa, A.; Cugat, R.; Ares, O.; Seijas, R.; Cusco, X.; Garcia-Balletbo, M. Infiltration of plasma rich in growth factors for osteoarthritis of the knee short-term effects on function and quality of life. Arch Orthop Trauma Surg, 2011, 131: 311-7.

27. Sánchez, M.; Delgado, D.; Sánchez, P.; Fiz, N.; Azofra, J.; Orive, G.; Anitua, E.; Padilla, S. Platelet Rich Plasma and Knee Surgery. BioMed Research International, 2014, 2014.

28. Nathan, C.; Ding, A. Nonresolving inflammation. Cell, 2010, 140: 871-82.

29. Sorokin, L. The impact of the extracellular matrix on inflammation. Nat Rev Immunol, 2010, 10: 712-23.

30. Lech, M.; Anders, H.J. Macrophages and fibrosis: How resident and infiltrating mononuclear phagocytes orchestrate all phases of tissue injury and repair. Biochim Biophys Acta, 2013, 1832: 989-97.

31. Wynn, T.A. Common and unique mechanisms regulate fibrosis in various fibroproliferative diseases. J Clin Invest, 2007, 117: 524-9.

32. Semple, J.W.; Italiano, J.E., Jr.; Freedman, J. Platelets and the immune continuum. Nat Rev Immunol, 2011, 11: 264-74.

33. Rock, K.L.; Kono, H. The inflammatory response to cell death. Annu Rev Pathol, 2008, 3: 99-126.

34. Ashley, N.T.; Weil, Z.M.; Nelson, R.J. Inflammation: mechanisms, costs, and natural variation. Annual Review of Ecology, Evolution, and Systematics, 2012, 43: 385-406.

35. Drake, W.T.; Issekutz, A.C. A role for alpha-thrombin in polymorphonuclear leukocyte recruitment during inflammation. In: ed.^eds., Seminars in thrombosis and hemostasis, 1991; pp. 333-340.

36. Brass, L.F. Did dinosaurs have megakaryocytes? New ideas about platelets and their progenitors. J Clin Invest, 2005, 115: 3329-31.

37. Hutchison, N.; Fligny, C.; Duffield, J.S. Resident mesenchymal cells and fibrosis. Biochim Biophys Acta, 2013, 1832: 962-71.

38. Mosser, D.M.; Edwards, J.P. Exploring the full spectrum of macrophage activation. Nat Rev Immunol, 2008, 8: 958-69.

39. Zheng, H.; Fu, G.; Dai, T.; Huang, H. Migration of endothelial progenitor cells mediated by stromal cell-derived factor-1alpha/CXCR4 via PI3K/Akt/eNOS signal transduction pathway. J Cardiovasc Pharmacol, 2007, 50: 274-80.

40. Gleissner, C.A.; Shaked, I.; Little, K.M.; Ley, K. CXC chemokine ligand 4 induces a unique transcriptome in monocyte-derived macrophages. J Immunol, 2010, 184: 4810-8.

41. Lee, C.H.; Shah, B.; Moioli, E.K.; Mao, J.J. CTGF directs fibroblast differentiation from human mesenchymal stem/stromal cells and defines connective tissue healing in a rodent injury model. J Clin Invest, 2010, 120: 3340-9.

42. Tidball, J.G.; Wehling-Henricks, M. Shifts in macrophage cytokine production drive muscle fibrosis. Nat Med, 2015, 21: 665-6.

43. Langer, H.F.; Gawaz, M. Platelets in regenerative medicine. Basic Res Cardiol, 2008, 103: 299-307.

44. Grounds, M.D. Complexity of extracellular matrix and skeletal muscle regeneration. In: ed.^eds., Skeletal Muscle Repair and Regeneration. Springer, 2008; pp. 269-302.

45. Martino, M.M.; Briquez, P.S.; Ranga, A.; Lutolf, M.P.; Hubbell, J.A. Heparin-binding domain of fibrin(ogen) binds growth factors and promotes tissue repair when incorporated within a synthetic matrix. Proc Natl Acad Sci U S A, 2013, 110: 4563-8.

46. Gilbert, P.M.; Havenstrite, K.L.; Magnusson, K.E.; Sacco, A.; Leonardi, N.A.; Kraft, P.; Nguyen, N.K.; Thrun, S.; Lutolf, M.P.; Blau, H.M. Substrate elasticity regulates skeletal muscle stem cell self-renewal in culture. Science, 2010, 329: 1078-81.

47. Discher, D.E.; Mooney, D.J.; Zandstra, P.W. Growth factors, matrices, and forces combine and control stem cells. Science, 2009, 324: 1673-7.

48. Wynn, T.A. Cellular and molecular mechanisms of fibrosis. J Pathol, 2008, 214: 199-210.

49. Rice, J.J.; Martino, M.M.; De Laporte, L.; Tortelli, F.; Briquez, P.S.; Hubbell, J.A. Engineering the regenerative microenvironment with biomaterials. Adv Healthc Mater, 2013, 2: 57-71.

50. Bentzinger, C.F.; Wang, Y.X.; Rudnicki, M.A. Building muscle: molecular regulation of myogenesis. Cold Spring Harb Perspect Biol, 2012, 4: doi 10.1101chsperspect.a008342.

51. Allen, J.E.; Sutherland, T.E. Host protective roles of type 2 immunity: parasite killing and tissue repair, flip sides of the same coin. Semin Immunol, 2014, 26: 329-40.

52. Klingberg, F.; Hinz, B.; White, E.S. The myofibroblast matrix: implications for tissue repair and fibrosis. J Pathol, 2013, 229: 298-309.

53. Ciciliot, S.; Schiaffino, S. Regeneration of mammalian skeletal muscle. Basic mechanisms and clinical implications. Curr Pharm Des, 2010, 16: 906-14.

54. Williams, G.C. Adaptation and natural selection: a critique of some current evolutionary thought. Princeton University Press 1966.

55. Serhan, C.N.; Savill, J. Resolution of inflammation: the beginning programs the end. Nat Immunol, 2005, 6: 1191-7.

56. Järvinen, T.A.; Kääriäinen, M.; Äärimaa, V.; Järvinen, M.; Kalimo, H. Skeletal muscle repair after exercise-induced injury. In: ed.^eds., Skeletal Muscle Repair and Regeneration. Springer, 2008; pp. 217-242.

57. Wynn, T.A.; Barron, L. Macrophages: master regulators of inflammation and fibrosis. Seminars in liver disease, 2010, 30: 245-257.

58. Willmer, P.; Stone, G.; Johnston, I. Environmental physiology of animals. John Wiley & Sons 2009.

59. Schaller, J.; Gerber, S.; Kaempfer, U.; Lejon, S.; Trachsel, C. Human blood plasma proteins: structure and function. John Wiley & Sons 2008.

60. Scott, A.; Khan, K.M.; Roberts, C.R.; Cook, J.L.; Duronio, V. What do we mean by the term "inflammation"? A contemporary basic science update for sports medicine. Br J Sports Med, 2004, 38: 372-80.

61. Marcus, A. Platelets: their role in hemostasis, thrombosis, and inflammation. Inflammation: basic principles and clinical correlates, 1999: 77-95.

62. Bendinelli, P.; Matteucci, E.; Dogliotti, G.; Corsi, M.M.; Banfi, G.; Maroni, P.; Desiderio, M.A. Molecular basis of anti-inflammatory action of platelet-rich plasma on human chondrocytes: mechanisms of NF-kappaB inhibition via HGF. J Cell Physiol, 2010, 225: 757-66.

63. Zhang, J.; Middleton, K.K.; Fu, F.H.; Im, H.J.; Wang, J.H. HGF mediates the anti-inflammatory effects of PRP on injured tendons. PLoS One, 2013, 8: e67303.

64. van Buul, G.M.; Koevoet, W.L.; Kops, N.; Bos, P.K.; Verhaar, J.A.; Weinans, H.; Bernsen, M.R.; van Osch, G.J. Platelet-rich plasma releasate inhibits inflammatory processes in osteoarthritic chondrocytes. Am J Sports Med, 2011, 39: 2362-70.

65. Homsi, E.; Janino, P.; Amano, M.; Saraiva Camara, N.O. Endogenous hepatocyte growth factor attenuates inflammatory response in glycerol-induced acute kidney injury. Am J Nephrol, 2009, 29: 283-91.

66. Okada, M.; Sugita, K.; Inukai, T.; Goi, K.; Kagami, K.; Kawasaki, K.; Nakazawa, S. Hepatocyte growth factor protects small airway epithelial cells from apoptosis induced by tumor necrosis factor-alpha or oxidative stress. Pediatr Res, 2004, 56: 336-44.

67. Hinz, B.; Phan, S.H.; Thannickal, V.J.; Galli, A.; Bochaton-Piallat, M.L.; Gabbiani, G. The myofibroblast: one function, multiple origins. Am J Pathol, 2007, 170: 1807-16.

68. Anitua, E.; Prado, R.; Sánchez, M.; Orive, G. Platelet-Rich Plasma: Preparation and Formulation. Operative Techniques in Orthopaedics, 2012, 22: 25-32.

69. Anitua, E.; Prado, R.; Azkargorta, M.; Rodriguez-Suarez, E.; Iloro, I.; Casado-Vela, J.; Elortza, F.; Orive, G. High-throughput proteomic characterization of plasma rich in growth factors (PRGF-Endoret)-derived fibrin clot interactome. J Tissue Eng Regen Med, 2015, 9: E1-E12.

70. Sanchez, M.; Anitua, E.; Delgado, D.; Sanchez, P.; Orive, G.; Padilla, S. Muscle repair: platelet-rich plasma derivates as a bridge from spontaneity to intervention. Injury, 2014, 45 Suppl 4: S7-14.

71. Borselli, C.; Storrie, H.; Benesch-Lee, F.; Shvartsman, D.; Cezar, C.; Lichtman, J.W.; Vandenburgh, H.H.; Mooney, D.J. Functional muscle regeneration with combined delivery of angiogenesis and myogenesis factors. Proc Natl Acad Sci U S A, 2010, 107: 3287-92.

72. Wohner, N. Role of cellular elements in thrombus formation and dissolution. Cardiovasc Hematol Agents Med Chem, 2008, 6: 224-8.

73. Rabai, G.; Szilagyi, N.; Sotonyi, P.; Kovalszky, I.; Szabo, L.; Machovich, R.; Kolev, K. Contribution of neutrophil elastase to the lysis of obliterative thrombi in the context of their platelet and fibrin content. Thromb Res, 2010, 126: e94-101.

74. Tidball, J.G. Inflammatory cell response to acute muscle injury. Med Sci Sports Exerc, 1995, 27: 1022-32.

75. Tidball, J.G. Inflammatory processes in muscle injury and repair. Am J Physiol Regul Integr Comp Physiol, 2005, 288: R345-53.

76. Pizza, F. Neutrophils and macrophages in muscle damage and repair. Skeletal Muscle Damage and Repair, 2008, 49: 57.

77. Grounds, M.D.; Sorokin, L.; White, J. Strength at the extracellular matrix-muscle interface. Scand J Med Sci Sports, 2005, 15: 381-91.

78. Anitua, E.; Zalduendo, M.; Troya, M.; Padilla, S.; Orive, G. Leukocyte inclusion within a platelet rich plasma-derived fibrin scaffold stimulates a more pro-inflammatory environment and alters fibrin properties. PLoS One, 2015, 10: e0121713.

79. McCarrel, T.M.; Minas, T.; Fortier, L.A. Optimization of leukocyte concentration in platelet-rich plasma for the treatment of tendinopathy. J Bone Joint Surg Am, 2012, 94: e143(1-8).

80. Barton, G.M. A calculated response: control of inflammation by the innate immune system. J Clin Invest, 2008, 118: 413.

81. Serrano, A.L.; Mann, C.J.; Vidal, B.; Ardite, E.; Perdiguero, E.; Munoz-Canoves, P. Cellular and molecular mechanisms regulating fibrosis in skeletal muscle repair and disease. Curr Top Dev Biol, 2011, 96: 167-201.

82. Ueha, S.; Shand, F.H.; Matsushima, K. Cellular and molecular mechanisms of chronic inflammation-associated organ fibrosis. Frontiers in immunology, 2012, 3.

83. Anitua, E.; Sanchez, M.; Zalduendo, M.M.; de la Fuente, M.; Prado, R.; Orive, G.; Andia, I. Fibroblastic response to treatment with different preparations rich in growth factors. Cell Prolif, 2009, 42: 162-70.

84. Anitua, E.; Andia, I.; Sanchez, M.; Azofra, J.; del Mar Zalduendo, M.; de la Fuente, M.; Nurden, P.; Nurden, A.T. Autologous preparations rich in growth factors promote proliferation and induce VEGF and HGF production by human tendon cells in culture. J Orthop Res, 2005, 23: 281-6.

85. Anitua, E.; Sanchez, M.; Nurden, A.T.; Zalduendo, M.; de la Fuente, M.; Orive, G.; Azofra, J.; Andia, I. Autologous fibrin matrices: a potential source of biological mediators that modulate tendon cell activities. J Biomed Mater Res A, 2006, 77: 285-93.

86. Anitua, E.; Sanchez, M.; Nurden, A.T.; Zalduendo, M.; de la Fuente, M.; Azofra, J.; Andia, I. Reciprocal actions of platelet-secreted TGF-beta1 on the production of VEGF and HGF by human tendon cells. Plast Reconstr Surg, 2007, 119: 950-9.

87. Sánchez, M.; Anitua, E.; Azofra, J.; Prado, R.; Muruzabal, F.; Andia, I. Ligamentization of tendon grafts treated with an endogenous preparation rich in growth factors: gross morphology and histology. Arthroscopy: The Journal of Arthroscopic & Related Surgery, 2010, 26: 470-480.

88. Fernandez-Sarmiento, J.A.; Dominguez, J.M.; Granados, M.M.; Morgaz, J.; Navarrete, R.; Carrillo, J.M.; Gomez-Villamandos, R.J.; Munoz-Rascon, P.; Martin de Las Mulas, J.; Millan, Y.; Garcia-Balletbo, M.; Cugat, R. Histological study of the influence of plasma rich in growth factors (PRGF) on the healing of divided Achilles tendons in sheep. J Bone Joint Surg Am, 2013, 95: 246-55.

89. Gong, R. Multi-target anti-inflammatory action of hepatocyte growth factor. Curr Opin Investig Drugs, 2008, 9: 1163-70.

90. Sanchez, M.; Anitua, E.; Azofra, J.; Andia, I.; Padilla, S.; Mujika, I. Comparison of surgically repaired Achilles tendon tears using platelet-rich fibrin matrices. Am J Sports Med, 2007, 35: 245-51.

91. Anitua, E.; Sanchez, M.; Merayo-Lloves, J.; De la Fuente, M.; Muruzabal, F.; Orive, G. Plasma rich in growth factors (PRGF-Endoret) stimulates proliferation and migration of primary keratocytes and conjunctival fibroblasts and inhibits and reverts TGF-beta1-Induced myodifferentiation. Invest Ophthalmol Vis Sci, 2011, 52: 6066-73.

92. Anitua, E.; Troya, M.; Orive, G. Plasma rich in growth factors promote gingival tissue regeneration by stimulating fibroblast proliferation and migration and by blocking transforming growth factor-beta1-induced myodifferentiation. J Periodontol, 2012, 83: 1028-37.

93. Assirelli, E.; Filardo, G.; Mariani, E.; Kon, E.; Roffi, A.; Vaccaro, F.; Marcacci, M.; Facchini, A.; Pulsatelli, L.

Effect of two different preparations of platelet-rich plasma on synoviocytes. Knee Surg Sports Traumatol Arthrosc, 2014.

94. Steinsvoll, S.; Halstensen, T.; Schenck, K. Extensive expression of TGF-b1 in chronically-inflamed periodontal tissue. Journal of clinical periodontology, 1999, 26: 366-373.

95. Ruiz-Moneo, P.; Molano-Munoz, J.; Prieto, E.; Algorta, J. Plasma rich in growth factors in arthroscopic rotator cuff repair: a randomized, double-blind, controlled clinical trial. Arthroscopy, 2013, 29: 2-9.

96. Sanchez, M.; Anitua, E.; Orive, G.; Padilla, S. A biological approach to orthopaedic surgery: are they lost in translation? Arthroscopy, 2013, 29: 969-70.

97. de Vos, R.J.; Weir, A.; van Schie, H.T.; Bierma-Zeinstra, S.M.; Verhaar, J.A.; Weinans, H.; Tol, J.L. Platelet-rich plasma injection for chronic Achilles tendinopathy: a randomized controlled trial. JAMA, 2010, 303: 144-9.

98. Bell, K.J.; Fulcher, M.L.; Rowlands, D.S.; Kerse, N. Impact of autologous blood injections in treatment of mid-portion Achilles tendinopathy: double blind randomised controlled trial. BMJ, 2013, 346: f2310.

99. Charousset, C.; Zaoui, A.; Bellaiche, L.; Bouyer, B. Are Multiple Platelet-Rich Plasma Injections Useful for Treatment of Chronic Patellar Tendinopathy in Athletes?: A Prospective Study. Am J Sports Med, 2014.

100. Janmey, P.A.; Miller, R.T. Mechanisms of mechanical signaling in development and disease. J Cell Sci, 2011, 124: 9-18.

101. Heisenberg, C.P.; Bellaiche, Y. Forces in tissue morphogenesis and patterning. Cell, 2013, 153: 948-62.

102. Huang, S. Cell fates as attractors - stability and flexibility of cellular phenotype. In: Press CU, ed.^eds., 2007; pp. 1761-1779.

103. Chazaud, B.; Brigitte, M.; Yacoub-Youssef, H.; Arnold, L.; Gherardi, R.; Sonnet, C.; Lafuste, P.; Chretien, F. Dual and beneficial roles of macrophages during skeletal muscle regeneration. Exerc Sport Sci Rev, 2009, 37: 18-22.

104. Aird, W.C.; Laubichler, M.D. Introductory essay: evolution, comparative biology and development. In: ed.^eds., Endothelial biomedicine. Cambridge University Press, 2007; pp. 23-28.

105. Endy, D. Foundations for engineering biology. Nature, 2005, 438: 449-53.

106. Marx, R.E.; Carlson, E.R.; Eichstaedt, R.M.; Schimmele, S.R.; Strauss, J.E.; Georgeff, K.R. Platelet-rich plasma: Growth factor enhancement for bone grafts. Oral Surg Oral Med Oral Pathol Oral Radiol Endod, 1998, 85: 638-46.

107. Anitua, E. Plasma rich in growth factors: preliminary results of use in the preparation of future sites for implants. Int J Oral Maxillofac Implants, 1999, 14: 529-35.

108. Maffulli, N. Autologous blood products in musculoskeletal medicine. BMJ, 2013, 346: f2979.

109. Padilla, S.; Orive, G.; Sanchez, M.; Anitua, E.; Westerlain, A.S.; Dragoo, J.L. Causality in biology has to answer 2 main questions--which and how: letter to the editor. Am J Sports Med, 2013, 41: NP22-3.

110. Padilla S.; Sánchez M.; Padilla I.; Orive G.; Anitua E.Healing or not healing. Current Pharmaceutical Biotechnology, 2016, 17, 419-430.

CHAPTER 4

Effects of Plasma Rich in Growth Factors on Cells and Tissues of Musculoskeletal System: from Articular Cartilage to Muscles and Nerves

AUTHORS

Padilla S.[1,2,4], Sánchez M.[3], Anitua E.[1,2,4]

[1] Eduardo Anitua Foundation for Biomedical Research, Vitoria-Gasteiz, Spain
[2] BTI-Biotechnology Institute, Vitoria-Gasteiz, Spain
[3] Arthroscopic Surgery Unit, Hospital Vithas San Jose, Vitoria-Gasteiz, Spain
[4] University Institute for Regenerative Medicine and Oral Implantology (UIRMI) from the University of Basque Country (UPV/EHU)

SUMMARY

An innovative approach to the treatment of acute and chronic sports injuries is the use of engineering biology assisted by the application of blood-derived biological drug delivery therapies (BDDTs) in their different formulations. The common ground of cartilage destruction and osteoarthritis (OA), tendinopathies, muscle and ligament strains, bone fracture or nerve compression or transection, among other tissue damage, is the sterile inflammation. Key processes in repairing the damaged tissues are inflammation, angiogenesis, macrophage activation and polarization, cell fates and progenitor stem cell differentiation, fibrogenesis as well as the active resolution of inflammation, angiogenesis, and fibrogenesis, which are essentially governed by cytokines, growth factors and other biological mediators The present chapter summarizes our current knowledge of effects of blood-derived biological drug delivery therapies (BDDTs) on tissues of the musculoskeletal system.

E. Anitua et al. (eds.), *Platelet Rich Plasma in Orthopaedics and Sports Medicine*,
https://doi.org/10.1007/978-3-319-63730-3_4

1. INTRODUCTION

Through the design and construction of synthetic biological materials, tissue engineering provides us with the best technically available scaffolds and replacement devices. However, the weakest point of the current orthopaedic surgical treatments lies not with these highly sophisticated biomaterials but with the quality of patient tissues at the site where the synthetic biomaterials will be attached or anchored. Therefore the field of regenerative medicine is moving away from more traditional synthetic biology toward increasingly complex and multimolecular biological drug delivery therapies (BDDTs). In fact, blood itself contains the basic ingredients to biologically engineer drug delivery devices that provide spatiotemporal control over the presentation of a wide range of bioactive agents including small molecules, cytokines and growth factors[1].

Blood contains a wide range of biological elements that influence the development of functional substitutes for damaged tissues. It contains the basic ingredients of the tissue engineering triad, that is, cells, growth factors and scaffold-forming elements[2]. Significantly, blood provides fibrin as a provisional scaffold for tissue growth. It also contains cell-signaling elements both in plasma and in platelets in the form of biochemical or environmental cues that affect the biological fate and phenotype of cells. Importantly, BDDTs need not be seeded with cells before administration, since blood-derived fibrin scaffolds are enriched in a patient´s own growth factors and cytokines providing cues to direct endogenous cells, including stem cells, to sites of repair[3]. The present chapter highlights our current knowledge of BDDTs in the therapeutic potential of their use in different relevant musculoskeletal tissue injuries including tendon, ligament, cartilage, muscle, and nerve.

2. BLOOD-DERIVED BIOLOGICAL DRUG DELIVERY THERAPIES

Platelets constitute one of the essential biological elements within the blood-BDDT. They are the first cells that accumulate at sites of injury and, after activation, release dozens of biologically active mediators into the microenvironment, including well-known chemokines, cytokines, and growth factors[4]. The multitude of released cues exerts complex biological effects that drive tissue repair and regeneration. For example, platelet-derived factors modulate activation of fibroblasts, induce proliferation and migration of cells critically involved in tissue repair, such as smooth muscle cells and mesenchymal stem cells (MSCs)[5], regulate angiogenesis, a pivotal process for recovery of tissue function[6], and may regulate apoptosis and survival of cells by means of released platelet microparticles[7]. Thus, blood-derived BDDTs, which are enriched in platelet secretome, may successfully be used as productive and autologous therapeutic tools, promoting the healing and repair of injured tissues.

The fibrin scaffold, which is generated from the blood-derived BDDT, consists primarily of enriched fibrinogen, thrombin, and calcium and coagulation factors (figure 1). Interestingly, it fulfills the critical capacities that a scaffold must have, including form, fixation, and formation[8]. For a scaffold to have form, it should be able to fill the space it is designed to fill. Blood-derived BDDT is used therapeutically to fill gaps in ulcers, bone defects or dental alveolus among others[9, 10]. Another key property is fixation: the ability of a scaffold to integrate and attach to the surrounding microenvironment. Autologous fibrin scaffolds are biocompatible and biodegradable, and they serve as delivery vehicles and as scaffolding matrices. Furthermore, they contain dozens of adhesive proteins, including fibronectin, vitronectin, and serpins, among others (all of them pivotal elements from the extracellular matrix). Following a high-throughput proteomic characterization and classifying the proteins into families and networks according to gene ontology, more than 40 proteins specifically involved in tissue regeneration and wound healing have been identified[11]. Finally, the fibrin scaffold is able to drive the formation of the intended tissue.

Interestingly, blood-derived biological drug delivery therapy is modernizing the ancient "art of healing" by providing dosage-form versatility over drug availability (Box 1). Current novel blood-based therapies can be administered topically, as an eye-drop or by subcutaneous, intradermal, and intramuscular injections. In addition, they can exist as a pure liquid, an in-situ gelling liquid, or a three-dimensional fibrin scaffold, thus enabling novel therapeutic strategies[1]. In general, all of these therapeutic formulations are administered locally. Once situated, the fibrin scaffold acts as a depot of bioactive mediators at any injury site, temporally controlling their presentation. The short half-lives of the autologous biological mediators, including growth factors, cytokines, and chemokines, emphasize the importance of this biology-mimicking delivery system (figure 1) .

Opponents to blood-derived BDDT hold that these therapies may show relevant but still poorly understood mechanisms of tissue repair. However, our accumulating knowledge of biology and molecular biology is alleviating some of these concerns[12]. For example, platelets within the BDDT release agents such as hepatocyte growth factor (HGF) and stromal-derived growth factor 1 (SFD-1), which are known to control proliferation, recruitment, and activation of cell types critically involved in wound healing and tissue regeneration (figure 1). In particular, HGF exerts antiapoptotic[13], proangiogenic[14], and immunosuppressive activity[15] and promotes recruitment of MSCs to human arterial endothelial cells[5]. SDF-1 stimulates progenitor cell recruitment to arterial thrombi and differentiation of the cells to endothelial progenitors in vivo[16, 17] .

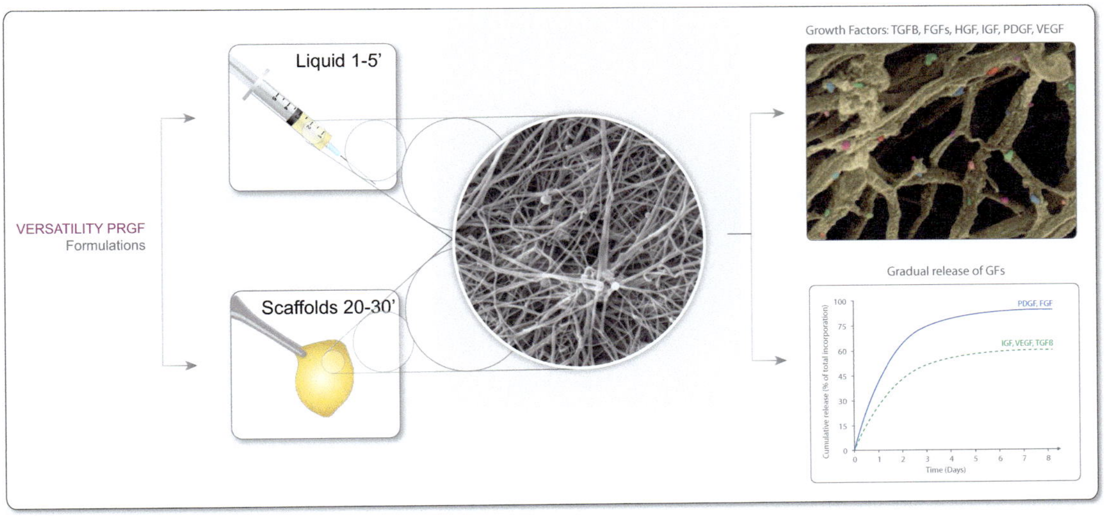

FIG. 1
Blood-derived biological drug delivery therapies (BDDTs) are based on a combination of naturally derived biomaterials such as fibrin and a pool of growth factors. For example, the three-dimensional fibrin scaffold obtained from fractionated human plasma represents a physiologically inspired solution to control the release of the wide range of plasma and platelet-derived mediators[64].

3. MECHANICS RULES CELL BIOLOGY

Virtually all the cells of the musculoskeletal tissues are mechano-sensitive and experience mechanical stress through the distortion of the extracellular matrix (ECM) complex. They respond to these stresses by changing their cellular biochemistry and physiology (mechanobiology and plastic adaptation) (figure 2)[18]. Moreover, mechanical forces are required to maintain the physical integrity of anatomical structures and homeostasis of the tissues by regulating cell functions, including gene induction, protein synthesis, and cell proliferation, differentiation, growth, survival and apoptosis[19].

However, the exposure of musculoskeletal cells to nonphysiological stimuli, either mechanical or biochemical, leads to swings of the tissue pendulum towards profound alterations of components of the extracellular matrix both cellular and acellular as well as the physical and chemical properties of the ECM. Such stimuli lead to cell microenvironment damage, degeneration and disease[20].

The exposure of cells (tenocytes, chondrocytes, fibroblasts, myofibres) to a novel cytoplasmic and extracellular microenvironment can modify their gene on-off state (gene switches) which might induce them to turn on previously silent genes, thereby altering their gene expression and gene products such as metalloproteinases (MMPs) and other molecules of the ECM (figure 2)[20, 21].

The common ground of cartilage destruction and osteoarthritis (OA), tendinopathies, muscle and ligament strains, bone fracture or nerve compression or transection, among other tissue damage, is the sterile inflammation. Key processes in healing the damaged tissues are inflammation, angiogenesis, macrophage activation and polarization, cell fates and progenitor stem cell differentiation, fibrogenesis as well as the active resolution of inflammation, angiogenesis, and fibrogenesis, which are essentially governed by cytokines, growth factors and other biological mediators (figure 3)[22].

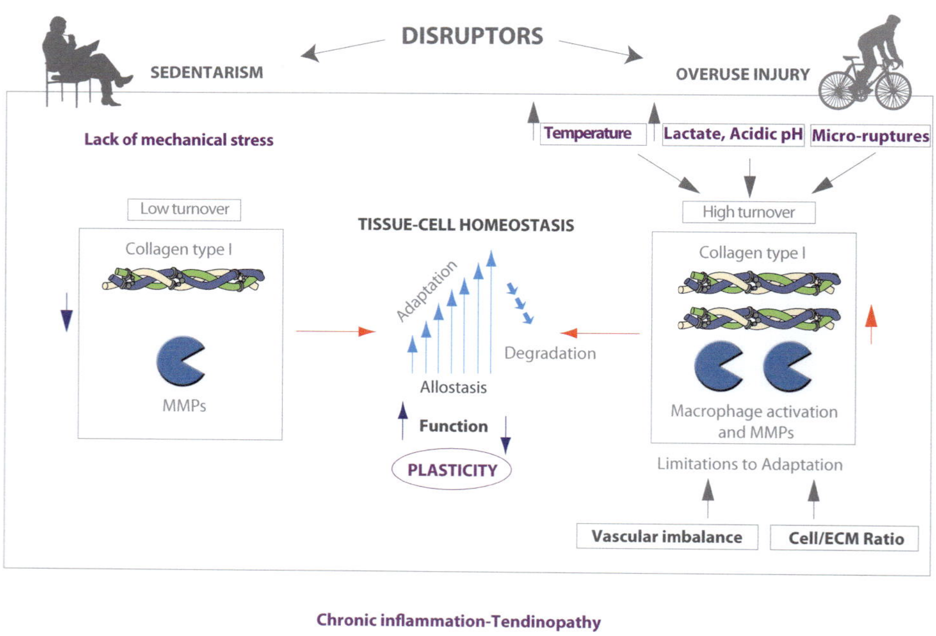

FIG. 2
The exposure of musculoskeletal cells to non-physiological stimuli, either mechanical or biochemical, leads to swings of the tissue pendulum towards profound alterations of cells and components of the extracellular matrix as well as the physical and chemical properties of the ECM. Such stimuli lead to cell microenvironment damage, low chronic inflammation and disfunction[20, 39].

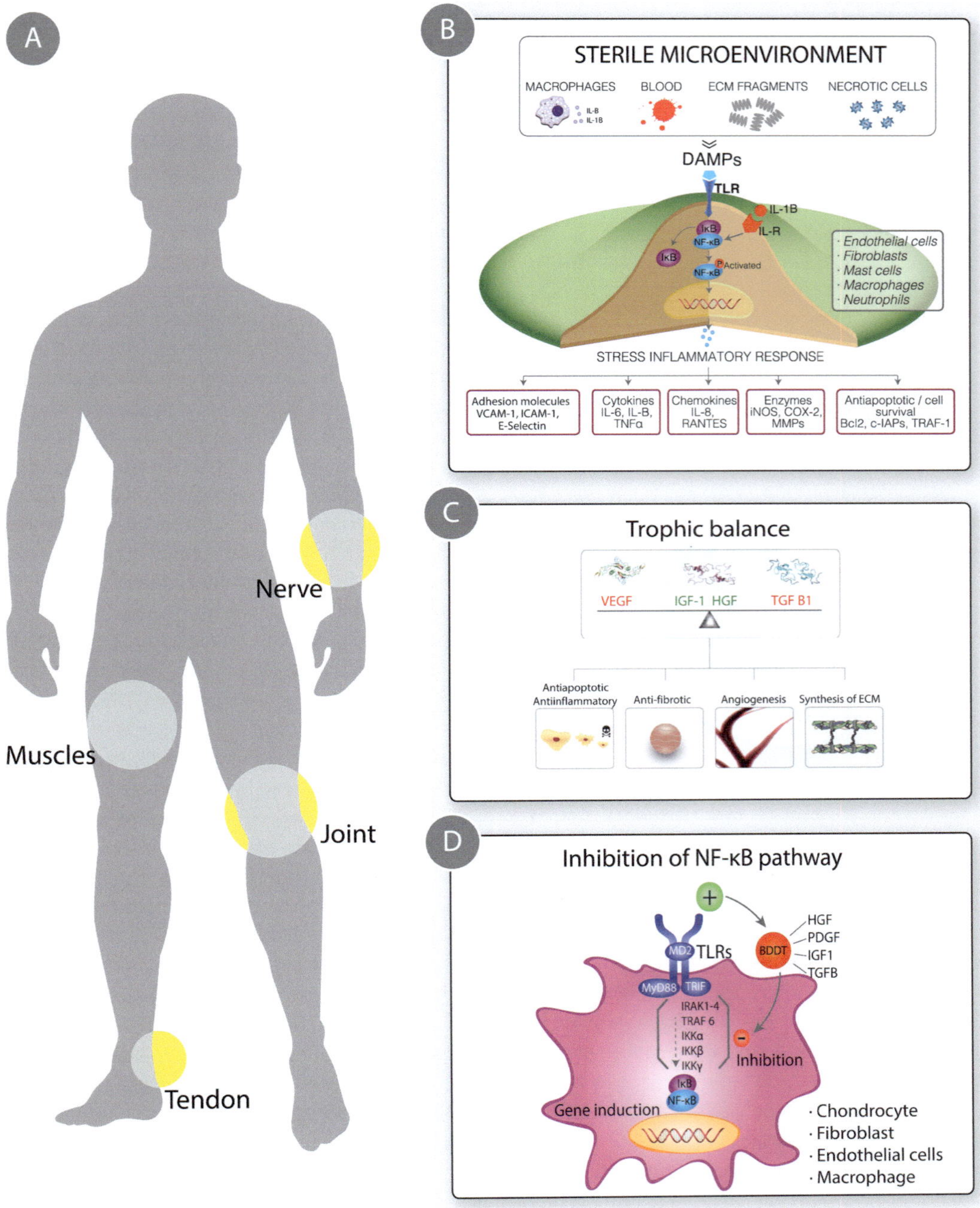

FIG. 3
The common ground of cartilage destruction and osteoarthritis (OA), tendinopathies, muscle and ligament strains, bone fracture or nerve compression or transection, among other tissue damage, is the sterile inflammation. B Tissue injury disrupts the chemical and physical composition of cell microenvironments, which prompts several cell lineages to respond with a pro-inflammatory gene expression through activation of the NFkB signaling pathway without any involvement of pathogens. C A hypothetical mechanism by which the concurrent presence and a balanced ratio between platelet-secreted TGFB1 and VEGF, and plasma growth factors such as IGF-1 and HGF all conveyed by blood-derived BDDT might exert some biological effects. D Blood-derived BDDT, GFs within it such us HGF, PDGF, IGF-1,TGFB1, and platelet microparticles have proven to exert an immunomodulatory effect and promote an antiinflammatory environment[22].
(Reprinted with permission from Padilla et al.[22])

4. EFFECTS OF BLOOD-DERIVED BDDT ON MUSCULOSKELETAL CONDITIONS

Thanks to a deeper understanding of molecular and cellular processes going on in musculoskeletal pathologies, orthopaedic surgery is going through a serious paradigm shift: instead of simply removing and replacing damaged tissue with artificial devices and materials, blood-derived biological drug delivery therapy application is aimed at triggering and enhancing the natural in vivo tissue morphogenesis and regenerative capacity of damaged tissue[23] (see chapter 3).

With this in mind, blood has always been present in the equation of healing therapies. Several lines of evidence derived either from systemic or local stem cell niche therapies, and represented by parabiosis or microfractures and tendon scarifications respectively, support the concept that factors stemmed from platelets or plasmatic proteins are candidates for mammalian tissue rejuvenation and healing[24-28].

Articular cartilage

The treatment of synovial joint pathologies such as traumatic osteochondral defects, osteochondritis disecans, osteonecrosis, bone marrow edema-like lesions, and osteoarthritis, whose ultimate victim appears to be the articular cartilage, with the subchondral bone as the culprit, remains daunting[29]. Current therapeutic strategies are oriented towards harnessing the endogenous repair response by stimulating bone marrow cells through drilling and microfracturing approaches, the transplantation of osteochondral autograft and osteochondral allograft, joint distraction, and the implantation of autologous chondrocytes. In this complex therapeutic landscape, blood-derived biological drug delivery therapies emerge as a promising adjuvant autologous biomaterial with trophic-anabolic, antiinflamatory, immunomodulatory, antioxidative, and analgesic effects on joint tissues (Box 2)[28]. Versatility makes these products optimal biomaterial, to be applied at the dysfunctional and deregulated injured site as a niche therapy[24, 28] (figure 4 B). They may be applied either alone, harnessing the proliferative, migratory, and chondrogenic effect on endogenous mesenchymal progenitor cells[30], or as a carrier of stem cells and/or extracellular components such as collagens and hyaluronic acid[31]. Animal model studies suggest that autologous blood-derived biological drug delivery therapies, whose fibrin is embedded with platelet-derived and plasmatic GFs, either alone or seeded with MSCs, have potential as a gel-scaffold for focal cartilage and osteochondral defects repair[32-35]. These BDDT products are minimally manipulated, conceived and prepared in situ and ready to be applied in the medical office or in the surgical theatre. Intraarticular injections of blood-derived BDDT have been proven to reduce pain and improve joint functionality in patients with knee or hip osteoarthritis[36, 37] (Figure 4 B, Box 2). Moreover, an increasing body of evidence indicates that blood-derived BDDT serves as a bone marrow stimulating approach, or combined with hydrogel, collagen and/or hyaluronic acid membrane, as a carrier of bone marrow-derived mesenchymal stem cells, resulting in structural and functional improvement in human focal cartilage defects[27, 30, 34]. A new strategy to safely deliver blood-derived BDDT to the damaged synovial joint–a strategy which circumvents systemic toxicity, offers an excellent bioavailability and does not present molecular size limitation–is the combination of intraarticular and intraosseous infiltrations of blood-derived BDDT as an in situ biological "joint centric" approach to treat traumatic osteochondral defects, osteochondritis disecans, osteonecrosis, bone marrow edema-like lesions, and osteoarthritis. Such clinical application opens new therapeutic avenues in treatment of joints pathologies[28, 38] (Box 2, Figure 4 B) (see chapter 9 and 11).

Tendon tissue

Musculoskeletal injuries are a growing medical problem associated with overuse and/or aged-related tissue alteration with an estimated annual \$30 billion spent on its management in the USA alone. Tendon and ligament represent 45% of these injuries and unfortunately none of the various therapeutics– including exercise-based physi-

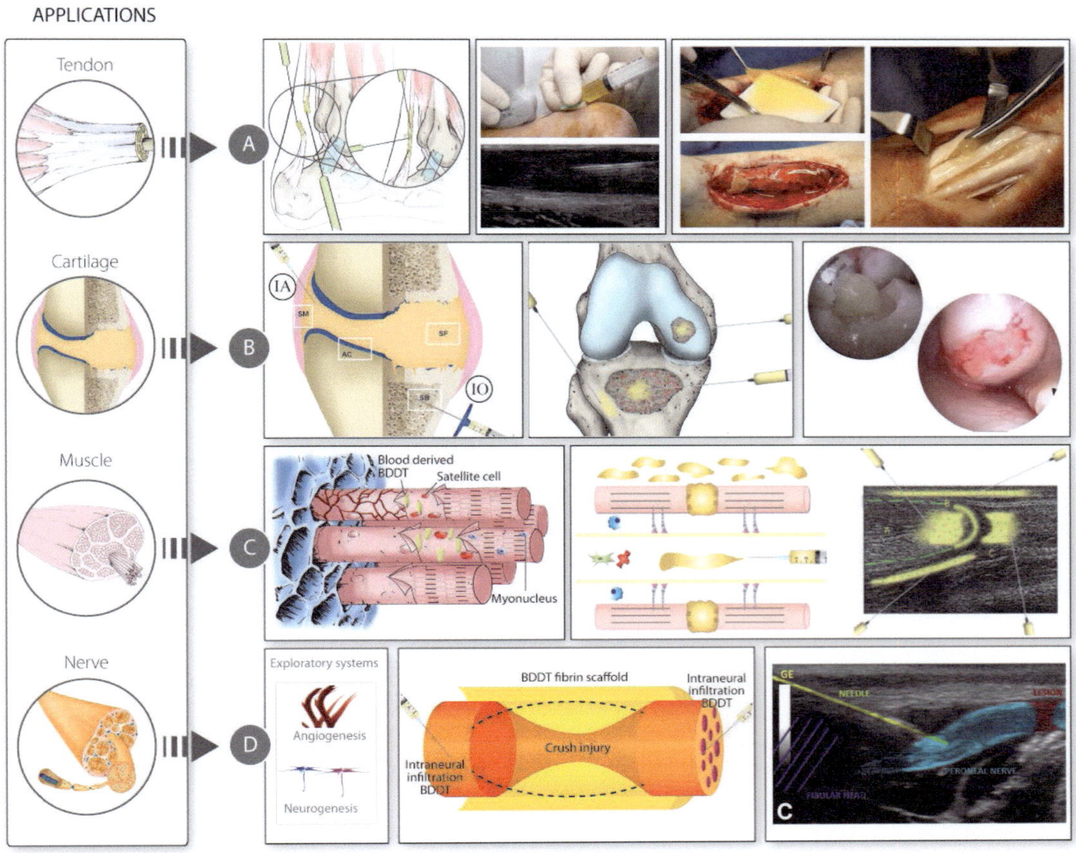

FIG. 4
Advances in regenerative orthopaedics based on the application of blood-derived BDDT. **A)** Intratendinous infiltrations and application of scaffolds obtained from blood-derived BDDT to assist surgical reconstruction of tendon ruptures. In chronic tendinopaties, intratendinous injections are applied under ultrasound guidance. **B)** A novel approach to treating severe knee osteoarthritis and osteochondral injuries by targeting synovial membrane, superficial articular cartilage, synovial fluid, and subchondral bone by combining intraarticular injections and intraosseous infiltrations of blood-derived BDDT. **C)** Blood-derived BDDT has been proposed as a bridge from spontaneity to molecular intervention in muscle tear repair. Early intramuscular injection performed with ultrasound guidance allocates the product into interfascicular and interfibrillar space, and into the injured site. Local fibrinolysis acts on fibrin scaffold gradually releasing GFs and cytokines. **D)** Peripheral nerve regeneration relies on angiogenesis and Schwann cell transdifferentiation, whose exploratory behavior drives spontaneous nerve regeneration. Ultrasound-guided intraneural infiltrations of blood-derived BDDT combined with the application of a fibrin scaffold wrap the injured area and enhance nerve regeneration[22]. (Reprinted with permission from Padilla et al.[22])

cal therapy, corticosteroid injections, non-steroidal anti-inflammatory drugs, extracorporeal shock wave therapy and surgical interventions–has provided a successful long-term solution[39]. Tendon is a hypo-cellular dynamic mechanosensitive composite structure that harbors immunocompetent and tendon multipotent stem/progenitor cells (TDSCs)[40], the key targets of blood-derived BDDTs (Figure 4 A, Box 3). The anabolic/catabolic balance of stromal and parenchymal cells shift according to its mechanical loading history (Figure 2). Together with other highly specialized biological structures, tendons are extremely effective at performing the roles for which they have evolved while yet remaining particularly delicate. The fragile balance that their cells maintain with the extracellular matrix can be disrupted in different ways. This is the case, for instance, for high level sports activities with high performance demands and damage from overuse, or, in the opposite sense, the case of a sedentary life style and the subsequent damage from disuse. Acute and chronic tendon injuries result in pain, focal tenderness, and a decrease in strength and movement stemmed from an inflammed and/or ruptured tendon. Blood-derived autologous bio-scaffolds have been used for a number of years as a raw material in tissue-engineered constructions, either alone in liquid or matrix formulations, or enriched with mechanical or chemical signals, and its application has been a product of in vitro and in vivo research which has provided a better understanding of tenocytes and TDSC response to blood-derived BDDT[41-43] (Box 3, Figure 4 A).

Blood-derived BDDT has been applied either as US-guided intratendinous or intraligament infiltrations on chronic patellar tendinopathy and acute ankle sprain[44, 45] respectively or as intratendinous infiltrations combined with fibrin scaffolds intraoperatively on surgically repaired Achilles tendons tears[43] (Figure 4 A). In both situations, results showed an improvement of symptoms and function, a return to normal architecture of tendon and syndesmosis assessed by MRI, and a shorter time in the recovery of motion and return to sporting activities[43]. Moreover, the application of blood-derived bio-scaffold on the tendon graft or the donor-site level after anterior cruciate ligament reconstruction was found to significantly reduce clinical symptoms and accelerate the process of remodelling and integration of the graft, in addition to satisfactorily filling the gap and reconstructing patella tendon and tibial and patella bone gap[46-48].

Muscle and Nerve tissues

Two other highly specialized tissues that form a functional unit in the musculoskeletal system are muscles and nerves, and several parallels can be drawn between their regeneration processes (Box 4). In acute muscle injuries, blood-derived BDDT liquid is infiltrated into the injury site, adjacent areas and peripheral healthy muscle under ultrasound guidance. In the ensuing 1-3 minutes, this liquid-to-gel transition 3D injectable scaffold allows a successful filling of the muscle gaps and defects and serves as a highway for mechanical energy to transit from the environment to the cell, thereby bridging cell-to-cell tissue transition, promoting multi-cellular assembly and targeting muscle stem and immunocompetent cells, providing chemical signals, mechanical support and plastic-elastic stiffness which not only has a drastic impact on fates of muscle stem cells, but also endows tissues with a suitable mechanical and chemical microenvironment for biological restoration[49] (Figure 1, and 4 C). This dynamic sponge-like fibrin-matrix biological drug delivery therapy is autologous, bio-reabsorbable, and biocompatible[12]. The application of blood-derived BDDT has been shown to shorten the recovery time and even to reduce pain in the case of human application[50]. Notable here is another recent study which reported no benefit of this therapeutic approach[51]. However, it is quite possible that the source of inconsistent clinical outcomes in muscle injuries treated with blood-derived BDDT could well be derived from the delayed administration, low dosage, and the heterogeneity of the blood-derived BDDT biological composition itself, for which there is yet no standard protocol[52]. In order to characterize, standardize, and tailor the composition of blood-derived BDDT to the specific cellular target and tissue repair processes, several in vitro and in vivo efforts are ongoing with an emphasis on applying only plasmatic factors or modifying its composition[53] by blocking TGFB as a fibrotic factor or depleting the myostatin (MSTN) with the goal of enhancing myoblast differentiation[54, 55].

In the management of peripheral nerve injury (PNI) and fuelled by the drawbacks posed by autologous nerve autografts, a great deal of biomedical engineering strategies have been applied, including nerve guidance conduits and scaffolds, incorporation and delivery of neurotrophic factors[56], incorporation of support cells into nerve guidance conduits (NGCs) or fibrin gels, and stimulation of target organs through intramuscular injections of GFs[56, 57]. In animals, platforms using fibrin scaffolds bathed in a cocktail of growth factors and injected or placed into the damaged area enhance the axonal growth necessary to achieve optimal functional recovery[56, 58].(Box 4). In humans, the molecular intervention with blood-derived BDDT is partially bridging the gap between the basic and clinical application, and in a double-blind, randomized, clinical trial, the application of US-guided blood-derived BDDT injections in tibial and ulnar nerves has shown sensory improvement in leprosy peripheral neuropathy[59]. In addition, several case studies applying blood-derived biological drug delivery therapies either as a filler of nerve conduits across nerve gaps post trauma[60] or by infiltrating intraneurally in a peroneal nerve palsy[61], have reported neurological recovery (Figure 4 D). Therefore, blood-derived BDDT applied in a combinatorial strategy as a filler, suturable membrane, and scaffold, stand out as a promising candidate for an adjuvant nerve repair approach which can be harnessed by surgeons in the operating room and in the clinical setting.[61, 62] (see chapter 16).

5. FUTURE DIRECTIONS

The daunting complexity of many musculoskeletal tissues targeted by blood-derived BDDT, coupled with misleading factors associated with the regulatory, clinical and commercial contexts, adds up to multiple barriers to further product development and progress. In the last few years, many aspects related to the technological, biological and pharmaceutical fields have been addressed, including strategies for in vitro characterization of drug release, regulatory processes for in-situ drug preparation[63], minimizing manipulation, and preparing devices that enhance safety and versatility of blood-based biological drug delivery therapies. Moreover, efforts in academia and the biotechnology industry to rapidly translate basic to clinical applications tend to overtake our basic-science understanding of the biological roles of this therapy.

Fortunately, there are reasons for optimism. Novel formulations and fabrication methods are likely to help broaden the catalogue of blood-based BDDT applications. Designing operator-free technologies for BDDT fabrication together with the use of new technologies of additive manufacturing, or 3D bioprinting, may help to control the final properties of the autologous preparations. Efforts must continue to expand the science behind the current generation of blood-derived BDDT. The exploration of its potential for the ex vivo expansion of mesenchymal stem cells, together with the value of fibrin scaffolds for stem cell handling and transplantation, may also reduce some of the challenges faced in the field. Finally, homologous blood-derived BDDT may become an alternative to patients whose blood components such as plasma, platelets, or fibrinogen lack several regenerative key inductors. As a result of these and other advances, the safe clinical implementation of blood-derived BDDT is expected to accelerate and expand.

BOX 1

Biopharmaceutical considerations about biological drug delivery therapies

The therapeutic success of a medicine does not only rely on the type and number of drugs (biologically active mediators) but also on the manner and timing of their delivery to the tissue. When drugs are released without control over their location or rate of delivery, large doses are needed to achieve the desired biological effects, leading to increased toxicity or undesirable side effects. Blood-derived biological drug delivery therapies (BDDT) are based on a combination of naturally derived biomaterials such as fibrin and a pool of growth factors. For example, the three-dimensional fibrin scaffold obtained from fractionated human plasma represents a physiologically inspired solution to control the release of the wide range of plasma and platelet-derived mediators[64]. In practice, the release profile is a combination of diffusion and degradation of the matrix. Diffusion controls the release of the biologically active agents when it is slow compared with the rate of drug dissociation from the material, yet it happens much faster than material degradation[65]. Matrix degradation is preferentially regulated by hydrolytic cleavage of the carrier body and by enzymatic degradation. In this way, growth factors are progressively released and the fibrin scaffold acts as a temporary matrix for the new growing tissue (figure 1).

BOX 2

Harnessing endogenous repair process of joint tissues

Articular cartilage (AC) is a tissue that is remarkably resilient to compressive and shearing forces. Yet it is highly fragile to alterations of the synovial membrane (SM) and subchondral bone (SCB), two well-vascularized tissues from where systemic and local inflammation insults arise[66]. These aggressions are mediated by pro-inflammatory cytokines and inflammatory macrophages and synoviocytes, which damage articular cartilage as in the case of rheumatoid arthritis or osteoarthritis[66]. However, SM and SCB are also the egress point and source of nutrients and mesenchymal progenitor cells for mounting a chondrogenic reparative response, which is driven by the recruitment and chemotactic homing of synovium and bone marrow-derived stem cells mediated by SDF-1, TGFB, and fibronectin. This is the case in microfracture techniques and in the combined strategy using intraarticular (IA) and intraosseous (IO) infiltrations of blood-derived BDDT[26, 28]. In doing so, this novel local BDDT tackles the four synovial joint tissues—AC, SF, SM, and SCB—and acts as a dynamic autologous liquid scaffold that, in a sustained and gradual manner, conveys chemotactic endogenous MSC homing and chondrogenic factors such as SDF-1, TGFB, and fibronectin[27, 28, 30, 67]. In addition, this BDDT dampens inflammatory stress at the level of joint tissues, by both inhibiting the NFkB on chondrocytes and macrophages[68] and up-regulating the antioxidant response element NF-E2-related factor 2 (NrF2-ARE) pathway in osteoblasts[69]. Improvements of clinical outcomes in patients with knee and hip OA were reported applying this strategy[28, 36], which might primarily be mediated by HGF, CTGF, IGF-1, PDGF, among others[68-71], thereby paving the way to cartilage regeneration, however elusive it may remain (figure 3).

BOX 3

Adaptation, inflammation, and homeostatic process in tendon.

There is increasing evidence showing that tendon and ligament adaptation, injury, and repair processes share several intracellular pathways, and although it is difficult to draw the line between the cellular and molecular responses that lead to either tissue adaptation or tissue damage, inflammatory process appear to be at the interface of tendon adaptation and damage (figure 2)[39, 68]. Repetitive mechanical loading, as is the case in early stages of tendinopathy, and tendon overuse induce the activation of NFkB and thereby the synthesis of matrix metalloproteinases (MMPs), two isoforms of cyclooxygenase (COX) COX-1 and COX-2, and PGE2 by inflammatory tenocytes, mast cells and other immunocompetent cells[39, 72-74]. PGE2 is a major systemic and local inflammatory mediator that decreases the production of collagen and causes aberrant differentiation of TDSCs into adipogenic and osteogenic lineages [74], which might partially account for the presence of fibrocartilage, calcifications and adipose tissue in injured and chronic degenerative tendons[39, 40, 72, 74].

An excellent series of in vitro and in vivo studies demonstrated that blood-derived BDDT induced tenocyte proliferation, stimulated the synthesis of type I collagen and the neovascularization [42], promoted differentiation of TDSCs into active tenocytes, but significantly, the addition of leukocytes into the releasate increased the synthesis of PGE2 and the gene expression of metalloproteinase-1 (MMP-1), MMP-13, interleukin-1B (IL-1B), and decreased the expression of alfa-SMA as a marker of active tenocytes[73-75]. Among the myriad mediators conveyed by blood-derived BDDT, hepatocyte growth factor (HGF), and lipoxin A4 (LX4) have been shown to exert an anti-inflammatory and pro-resolution of inflammation effect on injured tendons (Figure 1 D and Figure 2 A)[73, 76].

BOX 4

Blood-derived BDDT application on muscle and nerve pathologies

Early inflammation, muscle satellite and stem cell-like myelinating Schwann cell activation, angiogenesis, and macrophage polarization, are key drivers of full function recovery, where growth factors (GFs) and the fibrin scaffold are instrumental instructive and permissive factors[77-80]. In the full reconstruction of muscle tissue, endothelial and muscle satellite cells, together with macrophages and other myogenic progenitor cells, signal reciprocally primarily by VEGF, PDGF, IGF-1, and HGF, making angiogenesis, myogenesis and neurogenesis proceed concomitantly[77, 80]. In extensive in vitro and in vivo preclinical studies, the combination of the aforementioned GFs or the use of blood-derived BDDT promoted an earlier regeneration of damaged muscles mainly by the modulation of inflammatory response, a reliable angiogenic stimulus, a significant expansion of the myogenic pool, and a macrophage polarization from an inflammatory to a trophic phenotype[79-81]. These biological effects prevented the formation of aberrant repair and fibrosis, which would otherwise result in clinical muscle relapses (figure 4 C).

In the management of peripheral nerve injury (PNI) blood-derived BDDT has emerged as a novel and versatile adjuvant approach. Once infiltrated intraneurally as a liquid-to-gel injectable scaffold, or wrapped around the injured nerve gap as a matrix-like viscous and malleable structure, or both, [58] (Figure 4 D) tissue fibrinolysis breaks the fibrin down, thereby releasing cell signalling molecules such as neurotrophic (NGF, BDGF, IGF-1, PDGF, VEGF, HGF) and neurotropic factors (fibrin, fibronectin, and vitronectin)[82]. These biomolecules govern early inflammation, stem cell-like myelinating Schwann cell activation, angiogenesis, macrophage polarization, as well as the active resolution of inflammation, angiogenesis, and fibrogenesis, thereby acting as key drivers of full nerve function recovery[56, 77].

1. Anitua, E. et al. (2007) The potential impact of the preparation rich in growth factors (PRGF) in different medical fields. Biomaterials. 28, 4551-4560

2. Langer, R. and Vacanti, J.P. (1993) Tissue engineering. Science. 260, 920-926

3. Murphy, C.M. et al. (2013) Cell-scaffold interactions in the bone tissue engineering triad. Eur Cell Mater. 26, 120-132

4. Anitua, E. et al. (2004) Autologous platelets as a source of proteins for healing and tissue regeneration. Thromb Haemost. 91, 4-15

5. Langer, H.F. et al. (2009) Platelet derived bFGF mediates vascular integrative mechanisms of mesenchymal stem cells in vitro. J Mol Cell Cardiol. 47, 315-325

6. Stellos, K. et al. (2010) Platelets in regeneration. Semin Thromb Hemost. 36, 175-184

7. Gawaz, M. and Vogel, S. (2013) Platelets in tissue repair: control of apoptosis and interactions with regenerative cells. Blood. 122, 2550-2554

8. Hollister, S.J. and Murphy, W.L. (2011) Scaffold translation: barriers between concept and clinic. Tissue Eng Part B Rev. 17, 459-474

9. Anitua, E. et al. (2015) Clinical, radiographical, and histological outcomes of plasma rich in growth factors in extraction socket: a randomized controlled clinical trial. Clin Oral Investig. 19, 589-600

10. Anitua, E. et al. (2008) Effectiveness of autologous preparation rich in growth factors for the treatment of chronic cutaneous ulcers. J Biomed Mater Res B Appl Biomater. 84, 415-421

11. Anitua, E. et al. (2015) High-throughput proteomic characterization of plasma rich in growth factors (PRGF-Endoret)-derived fibrin clot interactome. J Tissue Eng Regen Med. 9, E1-12

12. Anitua, E. and Orive, G. (2012) Endogenous regenerative technology using plasma- and platelet-derived growth factors. J Control Release. 157, 317-320

13. Xiao, G.H. et al. (2001) Anti-apoptotic signaling by hepatocyte growth factor/Met via the phosphatidylinositol 3-kinase/Akt and mitogen-activated protein kinase pathways. Proc Natl Acad Sci U S A. 98, 247-252

14. Aoki, M. et al. (2000) Angiogenesis induced by hepatocyte growth factor in non-infarcted myocardium and infarcted myocardium: up-regulation of essential transcription factor for angiogenesis, ets. Gene Ther. 7, 417-427

15. Okunishi, K. et al. (2005) A novel role of hepatocyte growth factor as an immune regulator through suppressing dendritic cell function. J Immunol. 175, 4745-4753

16. Massberg, S. et al. (2006) Platelets secrete stromal cell-derived factor 1alpha and recruit bone marrow-derived progenitor cells to arterial thrombi in vivo. J Exp Med. 203, 1221-1233

17. Stellos, K. et al. (2008) Platelet-derived stromal cell-derived factor-1 regulates adhesion and promotes differentiation of human CD34+ cells to endothelial progenitor cells. Circulation. 117, 206-215

18. Wang, J.H. and Li, B. (2010) Mechanics rules cell biology. Sports Med Arthrosc Rehabil Ther Technol. 2, 16

19. Ingber, D.E. (2006) Cellular mechanotransduction: putting all the pieces together again. Faseb j. 20, 811-827

20. Kjaer, M. (2004) Role of extracellular matrix in adaptation of tendon and skeletal muscle to mechanical loading. Physiol Rev. 84, 649-698

21. Riley, G.P. (2005) Gene expression and matrix turnover in overused and damaged tendons. Scand J Med Sci Sports. 15, 241-251

22. Padilla S, S.M., Orive G, Anitua E. Human-based biological and biomimetic autologous therapies for muskuloskeletal tissue regeneration. Trends Biotechnol. In press. http://dx.doi.org/10.1016/j.tibtech.2016.09.008

23. Ivkovic, A. et al. (2011) Regenerative medicine and tissue engineering in orthopaedic surgery. Front Biosci (Elite Ed). 3, 923-944

24. Wagers, A.J. (2012) The stem cell niche in regenerative medicine. Cell Stem Cell. 10, 362-369

25. Cosgrove, B.D. et al. (2014) Rejuvenation of the muscle stem cell population restores strength to injured aged muscles. Nat Med. 20, 255-264

26. Steadman, J.R. et al. (1997) Microfracture technique forfull-thickness chondral defects: Technique and clinical results. Operative techniques in orthopaedics. 7, 300-304

27. Liu, H.Y. et al. (2014) Delayed animal aging through the recovery of stem cell senescence by platelet rich plasma. Biomaterials. 35, 9767-9776

28. Sanchez, M. et al. (2016) A new strategy to tackle severe knee osteoarthritis: Combination of intra-articular and intraosseous injections of Platelet Rich Plasma. Expert Opin Biol Ther. 16, 627-643

29. Campbell, T.M. et al. (2016) Mesenchymal Stem Cell Alterations in Bone Marrow Lesions in Patients With Hip Osteoarthritis. Arthritis Rheumatol. 68, 1648-1659

30. Kreuz, P.C. et al. (2015) Platelet-Rich Plasma Preparation Types Show Impact on Chondrogenic Differentiation, Migration, and Proliferation of Human Subchondral Mesenchymal Progenitor Cells. Arthroscopy. 31, 1951-1961

31. Zhu, Y. et al. (2013) Basic science and clinical application of platelet-rich plasma for cartilage defects and osteoarthritis: a review. Osteoarthritis Cartilage. 21, 1627-1637

32. Milano, G. et al. (2010) The effect of platelet rich plasma combined with microfractures on the treatment of chondral defects: an experimental study in a sheep model. Osteoarthritis Cartilage. 18, 971-980

33. Lee, H.R. et al. (2012) Platelet-rich plasma loaded hydrogel scaffold enhances chondrogenic differentiation and maturation with up-regulation of CB1 and CB2. J Control Release. 159, 332-337

34. Xie, X. et al. (2014) Biology of platelet-rich plasma and its clinical application in cartilage repair. Arthritis Res Ther. 16, 204

35. Chiang, C.-W. et al. (2014) Application of Synovial Fluid Mesenchymal Stem Cells: Platelet-rich Plasma Hydrogel for Focal Cartilage Defect. Journal of Experimental & Clinical Medicine. 6, 118-124

36. Sanchez, M. et al. (2012) Ultrasound-guided platelet-rich plasma injections for the treatment of osteoarthritis of the hip. Rheumatology (Oxford). 51, 144-150

37. Sanchez, M. et al. (2012) A randomized clinical trial evaluating plasma rich in growth factors (PRGF-Endoret) versus hyaluronic acid in the short-term treatment of symptomatic knee osteoarthritis. Arthroscopy. 28, 1070-1078

38. Sánchez, M. et al. (2016) Combination of Intra-Articular and Intraosseous Injections of Platelet Rich Plasma for Severe Knee Osteoarthritis: A Pilot Study. BioMed Research International. 2016

39. Dakin, S.G. et al. (2015) Inflammation activation and resolution in human tendon disease. Sci Transl Med. 7, 311ra173

40. Bi, Y. et al. (2007) Identification of tendon stem/progenitor cells and the role of the extracellular matrix in their niche. Nat Med. 13, 1219-1227

41. Crowe, C.S. et al. (2015) Tendon regeneration with a novel tendon hydrogel: in vitro effects of platelet-rich plasma on rat adipose-derived stem cells. Plastic and reconstructive surgery. 135, 981e-989e

42. Anitua, E. et al. (2006) Autologous fibrin matrices: a potential source of biological mediators that modulate tendon cell activities. J Biomed Mater Res A. 77, 285-293

43. Sanchez, M. et al. (2007) Comparison of surgically repaired Achilles tendon tears using platelet-rich fibrin matrices. Am J Sports Med. 35, 245-251

44. Charousset, C. et al. (2014) Are multiple platelet-rich plasma injections useful for treatment of chronic patellar tendinopathy in athletes? a prospective study. Am J Sports Med. 42, 906-911

45. Laver, L. et al. (2015) Plasma rich in growth factors (PRGF) as a treatment for high ankle sprain in elite athletes: a randomized control trial. Knee Surg Sports Traumatol Arthrosc. 23, 3383-3392

46. Sanchez, M. et al. (2010) Ligamentization of tendon grafts treated with an endogenous preparation rich in growth factors: gross morphology and histology. Arthroscopy. 26, 470-480

47. de Almeida, A.M. et al. (2012) Patellar Tendon Healing With Platelet-Rich Plasma A Prospective Randomized Controlled Trial. The American journal of sports medicine. 40, 1282-1288

48. Cervellin, M. et al. (2012) Autologous platelet-rich plasma gel to reduce donor-site morbidity after patellar tendon graft harvesting for anterior cruciate ligament reconstruction: a randomized, controlled clinical study. Knee Surg Sports Traumatol Arthrosc. 20, 114-120

49. Sanchez, M. et al. (2014) Muscle repair: platelet-rich plasma derivates as a bridge from spontaneity to intervention. Injury. 45 Suppl 4, S7-14

50. Hamid, M.S.A. et al. (2014) Platelet-rich plasma injections for the treatment of hamstring injuries a randomized controlled trial. The American journal of sports medicine. 42, 2410-2418

51. Reurink, G. et al. (2014) Platelet-rich plasma injections in acute muscle injury. N Engl J Med. 370, 2546-2547

52. Anitua, E. et al. (2014) More on platelet-rich plasma injections in acute muscle injury. N Engl J Med. 371, 1264

53. Anitua, E. et al. (2009) Fibroblastic response to treatment with different preparations rich in growth factors. Cell Prolif. 42, 162-170

54. Li, H. et al. (2016) Customized platelet-rich plasma with transforming growth factor beta1 neutralization antibody to reduce fibrosis in skeletal muscle. Biomaterials. 87, 147-156

55. Miroshmychenko, O. et al. (2016) The use of platelet-rich and platelet-poor plasma to enhance differentiation of skeletal myoblasts: Implications for the use of autologous blood products for muscle regeneration. AAOS. Stanford Sports Medicine. July 7-10. The Broadmoor, Colorado.

56. Lu, P. et al. (2012) Long-distance growth and connectivity of neural stem cells after severe spinal cord injury. Cell. 150, 1264-1273

57. Pfister, B.J. et al. (2011) Biomedical engineering strategies for peripheral nerve repair: surgical applications, state of the art, and future challenges. Crit Rev Biomed Eng. 39, 81-124

58. Sanchez, M. et al. (2015) Ultrasound-guided plasma rich in growth factors injections and scaffolds hasten motor nerve functional recovery in an ovine model of nerve crush injury. J Tissue Eng Regen Med. DOI: 10.1002/term.2079

59. Anjayani, S. et al. (2014) Sensory improvement of leprosy peripheral neuropathy in patients treated with perineural injection of platelet-rich plasma. Int J Dermatol. 53, 109-113

60. Kuffler, D.P. (2014) Promoting peripheral axon regeneration across nerve gaps post trauma. JSM Neurosurg Spine. 2, 1044

61. Sanchez, M. et al. (2013) Ultrasound-guided platelet-rich plasma injections for the treatment of common peroneal nerve palsy associated with multiple ligament injuries of the knee. Knee Surg Sports Traumatol Arthrosc.

62. Kuffler, D.P. (2014) An assessment of current techniques for inducing axon regeneration and neurological recovery following peripheral nerve trauma. Prog Neurobiol. 116, 1-12

63. Anitua, E. et al. (2015) Closing regulatory gaps: new ground rules for platelet-rich plasma. Trends Biotechnol. 33, 492-495

64. Ahmed, T.A. et al. (2008) Fibrin: a versatile scaffold for tissue engineering applications. Tissue Eng Part B Rev. 14, 199-215

65. Kearney, C.J. and Mooney, D.J. (2013) Macroscale delivery systems for molecular and cellular payloads. Nat Mater. 12, 1004-1017

66. Scanzello, C.R. and Goldring, S.R. (2012) The role of synovitis in osteoarthritis pathogenesis. Bone. 51, 249-257

67. Liu, H.Y. et al. (2011) The balance between adipogenesis and osteogenesis in bone regeneration by platelet-rich plasma for age-related osteoporosis. Biomaterials. 32, 6773-6780

68. Bendinelli, P. et al. (2010) Molecular basis of anti-inflammatory action of platelet-rich plasma on human chondrocytes: mechanisms of NF-kappaB inhibition via HGF. J Cell Physiol. 225, 757-766

69. Tohidnezhad, M. et al. (2014) Role of platelet-released growth factors in detoxification of reactive oxygen species in osteoblasts. Bone. 65, 9-17

70. Coudriet, G.M. et al. (2010) Hepatocyte growth factor modulates interleukin-6 production in bone marrow derived macrophages: implications for inflammatory mediated diseases. PLoS One. 5, e15384

71. Montaseri, A. et al. (2011) IGF-1 and PDGF-bb suppress IL-1beta-induced cartilage degradation through down-regulation of NF-kappaB signaling: involvement of Src/PI-3K/AKT pathway. PLoS One. 6, e28663

72. Yang, G. et al. (2005) Repetitive mechanical stretching modulates IL-1beta induced COX-2, MMP-1 expression, and PGE2 production in human patellar tendon fibroblasts. Gene. 363, 166-172

73. Zhang, J. et al. (2013) HGF mediates the anti-inflammatory effects of PRP on injured tendons. PLoS One. 8, e67303

74. Zhang, J. and Wang, J.H. (2010) Production of PGE(2) increases in tendons subjected to repetitive mechanical loading and induces differentiation of tendon stem cells into non-tenocytes. J Orthop Res. 28, 198-203

75. Zhou, Y. et al. (2015) The differential effects of leukocyte-containing and pure platelet-rich plasma (PRP) on tendon stem/progenitor cells - implications of PRP application for the clinical treatment of tendon injuries. Stem Cell Res Ther. 6, 173

76. Dakin, S.G. et al. (2012) Inflamm-aging and arachadonic acid metabolite differences with stage of tendon disease. PLoS One. 7, e48978

77. Cattin, A.L. et al. (2015) Macrophage-Induced Blood Vessels Guide Schwann Cell-Mediated Regeneration of Peripheral Nerves. Cell. 162, 1127-1139

78. Tidball, J.G. and Villalta, S.A. (2010) Regulatory interactions between muscle and the immune system during muscle regeneration. Am J Physiol Regul Integr Comp Physiol. 298, R1173-1187

79. Dimauro, I. et al. (2014) Platelet-rich plasma and skeletal muscle healing: a molecular analysis of the early phases of the regeneration process in an experimental animal model. PLoS One. 9, e102993

80. Anitua, E. et al. (2015) Infiltration of plasma rich in growth factors enhances in vivo angiogenesis and improves reperfusion and tissue remodeling after severe hind limb ischemia. J Control Release. 202, 31-39

81. Borselli, C. et al. (2010) Functional muscle regeneration with combined delivery of angiogenesis and myogenesis factors. Proc Natl Acad Sci U S A. 107, 3287-3292

82. Anitua, E. et al. (2015) High-throughput proteomic characterization of plasma rich in growth factors (PRGF-Endoret)-derived fibrin clot interactome. J Tissue Eng Regen Med. 9, E1-E12

CHAPTER 5

Molecular Intervention with Plasma-Rich Growth Factors to Enhance Muscle Perfusion and Tissue Remodeling in Ischemic Diseases

PRGF treatment of ischemic muscle and heart

AUTHORS

Pelacho B.[1], Pérez A.[1], Prósper F.[1,2]

[1] Cell Therapy Area, Center for Applied Medical Research (CIMA)
[2] Hematology and Cell Therapy, Clínica Universidad de Navarra, IdiSNA, University of Navarra, Spain

SUMMARY

Ischemic diseases remain the first cause of morbidity and mortality worldwide. Current standard approaches based on drug-therapy or surgery have a palliative but not a repairing effect, which leads to chronification and worsening of the disease. Novel alternative approaches based on protein and stem cell therapy have been thoroughly assessed in the last two decades. Platelet-rich plasma has been shown to act as a rich depot of pro-angiogenic, pro-survival and pro-myogenic growth factors that can be locally released in the diseased tissues. This chapter focuses on the therapeutic potential of platelet-rich plasma and growth factors for protective and regenerative treatment of muscle and cardiac ischemic pathologies. We discuss the experimental and clinical results obtained when PRP/PRGF were injected in animal models of limb ischemia and myocardial infarction or angina patients, together with the mechanisms involved in such effects. Finally, the combination of platelet-derivatives with stem cells is also described as a novel protein/cellular delivery platform with improved potential for treating ischemic disease.

E. Anitua et al. (eds.), *Platelet Rich Plasma in Orthopaedics and Sports Medicine*,
https://doi.org/10.1007/978-3-319-63730-3_5

1. EPIDEMIOLOGY AND PATHOLOGY OF CARDIOVASCULAR DISEASES

Ischemia defines a state in which blood flow is insufficient to meet metabolic demands. This condition occurs regularly but transiently in healthy humans, for example when they begin to exercise. On the pathological side, there are multiple mechanisms that impair the functional and structural responses of the vasculature to the metabolic demands of the muscle and cardiac tissue (among others), provoking ischemia. According to the World Health Organization, cardiovascular diseases represent the first cause of morbidity and mortality worldwide, with approximately 17 million deaths per year. Unfortunately, predictions are not favorable and it is estimated that by 2030 about 24 million people per year will die from these diseases, which represents 42% of deaths worldwide[1]. Risk factors associated with ischemia are multiple, the principal ones being hypertension, high cholesterol, obesity, diabetes, aging, family history of cardiovascular disease, gender and ethnic origin. External factors like physical inactivity, tobacco and alcohol consumption also have a great influence on the progress of these diseases.

Peripheral Artery Disease (PAD) is a common cause of great disability and morbidity. The annual incidence of this ischemic disease in Europe and the United States ranges from 500 to 1000 new cases per million people[2]. PAD is an occlusive atherosclerotic disease caused by blockage of the arteries by cholesterol plaques that cause compromised blood flow in the limbs. Following atherosclerosis and blood flow limitation, adaptation, maladaptation and injury in the distal vascular bed and skeletal muscle contribute to exacerbate the disease. Symptoms of PAD include intermittent claudication, which is defined as calf or buttock pain or cramping with walking caused by inadequate blood flow to the limb. The most severe symptomatic manifestation of PAD is Critical Limb Ischemia (CLI), defined as pain at rest due to reduced blood flow to the limb. CLI may further result in ischemic ulceration and gangrene formation. Patients with CLI have not only a high risk of amputation but also a high rate of cardiovascular death, often due to complications related to coronary artery (55%) and cerebrovascular atherosclerosis (10%)[3]. Despite the remarkable progress made in medical treatments and endovascular procedures for revascularization, patients with CLI have a very low quality of life. Nowadays, angioplasty, with or without stenting, and bypass surgery are widely used surgical interventions, and tangible results have been reported showing how they decrease mortality and limb loss while also increasing patency and improving wound healing[4].

Ischemic Heart Disease (IHD) is the leading cause of death in the developed world, representing 33% of deaths of patients aged over[3, 5]. It is estimated that each year cardiovascular diseases cause a total of about 4 million deaths in Europe alone, most due to coronary heart disease, representing 47% of all deaths. Worldwide, the annual incidence of heart failure has reached staggering numbers, culminating in 20 million cardiac-related deaths per year worldwide. Indeed, decompensated heart failure is now the primary indication for repeated hospitalization, resulting in an annual expenditure of US$120 billion worldwide and a 5-year mortality of around 50% (reviewed in[1,5]).

Myocardial ischemia generally develops when deposits of cholesterol particles accumulate on the walls of heart blood vessels and form plaques, which narrow or block the arteries that supply blood to the heart. As in ischemic limbs, the lack of blood supply leads to cell death and tissue necrosis, which activates heart tissue inflammation and remodeling responses. By these processes, necrotic cells are eliminated and replaced by a non-contractile fibrotic scar mainly composed of activated fibroblasts and extracellular matrix components[6]. These compensatory mechanisms initially prevent cardiac rupture but, with time, become a maladaptive response, leading to contractile dysfunction, arrhythmias and ultimately, heart failure.

Routine therapies driven to improve myocardial function in IHD include pharmacological treatment, percutaneous intervention and surgery.

However, these techniques are aimed at minimizing the symptoms and preventing the progression of the disease, but are not able to regenerate the tissue or to restore the heart function in a sustained manner. Therefore, the only real option for severe cases is heart transplantation with the concomitant limitations of the donor waiting lists and the need for an immunosuppressive regimen to prevent rejection. The failure of these therapies to rescue the damaged heart and the inconvenience of heart transplants have led to the emergence of alternative treatments, including protein (reviewed in[7]) and stem cell (SC)–based (reviewed in[8]) therapies. These novel strategies are directed to induce tissue revascularization as well as to intervene in the tissue remodeling processes, and are vital for treating IHC as well as PAD patients[9]. Protein-based therapies as examples of this type of treatment will be discussed in detail in the following pages.

2. TREATMENT WITH GROWTH FACTORS FOR RECOVERY OF ISCHEMIC TISSUES

Since Dr. J. Folkman first described the process of angiogenesis in 1971, much has been learned about the cells, the extracellular factors, and the signaling pathways that modulate the neovascularization process[10]. Neovascularization, the establishment of stable and functional blood vessel networks, involves multiple complex events that require several angiogenic factors to induce sprouting of pre-existing resident endothelial cells (angiogenesis), maturation and enlargement of size of pre-existing small vessels through vascular remodeling (arteriogenesis), and the recruitment of endothelial progenitor cells (vasculogenesis)[11].

Angiogenesis, arteriogenesis, and vasculogenesis are critical to the process of ischemic muscle regeneration, and they are closely related to inflammation and extracellular matrix remodeling. Although the complex interactions between these multiple cell types are still not totally understood, the major role that monocytes and macrophages play in the remodeling process is well known, as they are recruited at the injured sites and generate chemokines and growth factors that contribute to arteriogenesis and angiogenesis. These factors are important for the subsequent recruitment of leukocytes to the injured tissue as well as endothelial and smooth muscle progenitor cells, and also play a critical role in the activation of muscle-derived progenitor cells.

In recent years, many growth factors and cytokines have been identified and their function analyzed in different animal models of ischemia, including those for high limb ischemia and myocardial infarction. Among these factors, VEGF has been pointed out as a key stimulatory factor of angiogenesis[12], which strongly induces endothelial cell proliferation and migration. However, the combined action of other factors is necessary in order to induce vascular maturation and stabilization, as VEGF by itself promotes the formation of leaky and unstable capillaries[13]. Factors like PDGF-BB are essential for these processes, and the lack of this single factor leads to fragile neovasculature[14]. Morevoer, bFGF and HGF also cooperate with VEGF or PDGF-BB by acting as chemoattractans to smooth muscle cells and inducing their growth. Thus, their action favors the promotion and enlargement of collateral vessels, as it has been previously shown in several animal models of limb ischemia and myocardial infarction[15,16]. Furthermore, the anti-inflammatory and anti-fibrotic role of HGF has also been demonstrated[17]. Other factors like SDF-1 and IGF-1 have direct or indirect effects on endogenous angiogenesis. SDF-1 guides, together with VEGF, the recruitment and homing of endothelial progenitor cells to ischemic muscles, contributing to neovascularization[18], and IGF-1 also stimulates angiogenesis[19], although with a less potent effect than other angiogenic factors. Importantly, a robust anti-apoptotic and pro-myogenic role has been reported for IGF-1[20].

Positive results have been observed after treating different ischemic animal models with pro-angiogenic growth factors. For example, on this basis, therapeutic angiogenesis was proposed as a good treatment for PAD and IHD patients. However, clinical trials of single and solution forms of pro-angiogenic agents have proven to have little or no efficacy in patients with such disorders. Thus, despite Phase-I clinical trials demonstrating promising results in patients with either PAD or IHD treated with growth factors like FGF2, VEGF or HGF, multi-center, randomized, double-bind, placebo-controlled phase-II/III trials contradicted the previous results, showing no significant beneficial effects in any of the groups of ischemic patients who received single doses of recombinant proteins such as FGF2 or VEGF, among others (reviewed in[21]).

The major limitation found in these growth factors-based clinical trials is that a cocktail of growth factors and cytokines is likely to be required according to the complex intricacy of the angiogenic/arteriogenic and tissue remodeling processes; thus, administration of a single growth factor may not be sufficient to achieve a complete response[13,15]. In addition, the short half-life of the proteins due to their high instability and protease action when injected as a bolus may also counteract their beneficial effects. Also, the low local biodistribution and lack of dose control might reduce their possible benefit. To overcome these limitations, several technologies have been explored to ensure more protected, controlled and localized release of the growth factors. These new technologies, which have been thoroughly reviewed by others[22], include many biological and synthetic systems based on the preparation of functionalized scaffolds, liposomes, nano- or micro-particles, whose main function is to protect proteins from degradation and to preserve their bioactivity during their release into the damaged tissues. In that sense, the use of platelet-rich gels might be considered another release system for growth factors, and this will be described next.

3. NOVEL TREATMENTS FOR THE ISCHEMIC MUSCLE: IS PLATELET-RICH PLASMA AN ALTERNATIVE OPTION?

3.1 Platelet-rich plasma

As previously discussed, successful reperfusion of the ischemic tissue depends on stimulation of angiogenic and arteriogenesis activities[23]. Platelets are critical to hemostasis and subsequent angiogenesis in wound healing. Transfusion of platelets enhances the angiogenic recovery of blood flow in models of ischemia[24], while their depletion suppresses this process[25]. Platelets contain more than 20 growth factors that stimulate proliferation, survival, adhesion, and chemotaxis of different progenitor cells such as hematopoietic cells or endothelial cells, affecting both angiogenesis, restoration of blood flow and wound healing. Once activated, platelets release pro-angiogenic and also anti-apoptotic and pro-myogenic factors, including VEGF, SDF-1, PDGF, FGF-2, HGF, TGF and KGF (reviewed in[26]). Since platelets constitute a potential source of multiple autologous growth factors, proteins and chemokines involved in tissue regeneration, a product enriched in platelets was designed, the platelet-rich plasma (PRP) product (also termed autologous platelet)[27]. The initial rationale for PRP products was to replace the blood clot with a preparation enriched in platelets, which could, once activated, secrete a large pool of proteins and factors to the local milieu, driving the tissue regeneration mechanism. Later on, another technique was developed to obtain a type of plasma that is highly enriched with proteins and circulating growth factors and concentrated in a gelatinous form, which has been named PRGF (Plasma Rich in Growth Factor)[28]. PRGF presents the advantage over PRP that it does not need thrombin for coagulation, being produced by a simple calcium-based reaction. Finally, Platelet Rich Fibrin (PRF) has also been produced by a simplified preparation, with no manipulation of blood. A detailed description of the preparation of these three platelet-derived products and their main features and advantages for therapeutic use has been previously reviewed[29].

3.2 Application of PRP in ischemic peripheral disease

Effective restoration of blood flow by augmentation of the number of capillaries and mature vessels after PRP delivery has been demonstrated in mouse hind limb ischemia models[30,31]. Sustained release of PRP accelerates the homing of hematopoietic progenitor cells to the ischemic site, which might be explained by the presence of VEGF and SDF-1 in the PRP, inducing the arteriogenesis process. Growth factors present in PRP play bioactive roles in the proliferation and differentiation of endothelial cells and smooth muscle cells, which may contribute to the formation of functional collateral vessels and facilitate their maturation[32]. The transient fibrin scaffold, which is formed after PRP activation and polymerization, in addition to contributing to angiogenesis by sequestering and releasing different growth factors, may favor cell survival in ischemic legs through cell adhesion motifs[33]. Furthermore, this biological scaffold of fibrin contributes to wound healing of dermal tissue loss in patients affected by CLI. Platelet-derived fibrin scaffold guides the mesenchymal cells to migrate from the base and the margins of the wound, eventually maturing into a granulation tissue[34,35]. They also contain anti-bacterial proteins, which help to reduce bacterial colonization in foot ulcers[36], as well as being less invasive, painless, easier to apply, and tolerated better by the patients. In addition, in order to attain maximum therapeutic effects, the combination of platelet-rich preparations with biomaterials has made it possible to develop novel therapeutic alternatives, improving the preexisting ones and increasing their versatility. In this sense, PRP-containing-fragmin/protamine microparticles as a delivery system for proteins in PRP have been shown to induce local arteriogenesis and angiogenesis in a rabbit model of hind limb ischemia, suggesting its possible use as treatment for PAD and CLI[32].

In the full reconstruction of ischemic limb muscles, angiogenesis and myogenesis must proceed concomitantly. Vascular endothelial progenitor cells are probably essential for muscle repair, since satellite cells, the adult stem cells of the skeletal muscle, are pre-positioned near capillaries. Thus, satellite cells can easily interplay with endothelial cells to set up co-ordinated angio-myogenesis response in a functional manner[37]. It has been shown that PRGF facilitates recruitment, activation and mobilization of myogenic progenitor cells and resident macrophages, contributing to muscle repair process, in addition to the already activated endothelial cells, macrophages, and platelets in the injured area[38]. In an animal model of severe hind limb ischemia, PRGF increases blood perfusion recovery, while improving the weight and caliber of affected myofibres. PRGF, in addition to preventing accumulation of fibrous tissue, impedes the apoptotic response of endothelial and muscle progenitor cells to hypoxia, which may explain the angiogenic and myogenic activities after ischemia[30]. These results may be explained by the fact that upon activation, satellite cells accumulate and proliferate close to capillaries, receive efficient support from endothelial cells for their growth, are pro-angiogenic, and co-localize with the new vessels during their myogenic differentiation, which strongly suggests that angiogenesis and myogenesis signal reciprocally. In addition, myogenic cells undergoing differentiation secrete VEGF[39], while endothelial cells produce a series of mitogens for myogenic cells[40]. Thus, it is likely that angiogenesis and myogenesis share growth factors and cytokines contained in PRGF as co-regulatory factors. For example, VEGF effects extend to a variety of non-endothelial cell types, including myogenic cells[41]. VEGF stimulates myogenic cell growth and their migration[42], protects them from apoptosis[41,42], up-regulates myoglobin expression and promotes formation of regenerating myofibers[41]. Similarly, bFGF, IGF1, HGF, and PDGF-BB influence muscle progenitor cells growth[40]. Furthermore, SDF-1, as in endothelial cells, recruits satellite cells from their native position to damaged areas for muscle repair[43]. Thus, harmonious increase of myofiber capillarization and caliber ensues, allowing larger myofibers to benefit from an appropriately enhanced blood supply.

3.3 Application of PRP in ischemic heart disease

As well as in ischemic peripheral diseases, the therapeutic potential of PRP has also been tested in diverse experimental models of myocardial infarction (Table 1). Similarly, the angiogeneic factors present in the PRP play a key role in rescuing the ischemic heart. Other factors like SDF-1 involved in the attraction of endogenous progenitors, or IGF-1, a potent factor that favors cell survival and induces the activation and proliferation of cardiac progenitor cells[20], greatly contribute to the regeneration of heart tissue. In that sense, the application of PRP, which releases many of these factors, exerts a beneficial effect in the ischemic heart (Figure 1). Thus, in a first study performed in 2008 by the group of Dr. Li and colleagues, thrombin-activated PRP derived from rat blood was injected in a rat model of MI induced by the permanent ligation of the descendent coronary artery. A positive effect over tissue remodeling and accelerated healing was observed four weeks post-implant. In

Animal Model	Treatment	Post-implant time analysis	Analysis	Plasma-derivatives Effect	Reference
Rat AMI	Rat Allogenic-PRP	4 weeks	Histological	Angiogenesis activation Limitation of ventricular expansion Attenuation of myocardial hypertrophy	Li et al. (2008)
Mouse AMI Mouse I/R	Human-PRP (RevaTen)	3 weeks	Functional (MR) Histological	Functional improvement (higher EF) Limitation of scar formation	Mishra et al. (2011)
Rat AMI	Autologous Rat Platelet-gel	6 weeks	Functional (Echo) Histological	Preserved cardiac function Limitation of ventricular expansion Attenuation of myocardial hypertrophy Angiogenesis activation No immune-inflammatory reactions	Cheng et al. (2012)
Rabbit I/R	Nanosecond Pulsed Rabbit-PRP	2 weeks	Hemodynamics	Improved LV function Cardioprotection	Hargrave et al. (2012)
Sheep SubAcute MI	Autologous PRGF	9 weeks	Histological	No toxicity or Immune-inflammatory reactions Angiogenesis activation	Gallo et al. (2013)
Pig AMI	Autologous PRP +/- anti-oxidant & anti-inflammatory agents +/- Hidrogel	8 weeks	Functional (Echo) Hemodynamics Histological	Functional improvement (higher EF) and Limitation of ventricular expansion Higher dp/dtmax Angiogenesis activation *Greater effects with combined treatment	Vu et al. (2014)
Rat AMI	Rat Platelet Gel + CSC	3 weeks	Functional (Echo) Histological	Functional improvement (higher EF) Limitation of ventricular expansion Angiogenesis and myogenesis activation	Cheng et al. (2012)
Rat AMI	PRF + Autologous ADSC	6 weeks	Functional (Echo) Histological / WB	Preserved LV function Attenuated LV Remodeling Angiogenesis activation	Sun et al. (2014) Chen et al. (2015)
Rabbit dilated-CM (Doxorubicin-induced)	PRP + ADSC	15 days	Functional (Echo and Electro) Histological	Impaired function and no remodeling improvement	Mosbacher et al. (2016)
Angina Class III/IV Patients	TMR + Autologous PRP	6 months	Functional (Echo)	Lower/none angina episodes Functional improvement	Wehberg et al. (2009)

TABLE 1 Summary of studies performed with platelet-rich derivatives in ischemic heart disease.
AMI: Acute Myocardial Infarction; SubAMI: Subacute Myocardial Infarction; I/R: Ischemia-Reperfusion; CM: Cardiomyopathy; TMR: Transmyocardial Rvascularization; MR: Magnetic Resonance; Echo: Echocardiography; WB: Western Blot; Electro: Electrocardiography; EF: Ejection Fraction.

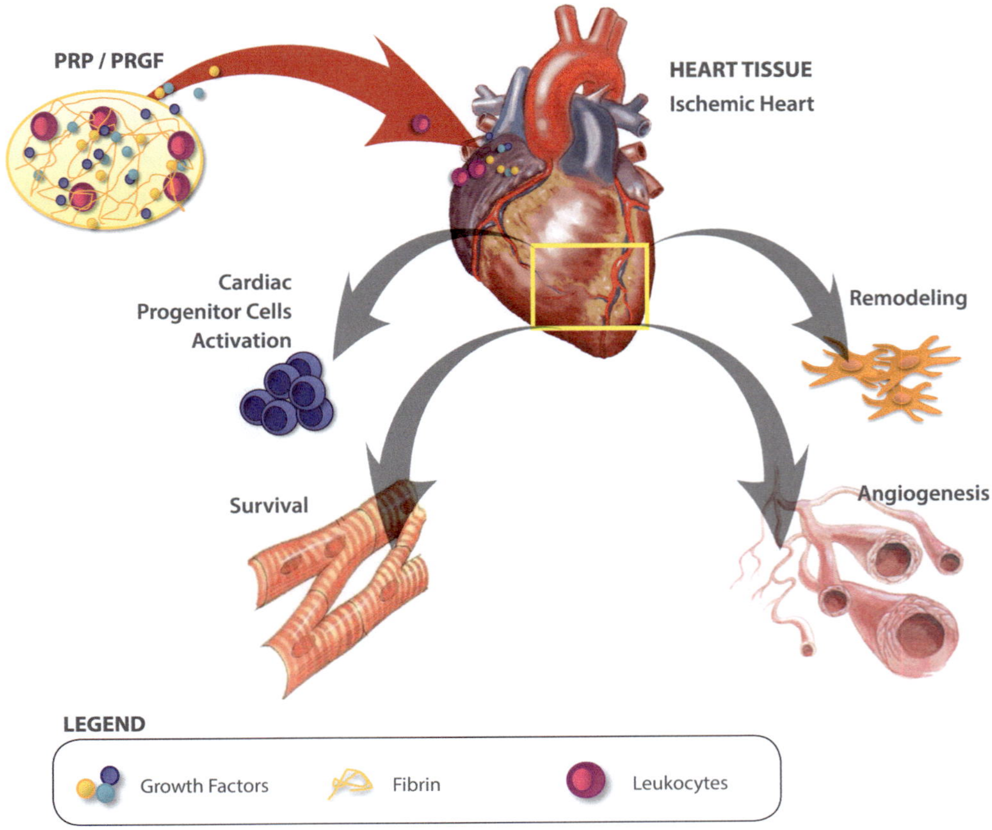

FIG. 1 Therapeutic potential of Platelet-rich plasma and growth factors in the ischemic heart.
Several mechanisms have already been described for PRP and PRGF action in ischemic diseases. The main one is by release of a cocktail of cytokines and growth factors (VEGF, PDGF, HGF or IGF among others) responsible to trigger several responses involved in anti-apoptotic signaling, cell proliferation, angiogeneic processes, fibrosis regulation or recruitment and activation of resident stem cells/progenitors able to reconstitute the damaged tissue. Also, leukocytes can immunomodulate and more robustly secrete growth factors and proteins also involved in regulating the aforementioned processes. Furthermore, fibrin content can give a robust mechanical support to the injured heart. Thus, to better know the key factors and optimal dose involved in such processes would help to improve the beneficial effect of this therapy.

more detail, the limitation of ventricular expansion, the attenuation of myocardial hypertrophy in the non-infarct region and the activation of the angiogeneic and arteriogeneic processes in the infarct area were also detected as consequence of the PRP-treatment[44]. Later on, another study was also performed in a rodent model of MI, induced either by permanent ligation or by 45 min-artery occlusion and following reperfusion[45]. Importantly, functional analyses performed by magnetic resonance were included in this study, demonstrating in both models a functional improvement 21 days after injection of human PRP (RevaTen). These functional results were later corroborated by a study performed by Chen and colleagues where an autologous platelet gel was also intra-myocardially injected in infarcted rats[46]. Deterioration in the cardiac function was evidenced in the vehicle-injected animals over the 6-week time course, while that was avoided in the platelet gel-injected animals. As in the previously described study, enhanced tissue protection together with an increment in capillary density and a lower compensatory myocyte hypertrophy were evidenced. In addition, the gel did not exacerbate inflammation in the heart whereas recruitment of endogenous cells involved in tissue regeneration was observed as a consequence of the gel injection.

Interestingly, a new way to activate the platelets based on the use of nanosecond pulsed electric fields (instead of thrombin addition) has recently been described[47,48]. This method also allows releasing growth factors stored in the platelets α-granules and has the advantages over the traditional PRP production that it can preserve the antioxidant properties of the platelets and avoid the putative adverse effects of thrombin. Moreover, an improvement in cardiac function at the mechanical and electrical level has been demonstrated in an ischemia-reperfusion model of MI in rabbit when treated with nano-pulsed PRP. The mechanisms behind these effects have been related to cardiac protection as an increase in the expression of the cardioprotective proteins Hsp27 and Hsp70, together with the stabilization of the mithocondria following diminished generation of free radicals has been demonstrated in vitro[48].

In view of the positive experimental results, the protective/regenerative potential of PRP has also been tested in two large animal models. In a first study performed in a chronic sheep model of MI, the promotion of vessel formation was histologically determined, confirming the pro-angiogenic capacity of PRP[49]. In more detail, a recent study performed in a pig preclinical infarct model, has shown the therapeutic benefit of PRP not only at the tisular but also at the functional level[50]. In this last study, infarct was induced by permanent ligation of the left circumflex coronary artery in animals randomized for intra-myocardial injection of the different treatments. Pigs received autologous PRP alone or combined with a hyaluronic acid-based hydrogel and anti-oxidant and anti-inflammatory factors, and the benefit then compared with a control group treated with saline, with the hydrogel alone or the hydrogel combined with the anti-oxidant and anti-inflammatory factors. Eight weeks after MI, a functional improvement was detected by echocardiography when treated with PRP, revealing an increase in the ejection fraction, a reduced left ventricular dilation and greater cardiac contraction. Also, an attenuated reverse remodeling and a positive impact in heart revascularization were evidenced. Interestingly, the combination of PRP with a cocktail of anti-inflammatory and anti-oxidant compounds together with a hydrogel that provided mechanical support to the heart has been shown to greatly improve heart performance. A smaller left ventricle size and better contractile function were shown with this combined treatment, demonstrating a boosting of PRP action.

Confirming all these experimental results, a clinical trial has been performed in 25 patients with refractory class III/IV angina who had no conventional revascularization options[51]. All patients underwent trans-myocardial revascularization and received PRP intra-myocardial injections or not. Interestingly, the patients that were also treated with PRP presented a lower or negligible angina score and an increase in the ejection fraction 6 months post-treatment, suggesting the clinical benefit of PRP treatment.

4. PLATELET-RICH FACTORS AND STEM CELLS FOR THE TREATMENT OF ISCHEMIC DISEASES

As well as with protein-based therapies, many efforts have been directed to develop novel therapies based on application of stem cells. As early as 1997, Asahara and colleagues isolated endothelial progenitor cells from human peripheral blood, and demonstrated that these cells retain the capacity to differentiate into mature and functional endothelial cells[52]. These findings had significant clinical implications and generated great optimism regarding offering new treatments for ischemic diseases: stem cell based approaches to promote angiogenesis and improve tissue function. However, although much progress has been made since Asahara´s findings, stem cell therapy has been slow to come to clinical use. A number of stem and progenitor cells have been examined since then for boosting angiogenesis and compensating the tissue remodeling processes within ischemic tissues, including endothelial progenitor cells, bone marrow-derived mononuclear cells, bone or adipose mechsenchymal cells and even pluripotent stem cell-derived endothelial cells. To date, more than 50 clinical studies have been reported on the treatment of PAD[53] and more than one hundred for the treatment of IHD with stem/progenitor cells[54], but with relatively limited success.

One of the main limitations of stem cell therapy is the fact that most therapeutic donor cells do not engraft and survive in the injured host tissues. The environment of ischemic tissues may have a deleterious effect on engraftment and survival of donor cells, which in turn may influence their stem cell function. Thus, making a more favorable environment in ischemic tissues by reducing the fibrotic content and the accumulation of inflammatory cells while improving the angiogenesis response of donor cells should improve the benefit of cell therapy for ischemic tissues. Therefore, a number of groups have developed approaches to enhance donor cell survival and function, along with paracrine factor delivery. In this sense, if the paracrine effects of growth factors can improve stem cell therapy, co-administering platelet-derived products could be of great relevance in this type of approach.

Few studies have been performed combining the platelet-derivatives with several populations of stem cells in order to boost the benefit of both treatments, but those that do exist hold considerable interest (Table 1). In 2012, the group of Dr. Marban, a well known expert in the isolation and characterization of cardiac derived stem cells, in particular a population named cardiosphere-derived cells (CDC), tested their potential in a rat model of acute MI when transplanted in a platelet-gel[46]. This study clearly showed the benefit of using transplanted cells pre-seeded in a platelet gel. A functional improvement three weeks post-implant was indeed observed in the animals implanted with the cellularized gel in comparison with the platelet gel alone. Also, greater recruitment of endogenous cells and the induction of neo-angiogenesis together with a positive impact on tissue remodeling were shown after treatment, in comparison with the control and only-gel implanted animals. This in vivo effect was explained by the fact that the cellularized-gel released a greater dose of "regenerative" cytokines, such as VEGF, IGF-1 and SDF-1, than the gel alone. Furthermore, although the contribution of CSC to heart tissue had been previously shown, the mechanism of action for tissue repair was mainly attributed to their trophic effect rather than to the exogenous cells' contribution through their own differentiation towards cardiovascular cells. On the other hand, a group implanted only with CDC was not included in this study and even though the benefit of the combined therapy was clearly demonstrated, it is not possible to evaluate the real impact the gel exerts over the transplanted cells in order to elucidate whether its addition significantly increases the benefit of the cells alone. In fact, the therapeutic benefit of the CDC has been experimentally (reviewed in[55]) and clinically demonstrated, as a Phase I/II clinical trial (CADUCEUS trial) was performed in patients with myocardial infraction[46]. Even though positive results are expected, it would be interesting to be able to quantify the real impact of combining the cells with the gel.

Also, the group of Dr. Yip, in two different studies, used a rat acute model of MI to test the potential of Platelet-rich fibrin (PRF)[29] combined with autologous ADSC. In both studies, 1 million cells were embedded in the platelet gel (also derived from the rat blood) and implanted in the heart one hour after MI induction. Other groups of animals were implanted only with ADSC[56] or only with PRF[57]. Six weeks after treatment, an improvement in cardiac function together with a reduction in ventricular remodeling and an induction of angiogenesis was detected in the animals implanted with the combined treatment when compared with a non-treated group. A superior effect was also detected when compared either with the PRF alone or the ADSC alone. Thus the known therapeutic effect of ADSC[58,59] was significantly boosted by the combination with PRF, probably due to greater engraftment and retention of the cells when implanted with the fibrin patch. Indeed, the advantage of transplanting cells with a matrix or scaffold has already been shown and explained as a consequence of their increased retention and the induction of adhesion-related survival pathways that increase their permanence in the tissue[60]. Moreover, the growth factors released by the PRF could exert a pro-survival effect (among other benefits) not only in the heart tissue but also in the implanted ADSC, heightening their beneficial effect even further.

Finally, a very recent manuscript has been published in which PRP combined with ADSC has been tested for the treatment of dilated cardiomyopathy. In this case, a rabbit model induced by doxorubicin was used. Surprisingly, a benefit was only observed after cell treatment alone, but not with the combination with PRP or PRP alone, when in fact, the disease was found to worsen. Functional examination was performed only 15 days post-infarct, so longer-term functional analyses to understand the impact of the treatment are missing. More detailed studies using this model would be of great interest in order to clarify the mechanisms behind these results[61].

5. CONCLUDING REMARKS AND FUTURE PERSPECTIVES

The therapeutic benefit of PRP/PRGF has already been demonstrated in several animal models of hind limb ischemia and myocardial infarction. The pro-angiogenic, pro-myogenic, immunomodulatory and anti-fibrotic effect induced by the released growth factors and the platelets/leukocyte action together with the mechanical support exerted by the fibrin matrix, justifies its therapeutic action in the ischemic tissues. Elucidation of the optimal platelet-rich formulation, dosage and delivery route for each disease will improve the potential benefits.

Moreover, safety is another advantage of this treatment. Low or negligible morbidity is associated with patient blood extraction for PRP/PRGF isolation and the autologous origin of the product avoids the viral risks of xenogeneic or allogenic products, antibody formation and risk of graft-versus-host disease[62]. Furthermore, the quick, easy protocol for preparing these products makes them a potentially cost-effective alternative compared to other novel therapies[63,64].

Finally, in view of the demonstrated benefit of PRP not only in experimental animal models but also in angina patients, and the potential of various stem cell populations like ADSC and CSC in infarcted patients, it would be of great interest to determine the therapeutic effect of PRP/PRGF in combination with stem cells and/or biomaterials, in these patients and in those suffering PAD diseases.

In conclusion, the striking functional benefits, together with the simplicity of manufacture and the autologous origin of PRP, make it an excellent candidate for the treatment of ischemic pathologies at the clinical level. Furthermore, since the actions of stem cells delivered in ischemic tissues are boosted when these are combined with PRP/PRGF, this approach opens up new therapeutic avenues for synergic treatment. In the future, the effect of such treatments is likely to be enhanced still further by fruitful combinations with bioengineering strategies.

1. Benjamin EJ, Blaha MJ, Chiuve SE, et al. Heart Disease and Stroke Statistics-2017 Update: A Report From the American Heart Association. Circulation. 2017;135:e146-e603.

2. Sigvant B, Lundin F, Wahlberg E. The Risk of Disease Progression in Peripheral Arterial Disease is Higher than Expected: A Meta-Analysis of Mortality and Disease Progression in Peripheral Arterial Disease. European journal of vascular and endovascular surgery : the official journal of the European Society for Vascular Surgery. 2016;51:395-403.

3. Tendera M, Aboyans V, Bartelink ML, et al. ESC Guidelines on the diagnosis and treatment of peripheral artery diseases: Document covering atherosclerotic disease of extracranial carotid and vertebral, mesenteric, renal, upper and lower extremity arteries: the Task Force on the Diagnosis and Treatment of Peripheral Artery Diseases of the European Society of Cardiology (ESC). European heart journal. 2011;32:2851-906.

4. Hiatt WR. Medical Treatment of Peripheral Arterial Disease and Claudication. New England Journal of Medicine. 2001;344:1608-21.

5. Sanchis-Gomar F, Perez-Quilis C, Leischik R, Lucia A. Epidemiology of coronary heart disease and acute coronary syndrome. Annals of translational medicine. 2016;4:256.

6. Thygesen K, Alpert JS, Jaffe AS, Simoons ML, Chaitman BR, White HD. Third universal definition of myocardial infarction. Global heart. 2012;7:275-95.

7. Rhim T, Lee M. Targeted delivery of growth factors in ischemic stroke animal models. Expert Opin Drug Deliv. 2016;13:709-23.

8. Sanganalmath SK, Bolli R. Cell therapy for heart failure: a comprehensive overview of experimental and clinical studies, current challenges, and future directions. Circulation research. 2013;113:810-34.

9. van Royen N, Piek JJ, Buschmann I, Hoefer I, Voskuil M, Schaper W. Stimulation of arteriogenesis; a new concept for the treatment of arterial occlusive disease. Cardiovascular research. 2001;49:543-53.

10. Folkman J, Merler E, Abernathy C, Williams G. Isolation of a tumor factor responsible for angiogenesis. The Journal of experimental medicine. 1971;133:275-88.

11. Conway EM, Collen D, Carmeliet P. Molecular mechanisms of blood vessel growth. Cardiovascular research. 2001;49:507-21.

12. Ferrara N, Gerber HP. The role of vascular endothelial growth factor in angiogenesis. Acta haematologica. 2001;106:148-56.

13. Cao R, Brakenhielm E, Pawliuk R, et al. Angiogenic synergism, vascular stability and improvement of hind-limb ischemia by a combination of PDGF-BB and FGF-2. Nature medicine. 2003;9:604-13.

14. Lindahl P, Johansson BR, Leveen P, Betsholtz C. Pericyte loss and microaneurysm formation in PDGF-B-deficient mice. Science. 1997;277:242-5.

15. Marui A, Kanematsu A, Yamahara K, et al. Simultaneous application of basic fibroblast growth factor and hepatocyte growth factor to enhance the blood vessels formation. Journal of vascular surgery. 2005;41:82-90.

16. Asahara T, Bauters C, Zheng LP, et al. Synergistic effect of vascular endothelial growth factor and basic fibroblast growth factor on angiogenesis in vivo. Circulation. 1995;92:Ii365-71.

17. Gallo S, Sala V, Gatti S, Crepaldi T. Cellular and molecular mechanisms of HGF/Met in the cardiovascular system. Clin Sci (Lond). 2015;129:1173-93.

18. Stellos K, Langer H, Daub K, et al. Platelet-derived stromal cell-derived factor-1 regulates adhesion and promotes differentiation of human CD34+ cells to endothelial progenitor cells. Circulation. 2008;117:206-15.

19. Haider H, Jiang S, Idris NM, Ashraf M. IGF-1-overexpressing mesenchymal stem cells accelerate bone marrow stem cell mobilization via paracrine activation of SDF-1alpha/CXCR4 signaling to promote myocardial repair. Circulation research. 2008;103:1300-8.

20. Suleiman MS, Singh RJ, Stewart CE. Apoptosis and the cardiac action of insulin-like growth factor I. Pharmacology & therapeutics. 2007;114:278-94.

21. Formiga FR, Tamayo E, Simon-Yarza T, Pelacho B, Prosper F, Blanco-Prieto MJ. Angiogenic therapy for cardiac repair based on protein delivery systems. Heart failure reviews. 2012;17:449-73.

22. Ungerleider JL, Christman KL. Concise review: injectable biomaterials for the treatment of myocardial infarction and peripheral artery disease: translational challenges and progress. Stem cells translational medicine. 2014;3:1090-9.

23. Helisch A, Schaper W. Arteriogenesis: the development and growth of collateral arteries. Microcirculation. 2003;10:83-97.

24. Anitua E, Andia I, Ardanza B, Nurden P, Nurden AT. Autologous platelets as a source of proteins for healing and tissue regeneration. Thrombosis and haemostasis. 2004;91:4-15.

25. Feng W, Madajka M, Kerr BA, Mahabeleshwar GH, Whiteheart SW, Byzova TV. A novel role for platelet secretion in angiogenesis: mediating bone marrow-derived cell mobilization and homing. Blood. 2011;117:3893-902.

26. Anitua E, Sanchez M, Nurden AT, Nurden P, Orive G, Andia I. New insights into and novel applications for platelet-rich fibrin therapies. Trends in biotechnology. 2006;24:227-34.

27. Inchingolo F, Tatullo M, Marrelli M, et al. Regenerative surgery performed with platelet-rich plasma used in sinus lift elevation before dental implant surgery: an useful aid in healing and regeneration of bone tissue. European review for medical and pharmacological sciences. 2012;16:1222-6.

28. Davis RL, Weintraub H, Lassar AB. Expression of a single transfected cDNA converts fibroblasts to myoblasts. Cell. 1987;51:987-1000.

29. Giannini S, Cielo A, Bonanome L, et al. Comparison between PRP, PRGF and PRF: lights and shadows in three similar but different protocols. European review for medical and pharmacological sciences. 2015;19:927-30.

30. Anitua E, Pelacho B, Prado R, et al. Infiltration of plasma rich in growth factors enhances in vivo angiogenesis and improves reperfusion and tissue remodeling after severe hind limb ischemia. Journal of Controlled Release. 2015;202:31-39.

31. Bir SC, Esaki J, Marui A, et al. Angiogenic properties of sustained release platelet-rich plasma: characterization in-vitro and in the ischemic hind limb of the mouse. Journal of vascular surgery. 2009;50:870-79.e2.

32. Fujita M, Horio T, Kishimoto S, et al. Effects of platelet-rich plasma-containing fragmin/protamine microparticles in enhancing endothelial and smooth muscle cell growth and inducing collateral vessels in a rabbit model of hindlimb ischemia. Journal of biomedical materials research. Part B, Applied biomaterials. 2013;101:36-42.

33. Martino MM, Briquez PS, Ranga A, Lutolf MP, Hubbell JA. Heparin-binding domain of fibrin(ogen) binds growth factors and promotes tissue repair when incorporated within a synthetic matrix. Proceedings of the National Academy of Sciences of the United States of America. 2013;110:4563-8.

34. Yotsu RR, Hagiwara S, Okochi H, Tamaki T. Case series of patients with chronic foot ulcers treated with autologous platelet-rich plasma. The Journal of dermatology. 2015;42:288-95.

35. Massara M, Barilla D, De Caridi G, et al. Application of autologous platelet-rich plasma to enhance wound healing after lower limb revascularization: A case series and literature review. Seminars in vascular surgery. 2015;28:195-200.

36. Bielecki TM, Gazdzik TS, Arendt J, Szczepanski T, Krol W, Wielkoszynski T. Antibacterial effect of autologous platelet gel enriched with growth factors and other active substances: an in vitro study. The Journal of bone and joint surgery. 2007;89:417-20.

37. Christov C, Chretien F, Abou-Khalil R, et al. Muscle satellite cells and endothelial cells: close neighbors and privileged partners. Molecular biology of the cell. 2007;18:1397-409.

38. Chazaud B, Brigitte M, Yacoub-Youssef H, et al. Dual and beneficial roles of macrophages during skeletal muscle regeneration. Exercise and sport sciences reviews. 2009;37:18-22.

39. Chazaud B, Sonnet C, Lafuste P, et al. Satellite cells attract monocytes and use macrophages as a support to escape apoptosis and enhance muscle growth. The Journal of cell biology. 2003;163:1133-43.

40. Hawke TJ, Garry DJ. Myogenic satellite cells: physiology to molecular biology. J Appl Physiol (1985). 2001;91:534-51.

41. Arsic N, Zacchigna S, Zentilin L, et al. Vascular endothelial growth factor stimulates skeletal muscle regeneration in vivo. Molecular therapy : the journal of the American Society of Gene Therapy. 2004;10:844-54.

42. Germani A, Di Carlo A, Mangoni A, et al. Vascular endothelial growth factor modulates skeletal myoblast function. The American journal of pathology. 2003;163:1417-28.

43. Bobadilla M, Sainz N, Abizanda G, et al. The CXCR4/SDF1 axis improves muscle regeneration through MMP-10 activity. Stem cells and development. 2014;23:1417-27.

44. Li XH, Zhou X, Zeng S, et al. Effects of intramyocardial injection of platelet-rich plasma on the healing process after myocardial infarction. Coronary artery disease. 2008;19:363-70.

45. Mishra A, Velotta J, Brinton TJ, et al. RevaTen platelet-rich plasma improves cardiac function after myocardial injury. Cardiovascular revascularization medicine : including molecular interventions. 2011;12:158-63.

46. Cheng K, Malliaras K, Shen D, et al. Intramyocardial injection of platelet gel promotes endogenous repair and augments cardiac function in rats with myocardial infarction. Journal of the American College of Cardiology. 2012;59:256-64.

47. Hargrave B, Li F. Nanosecond pulse electric field activation of platelet-rich plasma reduces myocardial infarct size and improves left ventricular mechanical function in the rabbit heart. The journal of extra-corporeal technology. 2012;44:198-204.

48. Hargrave B, Varghese F, Barabutis N, Catravas J, Zemlin C. Nanosecond pulsed platelet-rich plasma (nsPRP) improves mechanical and electrical cardiac function following myocardial reperfusion injury. Physiological reports. 2016;4.

49. Gallo I, Saenz A, Arevalo A, et al. [Effect of autologous platelet-rich plasma on heart infarction in sheep]. Archivos de cardiologia de Mexico. 2013;83:154-8.

50. Vu TD, Pal SN, Ti LK, et al. An autologous platelet-rich plasma hydrogel compound restores left ventricular structure, function and ameliorates adverse remodeling in a minimally invasive large animal myocardial restoration model: a translational approach: Vu and Pal "Myocardial Repair: PRP, Hydrogel and Supplements". Biomaterials. 2015;45:27-35.

51. Wehberg KE, Answini G, Wood D, et al. Intramyocardial injection of autologous platelet-rich plasma combined with transmyocardial revascularization. Cell transplantation. 2009;18:353-9.

52. Asahara T, Murohara T, Sullivan A, et al. Isolation of putative progenitor endothelial cells for angiogenesis. Science. 1997;275:964-7.

53. Rigato M, Monami M, Fadini GP. Autologous Cell Therapy for Peripheral Arterial Disease: Systematic Review and Meta-Analysis of Randomized, Non-Randomized, and Non-Controlled Studies. Circulation research. 2017.

54. Lerman DA, Alotti N, Ume KL, Peault B. Cardiac Repair and Regeneration: The Value of Cell Therapies. European cardiology. 2016;11:43-48.

55. Marban E, Cingolani E. Heart to heart: cardiospheres for myocardial regeneration. Heart rhythm. 2012;9:1727-31.

56. Sun CK, Zhen YY, Leu S, et al. Direct implantation versus platelet-rich fibrin-embedded adipose-derived mesenchymal stem cells in treating rat acute myocardial infarction. International journal of cardiology. 2014;173:410-23.

57. Chen YL, Sun CK, Tsai TH, et al. Adipose-derived mesenchymal stem cells embedded in platelet-rich fibrin scaffolds promote angiogenesis, preserve heart function, and reduce left ventricular remodeling in rat acute myocardial infarction. American journal of translational research. 2015;7:781-803.

58. Mazo M, Planat-Benard V, Abizanda G, et al. Transplantation of adipose derived stromal cells is associated with functional improvement in a rat model of chronic myocardial infarction. European journal of heart failure. 2008;10:454-62.

59. Mazo M, Hernandez S, Gavira JJ, et al. Treatment of reperfused ischemia with adipose-derived stem cells in a preclinical Swine model of myocardial infarction. Cell transplantation. 2012;21:2723-33.

60. Arana M, Gavira JJ, Pena E, et al. Epicardial delivery of collagen patches with adipose-derived stem cells in rat and minipig models of chronic myocardial infarction. Biomaterials. 2014;35:143-51.

61. Morschbacher PD, Alves Garcez TN, Paz AH, et al. Treatment of dilated cardiomyopathy in rabbits with mesenchymal stem cell transplantation and platelet-rich plasma. Veterinary journal. 2016;209:180-5.

62. Lacci KM, Dardik A. Platelet-rich plasma: support for its use in wound healing. The Yale journal of biology and medicine. 2010;83:1-9.

63. Mehrannia M, Vaezi M, Yousefshahi F, Rouhipour N. Platelet rich plasma for treatment of nonhealing diabetic foot ulcers: a case report. Canadian journal of diabetes. 2014;38:5-8.

64. Park KY, Kim IS, Yeo IK, Kim BJ, Kim MN. Treatment of refractory venous stasis ulcers with autologous platelet-rich plasma and light-emitting diodes: a pilot study. The Journal of dermatological treatment. 2013;24:332-5.

CHAPTER 6

Endoret® (PRGF®) Application in the Oral and Maxillofacial Field

AUTHORS

Anitua E. [1,2,3,4], Piñas L.[3,4], Alkhraisat H. M. [1,2,4]

[1] Eduardo Anitua Foundation for Biomedical Research. Vitoria-Gasteiz, Spain
[2] BTI-Biothecnology Institute. Vitoria-Gasteiz, Spain
[3] Private practice in oral implantology. Vitoria-Gasteiz, Spain
[4] University Institute for Regenerative Medicine and Oral Implantology (UIRMI) from the University of Basque Country (UPV/EHU)

SUMMARY

In 1995 the first intraosseous application of Endoret (PRGF) was reported in the regeneration of infected bone and soft tissue defect after tooth extraction. It is in the oral and maxillofacial surgery where the clinical use of Endoret (PRGF) was initiated and where its therapeutic formulations was designed. The oral and maxillofacial surgery (non-steril surgical field) also allows for the design of a split-mouth clinical trial. The safety, efficacy and predictability of this biological preparation trigged then its use in various medical fields including the orthopedics and sport medicine. In this chapter, we present a comprehensive review of the use of Endoret (PRGF) in oral and maxillofacial surgery. This review is evidence-based and provides guidelines for the use of the different therapeutic formulations of Endoret (PRGF). It will serve as a bridge of cross-talking between oral surgeons and orthopedic surgeons with the aim of approximating views and developing new ways of applying the various formulations in Endoret technology. In all its applications in oral and maxillofacial surgery, Endoret (PRGF) has improved the patient's quality of life, the healing of soft tissue and the regeneration of hard tissue. The preservation and handling of a grafting material has all improved once mixed with Endoret (PRGF).

E. Anitua et al. (eds.), *Platelet Rich Plasma in Orthopaedics and Sports Medicine*,
https://doi.org/10.1007/978-3-319-63730-3_6

1. INTRODUCTION

The development of Endoret (PRGF) technology started by the meticulous study of platelets and the optimal conditions under which they can be concentrated and maintain their properties unaltered. As a consequence, a simple, dynamic and versatile protocol has been developed that enables the clinician to obtain formulations of great therapeutic potential. Some of the properties that are peculiar to Endoret (PRGF) are:

- Endoret (PRGF) is autologous and biocompatible.

- It is more precise to speak of Endoret (PRGF) technology, as it is not a unique preparation, but rather a set of formulations with a therapeutic action, easily obtained from the patient's own blood. The formulations that constitute Endoret (PRGF) technology are:

- Endoret (PRGF) supernatant: this is an excellent culture medium to maintain primary cells and autologous bone. It contains platelet- and plasma-derived proteins and factors (fig. 1a).

- Activated liquid Endoret (PRGF): The activation of Endoret (PRGF) using calcium chloride as an activator starts the release of contents of the platelets, giving rise to a liquid formulation rich in proteins and growth factors. This formulation is used to inject Endoret (PRGF) in tissues such as muscle, tendon, skin and joints. It also used to biofunctionalize implant surface (fig. 1b).

- Endoret (PRGF) clot: In 3-5 minutes, the activated liquid Endoret (PRGF) becomes a three dimensional matrix of fibrin rich in cellular components and growth factors. This formulation can be used in various applications, from the regeneration of extraction socket to the treatment of muscular, skeletal or vascular pathologies. (fig. 1c)

- Fibrin membrane: The retraction of the clot obtained by the activation of fraction 1 (F1) of Endoret (PRGF) results in a dense and elastic membrane. This fibrin membrane is biocompatible and is used as a biological membrane. (fig. 1d)

This chapter gives an overall view of Endoret (PRGF) applications in oral surgery. Oral surgery has been used as an experimental model where different aspects of wound healing with Endoret (PRGF) have been assessed. Many randomized clinical trials, some of them split-mouth designed, have been performed and published.

2. USE OF ENDORET® (PRGF®) IN THE TREATMENT OF EXTRACTION SOCKET

Extraction socket is the defect that remains in the alveolar ridge after tooth extraction. Endoret (PRGF) and autologous fibrin are optimal biomaterials for the treatment of extraction socket. They are autologous, easy to prepare, completely re-absorbable, and cost-effective. The biological technique of Endoret (PRGF) has no side effects or harmful consequences. All these characteristics are the basis on which Endoret (PRGF) is recommended even for the treatment of dry socket (inflammation of the extraction socket), the most common complication after tooth extraction. Various studies have reported that the use of platelet concentrates have been effective in reducing the occurrence of dry socket[1,2].

The protocol for the management of tooth extraction with Endoret (PRGF) include several important aspects[3,4]. Atraumatic tooth extraction minimizes trauma to the surrounding bone and gingival tissue. The socket is filled with a clot prepared from the fraction 2 (F2) of the Endoret (PRGF). Then, the fibrin membrane, prepared from the fraction 1 (F1) of the Endoret (PRGF), is placed to cover the socket. A suture is finally applied to retain the clot and membrane in the socket.

The outcomes of applying this protocol are less pain and inflammation after tooth extraction[4]. This has contributed to accelerate healing and regeneration of the extraction socket[4]. Figure 2 shows an example of an extraction socket that has been treated with Endoret (PRGF). Here we can observe the absence of inflammation, Endoret (PRGF) remodeling and the closure of the defect with a new keratinized mucosa.

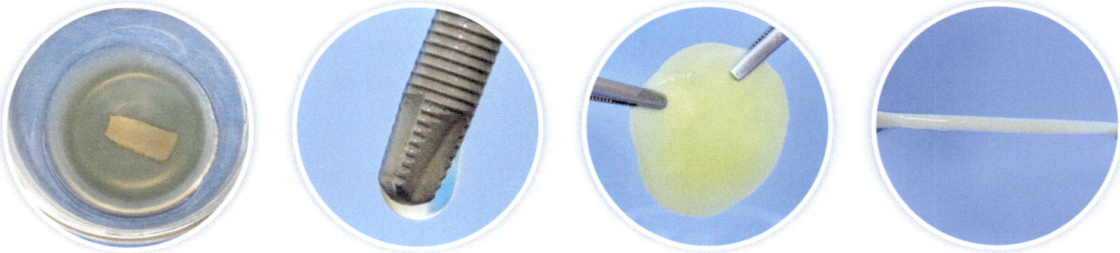

FIG. 1
Therapeutic formulations of Endoret (PRGF).

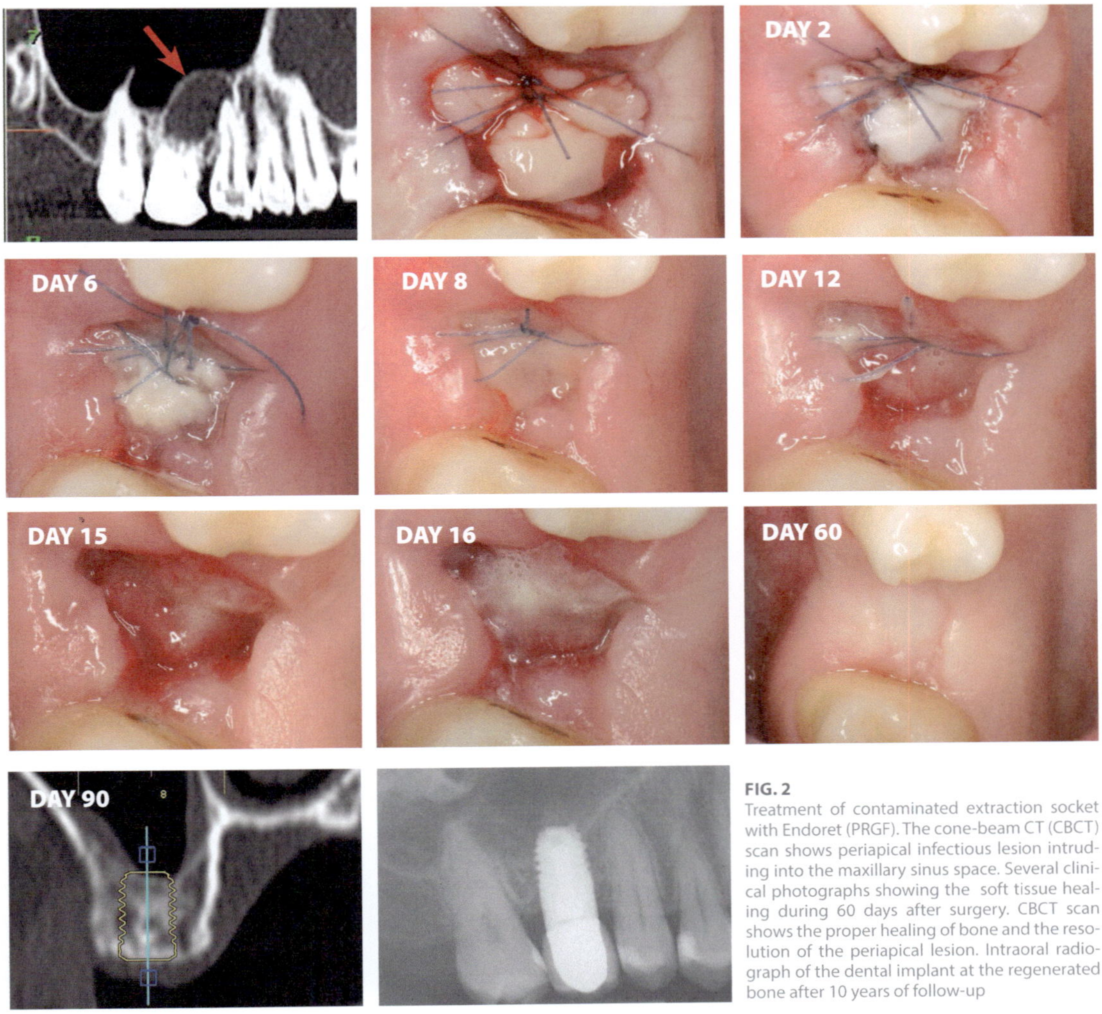

FIG. 2
Treatment of contaminated extraction socket with Endoret (PRGF). The cone-beam CT (CBCT) scan shows periapical infectious lesion intruding into the maxillary sinus space. Several clinical photographs showing the soft tissue healing during 60 days after surgery. CBCT scan shows the proper healing of bone and the resolution of the periapical lesion. Intraoral radiograph of the dental implant at the regenerated bone after 10 years of follow-up

Therapeutic potential of Endoret (PRGF) in the treatment of extraction socket: Experimental studies in animals

In 2000, we performed animal studies to investigate the regenerative potential of Endoret (PRGF)[4,5]. The experimental animal model was bone defect 5 mm in diameter produced in the tibia of goats. These defects were filled with Endoret (PRGF) in the experimental group and blood clot in the control group. After 8 weeks, bone samples were harvested and prepared for histological and histomorphometric analysis.

The defects treated with Endoret (PRGF) showed the presence of newly formed trabecular bone that was surrounded by a dense and highly vascularised connective tissue. The control defects were filled by a connective tissue with high cellularity and some small area of new bone formation (fig. 3).

Therapeutic potential of Endoret (PRGF) in the management of extraction socket: Preparation of future sites for dental implant and the first randomized controlled clinical study of a PRP in extraction socket

The first clinical study on the potential of Endoret (PRGF) to regenerate extraction socket for the future insertion of dental implants was reported in 1997, and published in 1999[4]. In that study, 20 patients in need of tooth extraction were recruited and randomized to receive Endoret (PRGF) or blood clot. The soft tissue healing of the defect was evaluated at day 3, day 7 and day 15 after tooth extraction. A dental implant was inserted at the site of extraction site after 10-16 weeks of tooth extraction. Before implant site preparation, a 6 mm long bone biopsy was obtained from the centre of the socket with a trephine bur.

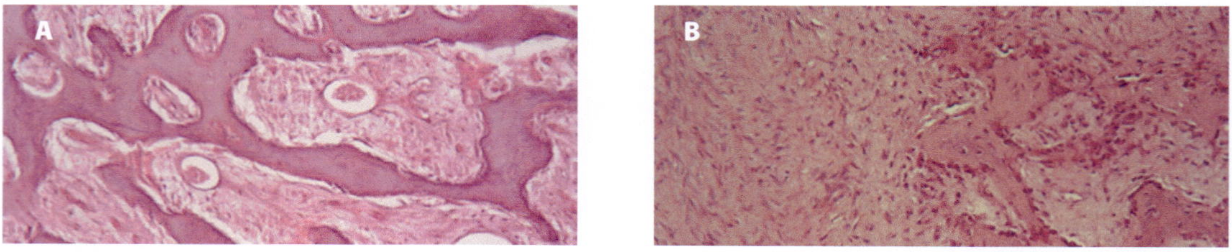

FIG. 3
The histological images of bone biopsy obtained from: A) The socket treated with Endoret (PRGF). B) The socket treated with blood clot.

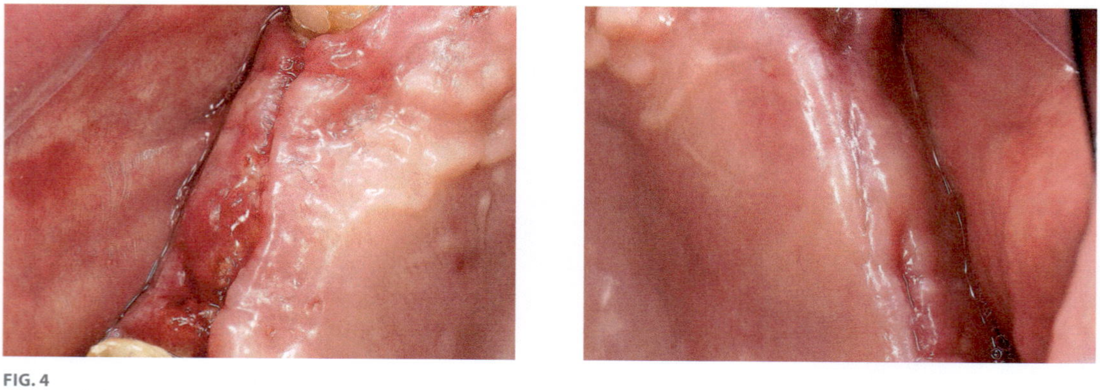

FIG. 4
Split-mouth design adopted to study the potential of Endoret (PRGF) in the treatment of extraction socket. Endoret (PRGF) was applied on the left side and the right side served as control. We can observe the differences in soft tissue healing between both groups after 14 days of surgery.

The soft tissue healing was excellent in the 10 patients treated with Endoret (PRGF). Three patients underwent bilateral tooth extractions, and thus a split-mouth study design was possible. This design permitted the comparison of the two treatments under the same biological conditions. Figure 4 shows the difference in soft tissue healing in the same patient who received Endoret (PRGF) on one side, and blood clot on the other side.

The histological analysis of the bone samples showed a difference in the degree of trabecular organization. More bone regeneration and better trabecular organization were observed at the sites treated with Endoret (PRGF) (fig. 5).

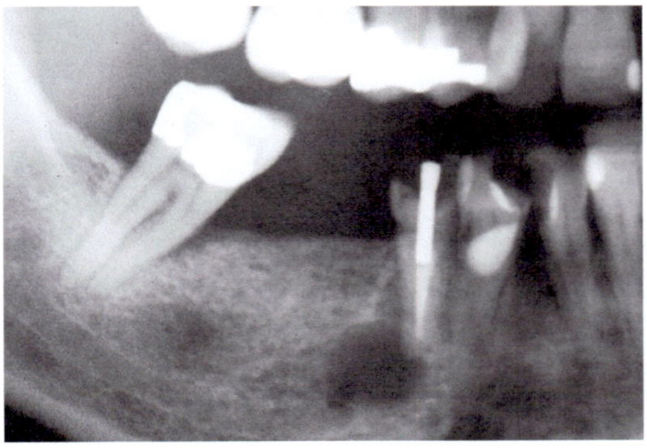

FIG. 5a
Radiographic image showing vertical fracture of the lower right first molar and the presence of periapical granuloma.

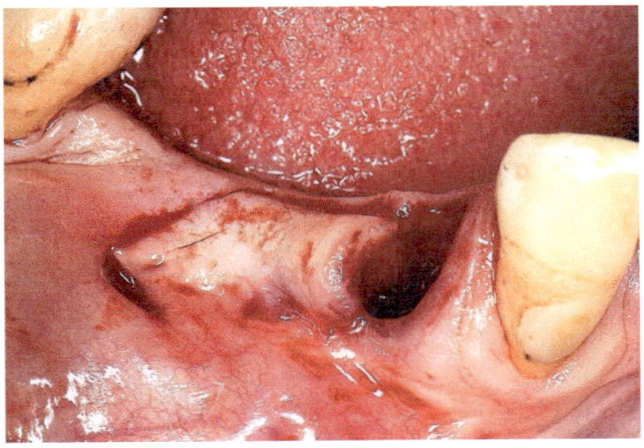

FIG. 5b
After flap elevation, atraumtic tooth extraction was performed and the socket was treated with Endoret (PRGF).

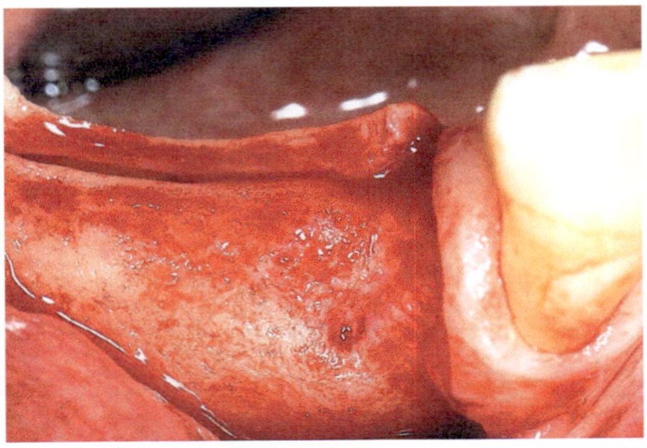

FIG. 5c
The Endoret (PRGF) stimulation of bone regeneration permitted the insertion of dental implant after 14 weeks of tooth extraction.

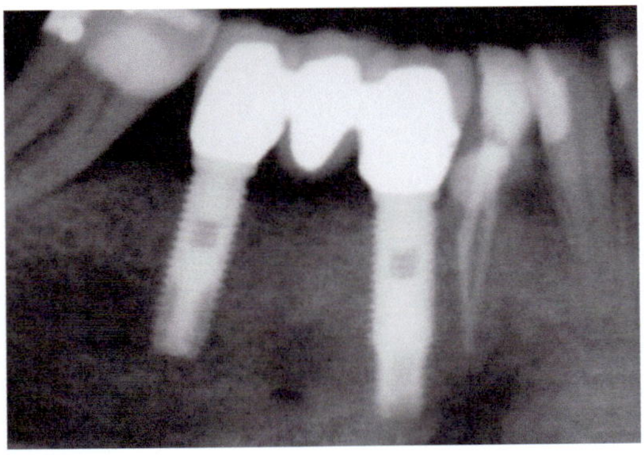

FIG. 5d
The clinical status of the dental implant after 4 years of insertion.

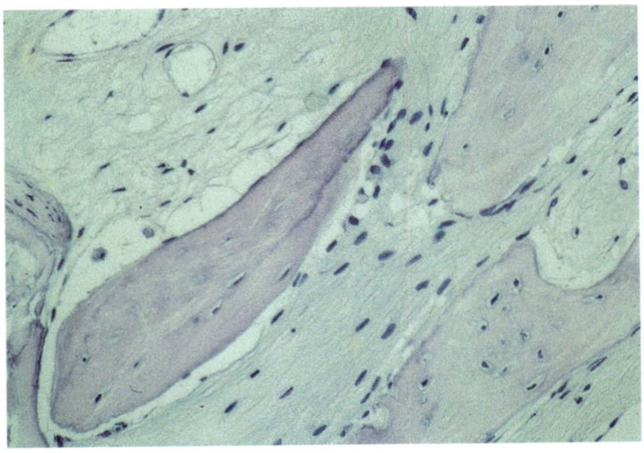

FIG. 5e
The histological analysis of bone biopsy obtained 14 weeks post-operatively. New formation of bone trabeculae with osteocytes was observed.

Therapeutic potential of Endoret® (PRGF®) in the treatment of extraction socket: Split-mouth clinical study to evaluate bone regeneration

In 2010, a split-mouth clinical study was performed to evaluate bone regeneration in the extraction socket treated with Endoret (PRGF)[6]. The study was performed in 14 patients and blood clot served as the control treatment.

A cone-beam CT (CBCT) scan was obtained for each patient at 11-14 weeks postoperatively. These scans were later analyzed to retrieve data about the volume of regenerated bone as well as the bone density expressed in Hounsfield units. To measure the density, a cylinder resembling an implant was placed inside the defect. The visualizing software (BTI scan) gave two measurements of the density, one for the area located within the cylinder, and the second for area outside the limit of the cylinder.

The values of both densities and the one measured at the centre of the defect were all statistically higher in the Endoret (PRGF) group (fig. 6). Figure 7 shows a clinical case where complete soft tissue healing and bone regeneration were obtained in a patient in whom Endoret (PRGF) had been used.

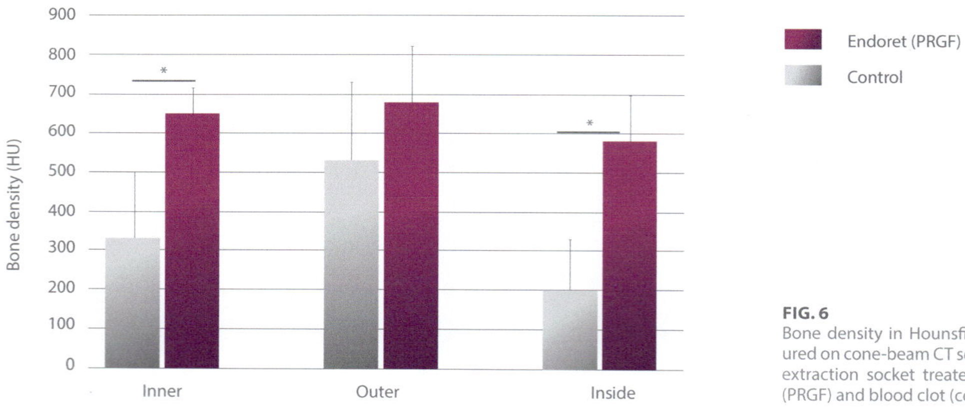

FIG. 6
Bone density in Hounsfield units measured on cone-beam CT scan obtained for extraction socket treated with Endoret (PRGF) and blood clot (control).

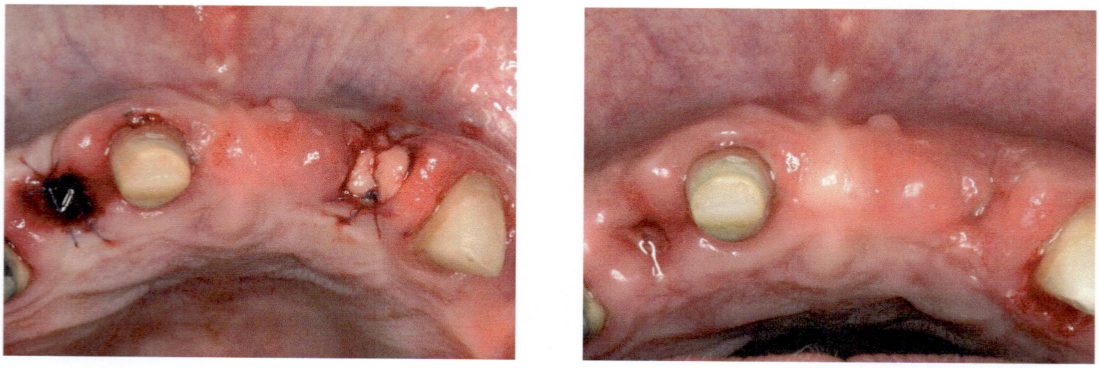

FIG. 7
The status of the extraction socket after application of the assigned treatment (Endoret (PRGF) or blood clot). A significant differences in soft tissue healing could be observed after 5 days of tooth extraction between both groups.

Therapeutic potential of Endoret (PRGF) in the treatment of extraction socket: assessor-blinded, parallel group, randomized controlled clinical trial

A single center, assessor-blinded, parallel group, randomized controlled clinical trial was conducted. Sixty patients with a simple one molar extraction in the mandible were randomized to receive Endoret (PRGF) or blood clot[7]. Thirty six patients were treated with Endoret (PRGF) and 24 with blood clot. A cross-stitch suture was placed in both groups. Clinical, radiographical and histological assessments were performed during 10-12 weeks of follow-up. The primary outcome was the percentage of patients having their sockets regenerated by ≥ 75% (from baseline to week 10-12). For measuring the primary outcome, CBCT scans at baseline and after 10-12 weeks of healing were imported into a software (BTI Scan II, BTI Biotechnology institute, Vitoria, Spain) and analyzed. The secondary variables were bone density, soft tissue healing index, thickness of regenerated keratinized mucosa, pain and inflammation. Additionally, histological analyses were performed for soft and hard tissue biopsies obtained before dental implant insertion.

After tooth extraction, the socket was examined for the presence/absence of bone septum. About 54% of the extraction sockets in the control group preserved the boney septum, while 39% of the experimental groups had the septum. The comparison of the extraction sockets showed that sockets in the experimental group had higher initial volume than in the control group (fig. 8).

Cone beam CT analysis has shown that the percentage of patients where the sockets are regenerated at ≥ 75% of the baseline volume was significantly higher in the Endoret (PRGF) group (96.7%) than the control group (45.5%) (fig. 9).

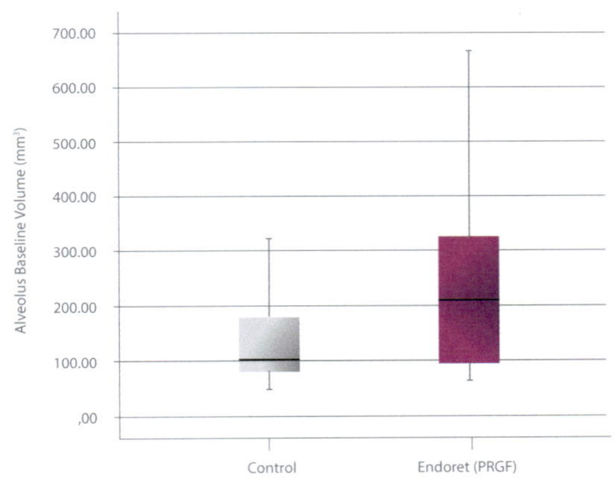

FIG. 8
Comparison of the volume of extraction socket between the Endoret (PRGF) group and blood clot group.

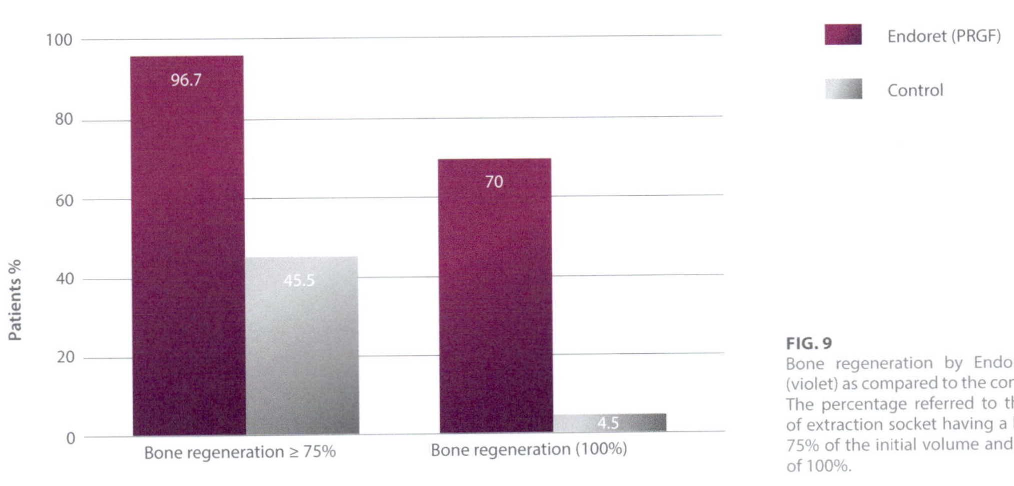

FIG. 9
Bone regeneration by Endoret (PRGF) (violet) as compared to the control (grey). The percentage referred to the fraction of extraction socket having a bone fill of 75% of the initial volume and a bone fill of 100%.

Histological analysis indicated the presence of significantly higher newly formed bone in the Endoret (PRGF) group (63.08% Vs. 35.56%) (fig. 10). No serious adverse events occurred in either group. Bone density was significantly higher in the Endoret (PRGF) group (450 HU Vs. 318 HU) (fig. 11).

Pain and inflammation (day 3 and day 7) were significantly lower in the PRGF group than the control group, but not at day 15 (figs. 12 and 13). Soft tissue healing scores were significantly higher in the test group at days 3, 7 and 15. Figure 14 showed the difference in tissue healing between the sockets treated with Endoret (PRGF) and blood clot.

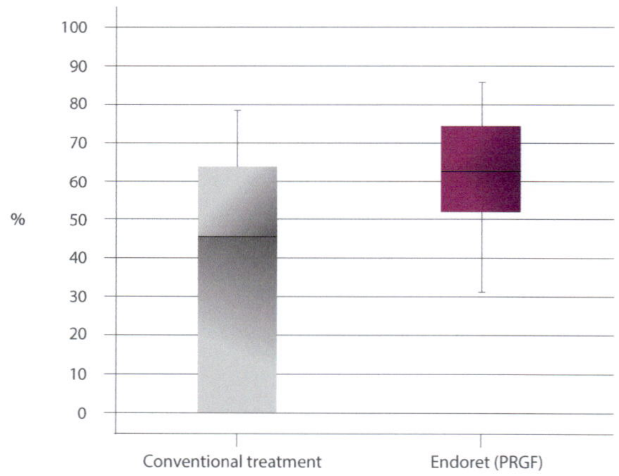

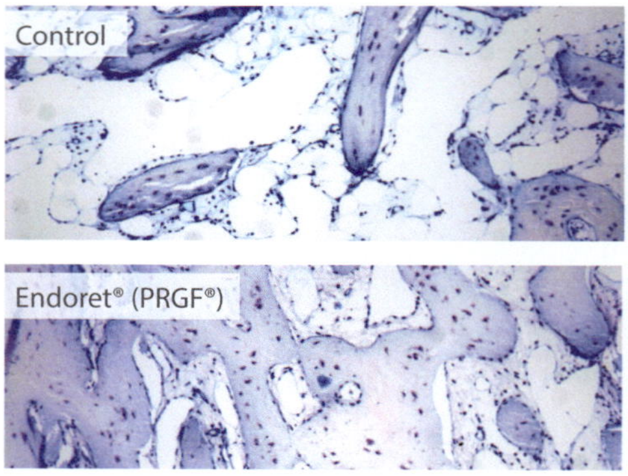

FIG. 10
Histological and histomorphometric analysis of newly formed bone in Endoret (PRGF) and control groups.

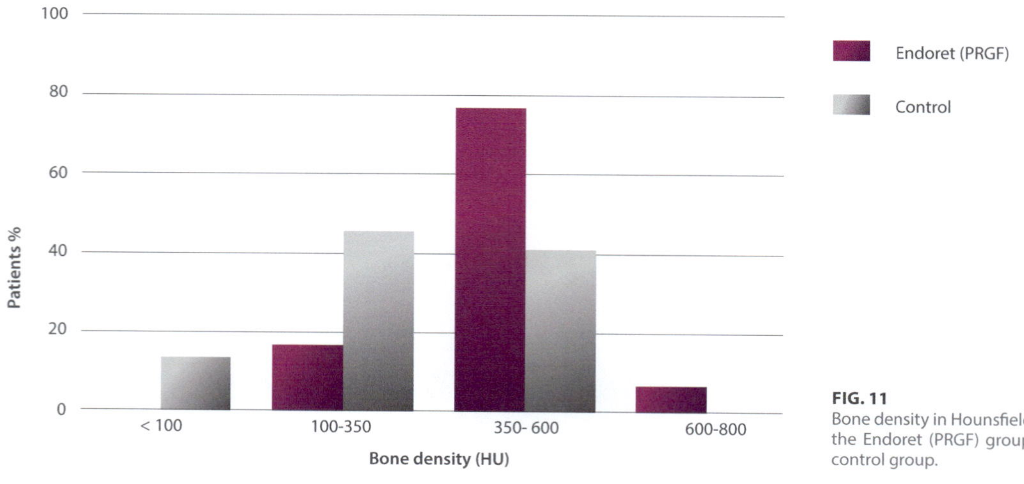

FIG. 11
Bone density in Hounsfield units for the Endoret (PRGF) group and the control group.

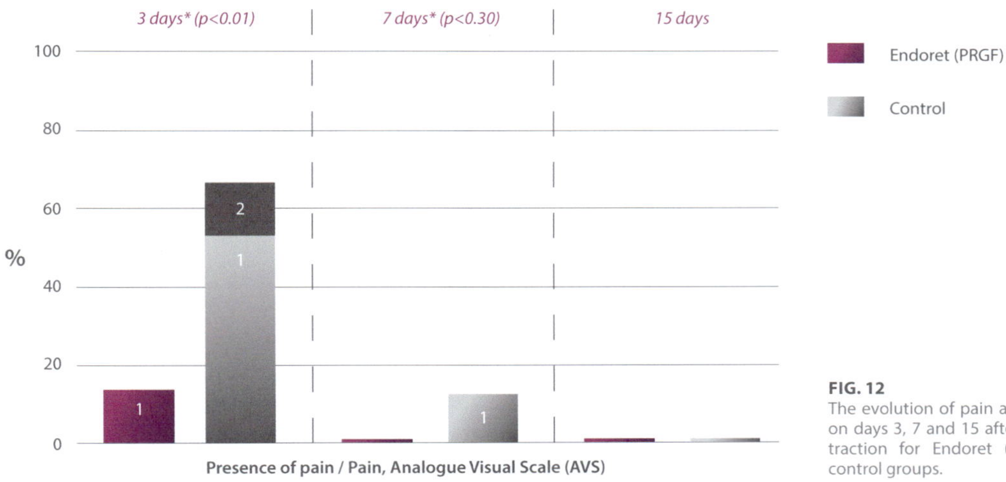

FIG. 12
The evolution of pain as measured on days 3, 7 and 15 after tooth extraction for Endoret (PRGF) and control groups.

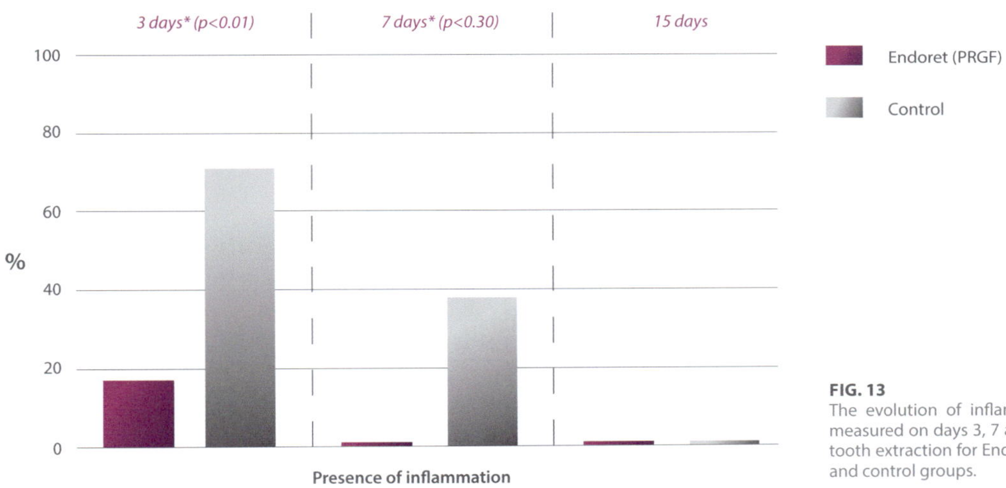

FIG. 13
The evolution of inflammation as measured on days 3, 7 and 15 after tooth extraction for Endoret (PRGF) and control groups.

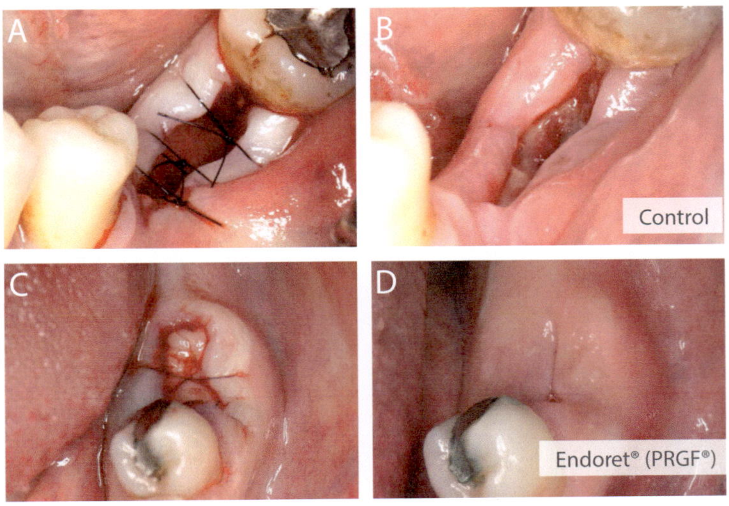

FIG. 14
A) Tooth extraction in the control group. B) Socket regeneration in the control group after 15 days. C) Tooth extraction in the Endoret (PRGF) group. D) Socket regeneration in the Endoret (PRGF) group after 15 days.

Histological analysis indicated the presence of significantly thicker keratinized epithelium in the Endoret (PRGF) group. The thickness was almost double in the Endoret (PRGF) group in comparison the control group (fig. 15).

The main conclusions we obtained from this study are:

1. The use of Endoret (PRGF) resulted in statistical significant differences for the following variables:
   - Defect fill by ≥ 75% of the initial volume.
   - Bone density
   - Histomorphometric analysis

2. Endoret (PRGF) produced statistically significant better soft tissue healing and higher thickness of the regenerated keratinized mucosa.

3. The use of Endoret (PRGF) produced statistically significant lower pain and inflammation.

4. The absence of surgical and post-operative complications indicates that Endoret (PRGF) is safe and effective.

3. THE USE OF ENDORET® (PRGF®) IN MAXILLARY SINUS FLOOR AUGMENTATION

In 1970 Tatum[8] described the first technique for sinus floor elevation through the removal of bone block from the lateral wall of the maxillary sinus. The Schneiderian membrane is then carefully elevated to create space above the alveolar ridge. This space was then filled with a bone graft. The objective of this technique was to obtain vertical bone augmentation in the posterior regions of the maxillary alveolar ridge. In 1980, the technique was modified by Boyne and James[9] to extend their use to permit the insertion of dental implants. In 1996, Anitua[10] described the use of Endoret (PRGF) in combination with bone grafts obtaining very good results for graft integration and reduced post-operative inflammation.

Lateral sinus floor elevation with Endoret® (PRGF®)

In this technique, a bone block is removed from the lateral wall of the maxillary sinus to produce a window and access the Schneiderian membrane.

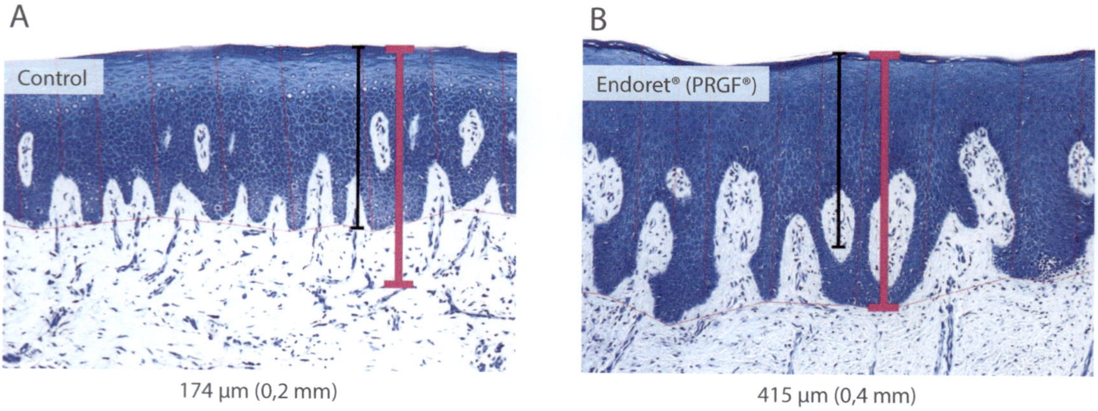

FIG. 15
Histological images of biopsies of the regenerated gingiva harvested at the centre of socket of the control (A) and Endoret (PRGF) (B) groups. The thickness was almost the double in the Endoret (PRGF) group.

Conventionally, this window is produced using a tungsten carbide or diamond bur connected to a hand piece. Heating and vibration of the drilling bur frequently resulted in perforations of the Schneiderian membrane that impaired the performance of sinus floor elevation. We have pioneered in 1994-1995 the use of ultrasonic surgery to create this window and avoid such complication. This new technique also avoided injury to the soft tissues during cutting.

Once the bone block is removed, it is conserved in the Endoret (PRGF) liquid to increase the possibility of cell survival. This is motivated by the fact that after completing the sinus elevation procedure, the block is repositioned to cover the lateral window and enhance bone regeneration.

The Schneiderian membrane is then carefully elevated by angled periotomes. The angulation of these periotomes is specifically designed to permit access to all borders of the opened window. Once the membrane is elevated, bone graft mixed with activated F2 of the Endoret (PRGF) is implanted to fill the created space below the membrane. The graft mixture with the Endoret (PRGF) will result in the formation of cohesive mass, facilitating its application to the sinus. The procedure is completed by repositioning the bone block. For this, the block is rotated 30º. Endoret (PRGF) membrane prepared from F1 is then applied to cover the surgical area, and the flap is repositioned and sutured (fig. 16).

Clinical outcomes of the use of Endoret® (PRGF®) in sinus floor elevation: A split-mouth clinical trial[11]

To study the advantages of Endoret (PRGF) use in lateral sinus floor elevation, 5 patients who needed bilateral sinus floor elevation were recruited. The procedure on one side was performed using Endoret (PRGF) and on the other was performed without Endoret (PRGF). Endoret (PRGF) was mixed with bovine bone graft only on the experimental side. The survival of the implants placed after sinus floor elevation was 100% during the observation period.

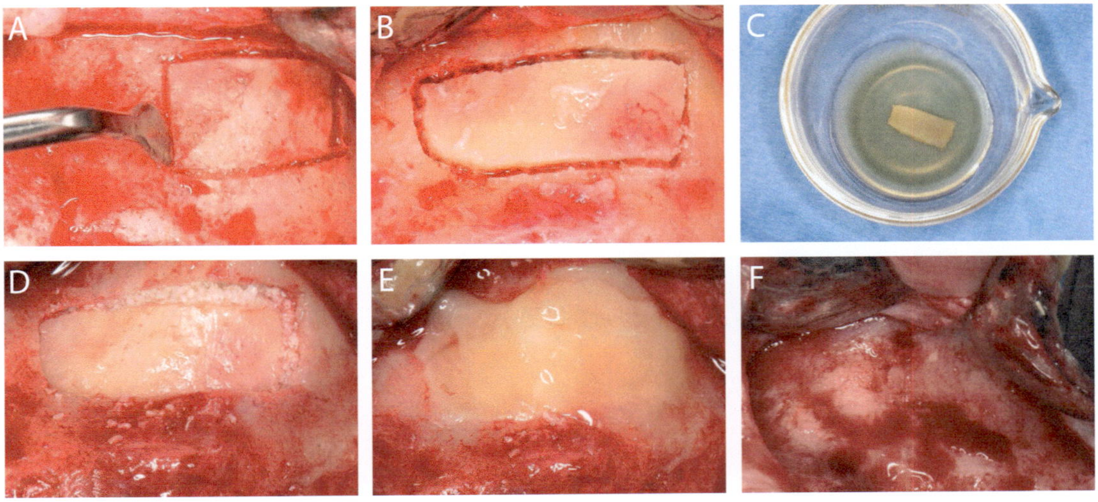

FIG. 16
Lateral sinus floor augmentation: a) Creating a window to access the sinus floor. b) After finishing bone cutting. c) The removed bone block maintained in Endoret (PRGF) liquid. d) the bone block was repositioned after grafting the sinus floor. e) Fibrin membrane prepared from F1 of Endoret (PRGF) covering the surgical area. f) The osseointegration of the bone block at the surgical re-entry.

At clinical examination, there was greater tissue inflammation and pain in the control side. Histological analysis of bone biopsies obtained before implant insertion showed more new bone formation and more blood vessels in the Endoret (PRGF) group (fig. 17).

Thus, the association of lateral sinus floor elevation with Endoret (PRGF) is safe and efficient for vertical bone augmentation. Endoret (PRGF) resulted in greater new bone formation and better vascularization of the graft.

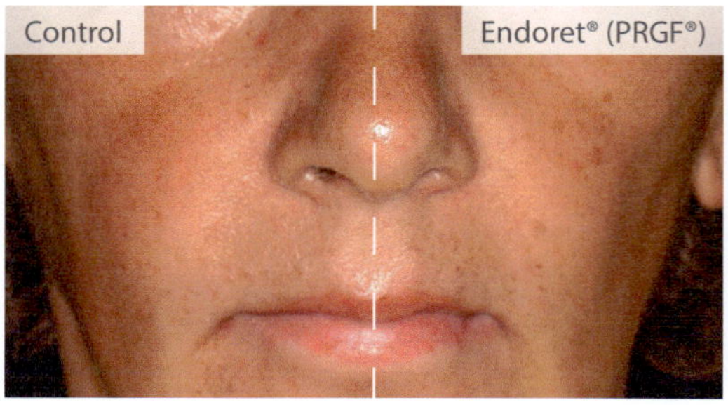

FIG. 17a
Clinical picture of split-mouth case showing more inflammation in the control group than the Endoret (PRGF) group.

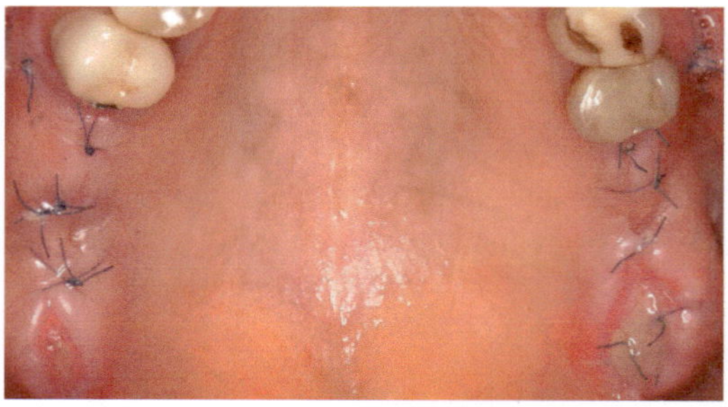

FIG. 17b
Comparison of soft tissue healing between Endoret (PRGF) and control groups.

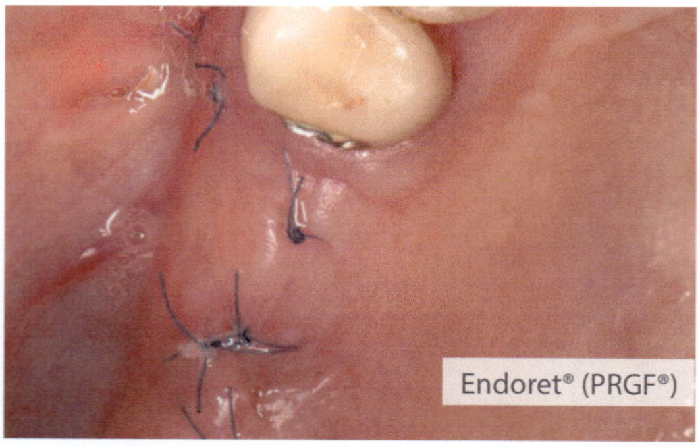

FIG. 17c
Image at higher magnification of extraction socket treated with Endoret (PRGF). The image was taken after 7 days of surgery to show the complete healing of the gingival tissue.

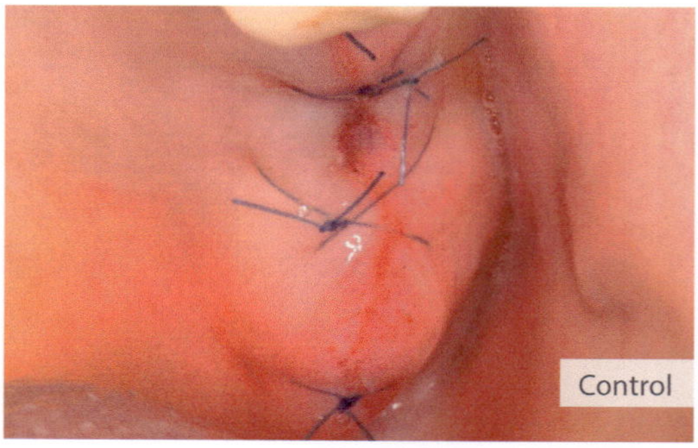

FIG. 17d
Image at higher magnification of tissue healing in the control side after 7 days of surgery. The healing was not complete due to the presence of dehiscence in the posterior region.

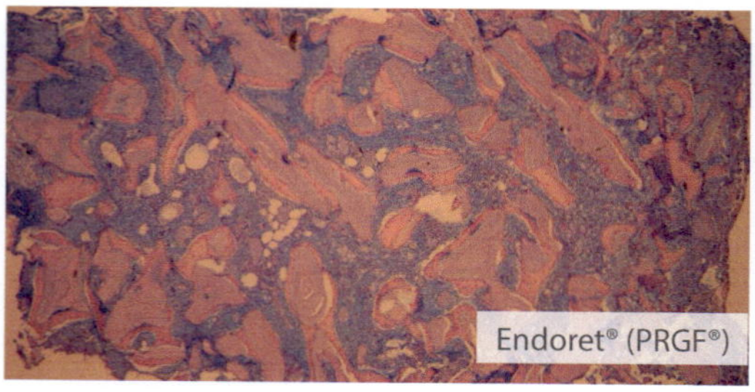

FIG. 17e
Histological image showing the formation of more bone tissue in the Endoret (PRGF) group. The goof quality of the tissue preserved the biopsy during processing.

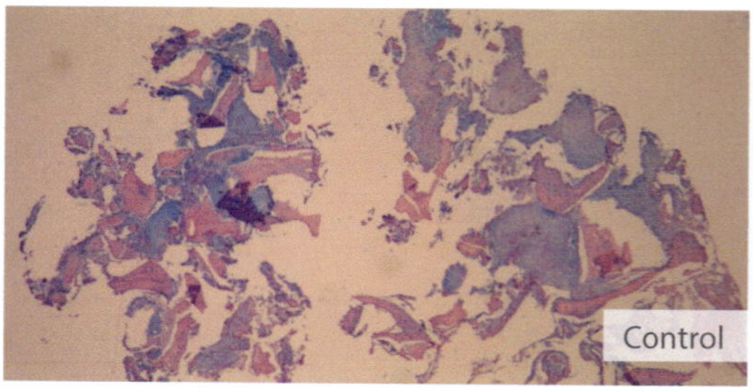

FIG. 17f
Histological image showing the formation of less bone tissue in the control group. The low quality of the tissue could not preserve the biopsy during processing.

Use of Endoret (PRGF) in the management of temperomandibular joint osteoarthritis and TMJ chronic pain

Temperomandibular joint (TMJ) disorders are a principal aetiological factor for chronic facial pain. TMJ disorders affect one third of adolescents and young adults and thus are not limited to older patients[12]. TMJ chronic pain would influence the patient's quality of life by limiting daily activities such as talking, smiling, and mastication. Generally, treatment of pain in such cases will be manifested in improving the functionality of TMJ and the patient's quality of life.

Several randomized clinical trials have shown the efficacy of Endoret (PRGF) in the treatment of knee osteoarthritis and has been better than hyaluronic acid[12-15]. In a recent publication, the use of Endoret (PRGF) has been shown to be efficient in the treatment of osteoarthritis of TMJ associated to chronic pain16. The visual analogue scale score of pain was 7.69 ± 1.9 at baseline, 1.54 ± 1.74 at 1 months and 0.23 ± 0.65 at 6 months. These differences in the results are statistically highly significant. In terms of maximum mouth opening, it was 30.15 ± 4.44 mm at baseline, 37.54 mm ± 5.10 at 1 month, and 39.54 ± 4.55 mm at 6 months. These differences were statistically significant ($P < 0.0001$ and $P < 0.01$, respectively). For that, articular injections of Endoret (PRGF) in the TMJ represent a an effective tool to control pain and to improve TMJ mobility.

A recent randomized clinical trial[17] analyzed the adjuvant use of Endoret (PRGF), in comparison to hyaluronic acid, in the surgical treatment of patients with anterior disc displacement without reduction who did not respond well to conservative treatment. These patients suffer pain and TMJ mobility limitations. The aims of the surgical treatment were to improve pain and TMJ function. Treatment success in this pathology (arthroscopic lavage and lysis and an anterior disc insertion coblation and part of the lateral pterygoid muscle) is based on reducing pain below 20 (on a visual analog scale from 0 to 100) and to get a maximum mouth opening of ≥ 35 mm. Based on these criteria, the results of this clinical trial show that the use of Endoret (PRGF) has significantly shortened the time required to achieve these fundamental goals.

- Patients in the control group still feel pain with a VAS ≥ 5 about a year after treatment and it took 18 months to get a VAS value close to 1, while patients in the Endoret (PRGF) group already have a pain VAS value ≤ 2 at 6 months after surgery.
- Considering the maximum opening, patients in the control group have taken 12 months to have a maximum opening ≥ 35 mm while patients treated with Endoret (PRGF) have achieved it in 6 months.
- Another interesting aspect of the study is that the technique used has resulted in a significant improvement in osteoarthritis, since 12 patients no longer show signs of osteoarthritis in the MRI performed 2 years after the treatment. But 10 of these 12 patients have been treated with Endoret (PRGF).

In another RCT[18], the effectiveness of the injection of Endoret (PRGF) was compared to hyaluronic acid (HA) following arthroscopic surgery in patients diagnosed with internal derangement of the temporomandibular joint (TMJ) with osteoarthritis (OA). In the study, 50 patients received an injection of Endoret (PRGF), and 50 received an injection of HA. The pain intensity and the maximum mouth opening before and after the procedure were compared. Endoret (PRGF) resulted in better results than hyaluronic acid, with a significant reduction in pain at 18 months, compared with HA treatment. The study concluded that the injection of Endoret (PRGF) following arthroscopy is more effective than the injection of HA with respect to pain in patients with advanced internal derangement of the TMJ.

4. ENDORET® (PRGF®) IN MEDICALLY COMPROMIZED PATIENTS

Hematological diseases and coagulopathies

In a randomized controlled clinical trial[19], Mozzati et al. have compared the effectiveness of autologous Endoret (PRGF) to that of a fibrin glue (Tisseel) as local measure in the management of patients with bleeding disorders and in need of dental extractions. The study was motivated by the risk of secondary bleeding and the possible need of repeated surgical and hematological interventions in these patients. Moreover, fibrin glue, with recognized efficacy, has the risk of viral infection transmission.

The study sample included 120 patients with different blood disorders who needed dental extraction without hospitalization. All patients received systemic hematological treatment. The main outcome was the secondary bleeding after the 7-day follow-up period or protracting after the repair procedure. The systemic treatment included tranexamic acid as oral antifibrinolytic agents. The treatment was complemented with desmopressin (a dose of 0.3 mg/kg in single subcutaneous injection about 30-60 minutes before the dental procedure) in patients with mild/moderate hemophilia A or type I von Willebrand's disease with a prior favorable response. However, in severe congenital bleeding disorders, desmopressin was replaced by a specific replacement therapy with a plasma-derived or recombinant form of the deficient factor. The dosage of the deficient factor was calculated to ensure a peak value greater than 50% in the peri-operative period and in the 3 days following tooth extraction. In patients with hemophilia A with inhibitors, recombinant activated factor VII (rFVIIa) was administered as a bolus dose of 90 mg/kg in close temporal proximity with respect to the single dental extraction.

In the group managed with fibrin glue, 106 extractions (7 retained third molars) were performed. Secondary bleeding occurred 3/60 patients (5%) on the third day after extraction. These patients necessitated additional surgery and systemic treatment (in one case the procedure had to be repeated on the seventh day) to control bleeding.

In the group managed with Endoret (PRGF), 98 extractions (23 retained third molars) were performed. Secondary bleeding occurred in two patients (3.3%) on the first day after extraction. Bleeding was effectively controlled with surgery but without systemic treatment.

Notably, 4 out of the five secondary bleeds occurred in patients with hemophilia A. Concomitant diabetes or liver disease significantly increased the bleeding risk.

Endoret (PRGF) was as effective as the fibrin glue as a local haemostatic measure. Endoret (PRGF) has the advantages of the autologous origin, no need for additional systemic treatment in post-extraction repair surgery, earlier onset of neo-angiogenesis and, overall, reducing patients' distress and costs to the health system.

Patients with insulin-dependent diabetes mellitus

Endoret (PRGF) has been tested in a RCT that recruited patients affected by insulin-dependent diabetes mellitus[20]. The study was conducted in a split-mouth design and evaluated the healing Index, residual socket volume, visual analogue scale, postsurgical complications, and outcome of a patient questionnaire. During follow-up period of 21 days, patients were evaluated at 4 time points. Finally, 34 patients affected by insulin-dependent diabetes mellitus were included. Endoret (PRGF) resulted in significantly smaller residual socket volumes and better Healing Indices from days 3 to 14. The patients' questionnaire outcomes were unanimously in favor of PRGF treatment. The study also reported that small sample of patients with glycemia values of at least 240 mg/dL showed worse healing index. The study concluded that Endoret (PRGF) is efficient in improving tissue healing (closure of the extraction socket) and the differences between PRGF and control groups have been statistically significant.

5. PREVENETION AND TREATMENT OF MEDICATION-RELATED OSTEONECROSIS OF THE JAW

Bisphosphonates

Bisphosphonates are analogues of pyrophosphate, and are used as medication to inhibit bone resorption in numerous pathologies such as osteoporosis, Paget disease, multiple myeloma, malignant hypercalcemia, and metastasis related to breast and prostate cancers[21,22]. They are seekers of bone, the tissue where they act and accumulate. Bisphosphonates are not metabolized, and are eliminated in the urine.

The clinical use of bisphosphonates is based on the fact that the dose necessary to have an antiresorptive effect is several times lower than the dose needed to inhibit bone mineralization. Several studies have reported that bisphosphonates improve the mechanical properties of osteoporotic bone and reduce the risk of bone fracture[21,22].

The potency of bisphosphonates depends on their affinity to hydroxyapatite and their potency to inhibit the enzyme farnesyl diphosphate synthase[21]. The inhibition of bone remodeling also varies between bone sites. This inhibition is higher in the trabecular bone than the cortical bone. It also seems that these drugs do not inhibit the bone remodeling at the periosteal surface of bone. The recovery of the bone remodeling rate is not immediate after discontinuing the treatment with bisphosphonates.

Bisphosphonates-related osteonecrosis of the jaw (BRONJ) is the most relevant side effect of bisphosphonates in the oral and maxillofacial field. For the diagnosis of BRONJ, the following criteria should be fulfilled: the presence of exposed necrotic bone for more than 8 weeks, an evidence of treatment with bisphosphonates, and the absence of a history of radiotherapy.

The first cases of BRONJ were described by Marx and Ruggiero[23,24]. Since then, the management of patients positive for treatment with bisphosphonates is a question of debate given the absence of effective protocol for the prevention and treatment of BRONJ[24]. For this reason, dentists and maxillofacial surgeons have a great interest in having such an effective protocol. An important reference in this aspect is the guide of the American Association of Oral and Maxillofacial surgeons (AAOM)[25]. The main objective of this guide is to minimize the risk of development of BRONJ, alleviate the symptoms of BRONJ (pain and infection) and minimize the disease progression[26].

Several longitudinal studies have identified risk factors associated with the occurrence of BRONJ. Of the most important is dentoalveolar trauma (tooth extraction), prolonged time of treatment with bisphosphonates, and the use of intravenous potent bisphosphonates (0.8%-12%)[27]. Although the risk is low, BRONJ has been described in patients who received oral bisphosphonates (0.01%-0.04%).

Why Endoret® (PRGF®)?

Several theories have been suggested to explain the occurrence of BRONJ. Of these are the bacterial infection, anti-angiogenic effect of bisphosphonates, accumulation of micro-fractures within the bone, and the effect of bisphosphonates on bone remodeling.

The Endoret (PRGF) family presents several properties that could reduce the risk of MRONJ and be useful in its treatment. Endoret (PRGF) stimulates neo-angiogenesis, cellular proliferation and migration, and inhibits inflammation[28]. Endoret (PRGF) also has antimicrobial properties against Candida albicans, Entrecoccus Faecalis, Streptococcus agalactiae, Streptococcus oralis, Staphylococcus aureus and Staphylococcus epidermis[29,30]. The biodegradation of Endoret (PRGF) does not require osteoclastic activity but it is resorbed by circulating macrophages.

6. ENDORET® (PRGF®) IN THE PREVENTION OF BRONJ

Tooth extraction is the main risk factor for the occurrence of BRONJ. This has motivated Mozzati et al. to study the efficacy of Endoret (PRGF) in the prevention of BRONJ in patients treated with zoledronic acid[31]. One hundred seventy six patients were recruited and randomized to Endoret (PRGF) group and control (blood clot) group. The Endoret (PRGF) group had 91 patients and the control group had 85. The Endoret (PRGF) clot prepared from the F2 of Endoret (PRGF) was first introduced into the socket after atraumatic tooth extraction. The socket was then covered by a fibrin membrane prepared from F1 of Endoret (PRGF).

The results showed the occurrence of BRONJ in 5 patients in the control group where 267 tooth extractions were performed. Endoret (PRGF) was effective in preventing the occurrence of BRONJ in all patients where 542 extractions had been performed[31].

Scoletta et al. performed another clinical study where Endoret (PRGF) was used to manage the extraction socket in patients treated with intravenous bisphosphonates[32]. The results showed correct soft tissue healing in 62 out of 63 patients. The radiographical analysis showed normal bone regeneration after 6 months of tooth extraction[32].

Treatment of medication-related osteonecrosis of the jaw by Endoret® (PRGF®)

We recently reported the outcomes of patient treatment with BRONJ by Endoret (PRGF)[26]. The patient was 50 years old and attended the clinic for the first time in April, 2008. Upon clinical examination, the presence of exposed necrotic bone was observed in the fourth quadrant. The lesion was associated with a history of tooth extraction and treatment with intravenous bisphosphonates. The patient was suffering from severe pain, halitosis, and difficulty to masticate and to open the mouth (fig. 18).

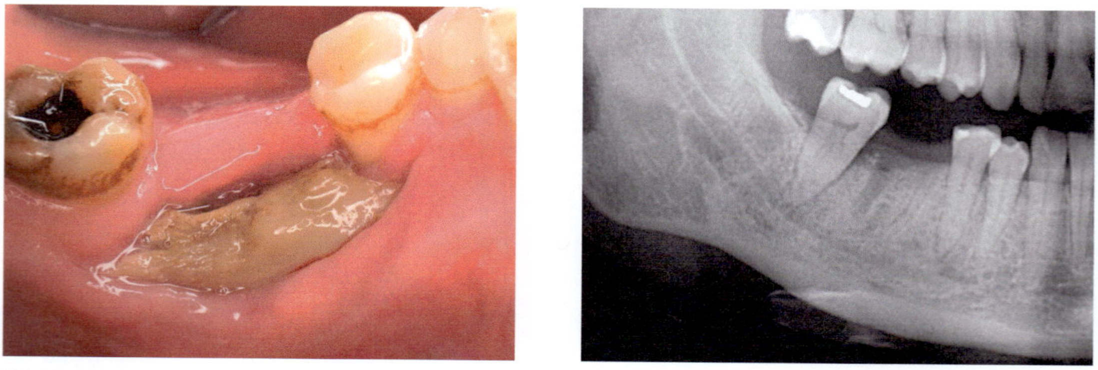

FIG. 18
The presence of soft tissue ulcer and bone exposure on the lower right posterior sector of the mouth. The lesion was associated with a recent tooth extraction. The diagnosis was bisphosphonates-related osteonecorsis of the jaw.

Following the AAMOS guide, conservative treatment that included lesion cleaning with chlorhexidine, analgesics and antibiotics was undertaken. The patient was seen in April, June, and September 2009. Hyperbaric oxygen treatment was also performed.

However, the progression of the lesion did not stop, with increase in the size of the ulcer and the occurrence of bone sequestration (fig. 19). The patient started to suffer from hemiparesthesia of the mandible at the side of the lesion[26].

Facing this situation, we developed a protocol to resolve the problem of the patient. This protocol consisted of the resection of the necrotic bone area and the bio-stimulation of tissue regeneration with Endoret (PRGF). This protocol was applied using piezoelectric surgery to remove the necrotic bone. The defect was then filled by Endoret (PRGF) clot prepared from F2 and the surgical area was then covered by a fibrin membrane prepared from F1 of the Endoret (PRGF). The flap was repositioned and sutured. Activated F2 of Endoret (PRGF) was then injected at the incision borders (fig. 20).

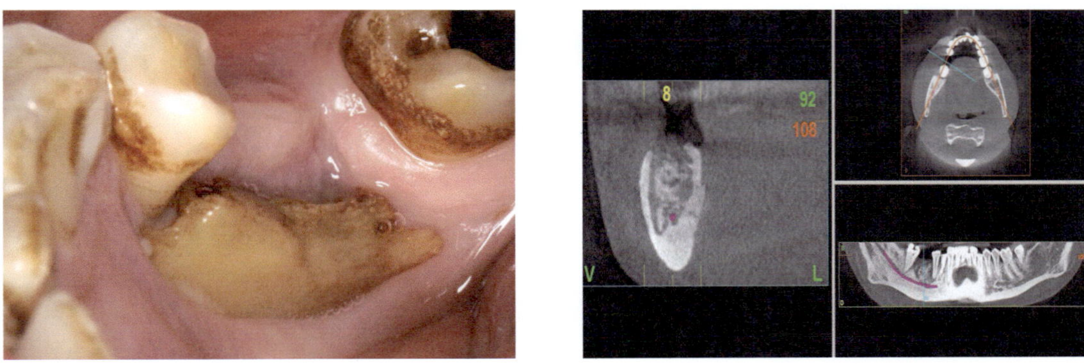

FIG. 19
The progression of the lesion of bisphosphonates-related osteonecorsis of the jaw. The lesion increased in size although a conservative approach and hyperbaric oxygen therapy were applied to control the pain and infection.

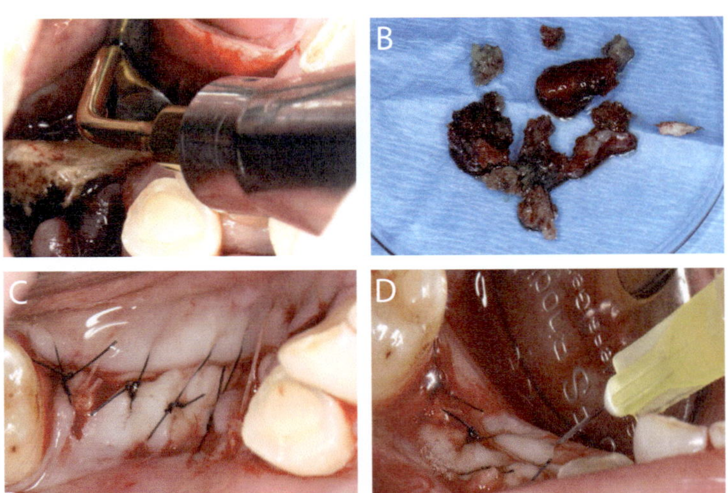

FIG. 20
The biological protocol developed to treat the bisphosphonates-related osteonecorsis of the jaw include the resection of necrotic bone, filling the defect with Endoret (PRGF) clot and covering the area with fibrin membrane. Activated Endoret (PRGF) liquid were injected at the borders of the flap after suturing.

At follow-up, the patient reported suffering from less pain, and the recovery of inferior alveolar nerve function was apparent[26]. The application of Endoret (PRGF) was effective in the stimulation of soft tissue healing and the closure of the defect, although bone filling is not evident at that time (fig. 21). Recovery of nerve function and no pain was complete after one month of treatment.

Bone regeneration was favorably progressing as evidenced by the recovery of tissue volume at the central area of the defect after 20 months of treatment (fig. 22).

Cone-beam CT scan was obtained at 1, 6, 12, 18 and 32 months postoperatively to assess the bone regeneration (fig. 23). Reduction of the residual volume of the defect and bone regeneration were observed after 6 months of treatment. The volume of the residual bone defect was 25% and 10% after 12 and 18 months of treatment (fig. 23). The bone healing started from the borders of the defect and continued toward its centre as evidenced from serial radiographs. Bone regeneration facilitated the elimination of tissue invagination initially seen at the centre of the defect. Figures 21 and 22 show the evolution of the soft tissue healing.

After 32 months, the CBCT showed complete bone regeneration indicating the viability of bone defect regeneration in patients having BRONJ (fig. 23). Thus, the bio-stimulation of tissue healing with Endoret (PRGF) is effective in the regeneration of hard and soft tissues lost from drug-related osteonecrosis of the jaw.

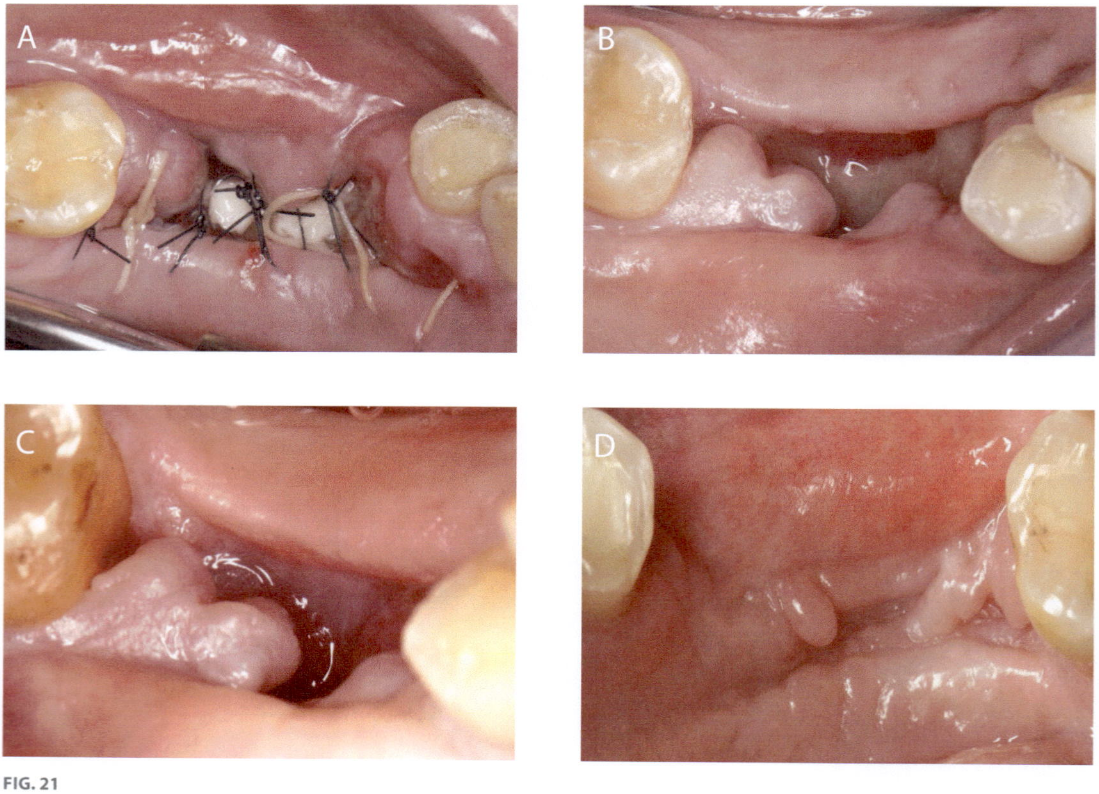

FIG. 21
The healing of the soft tissues after the application of Endoret (PRGF) treatment and the achievement of complete closure the ulcer. A) immediately after surgery.
B) one week postoperatively.
C) 3-4 weeks postoperatively.
D) 6 months postoperatively.

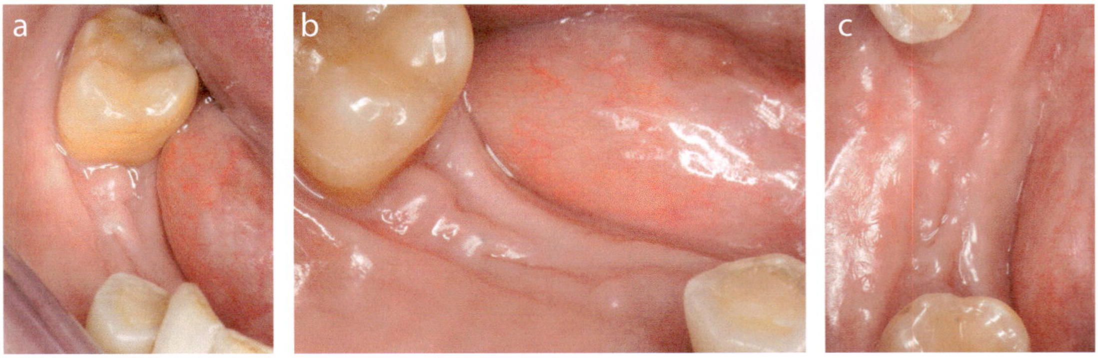

FIG. 22
Recovery of the volume of the residual alveolar ridge after 20 months of receiving PRGF (Enodret) therapy.

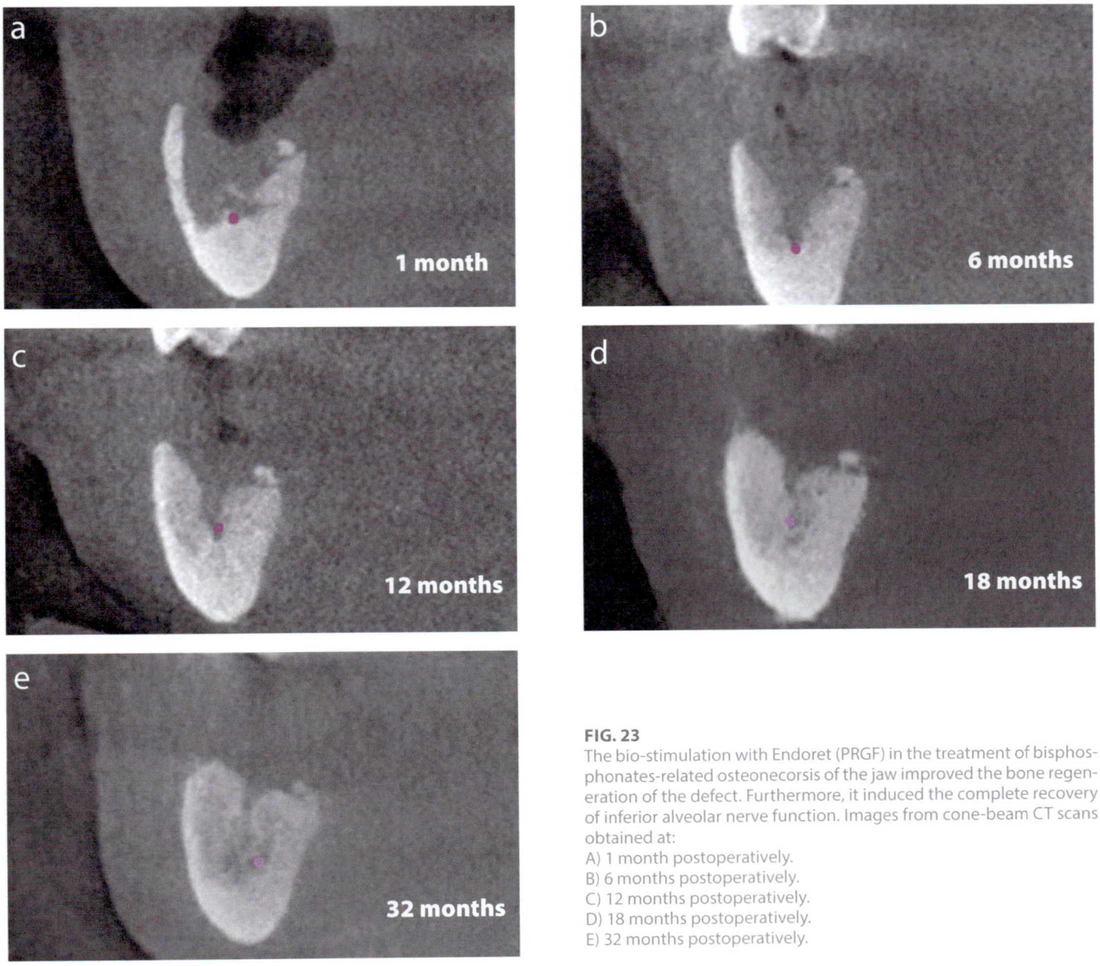

FIG. 23
The bio-stimulation with Endoret (PRGF) in the treatment of bisphosphonates-related osteonecorsis of the jaw improved the bone regeneration of the defect. Furthermore, it induced the complete recovery of inferior alveolar nerve function. Images from cone-beam CT scans obtained at:
A) 1 month postoperatively.
B) 6 months postoperatively.
C) 12 months postoperatively.
D) 18 months postoperatively.
E) 32 months postoperatively.

A surgery was planned to place 2 dental implants in the regenerated alveolar bone. Figure 24 shows the placed implants which were immediately loaded. Two biopsies were obtained at the implant sites before drilling with a trephine bur. The histological analysis confirmed the neoformation of bone tissue in the area previously affected by BRONJ (fig. 25). In the same surgery, the lower right second molar was extracted due to a vertical fracture. The extraction sockets were successfully regenerated by PRGF (Endoret). The patient follow-up indicated the absence of any adverse effects and the correct function and integration of the implants a year after the placement of the definite prosthesis (fig. 26).

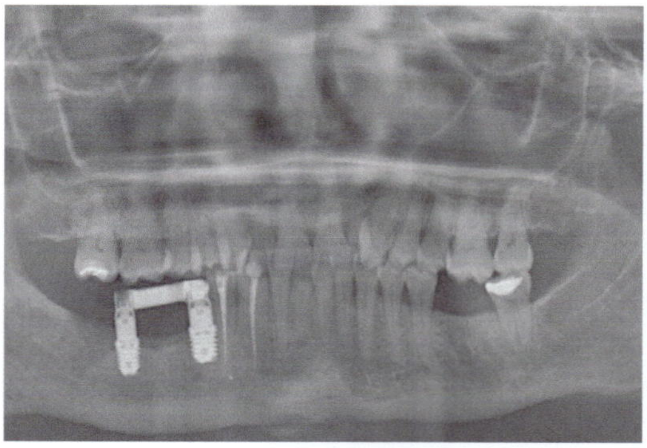

FIG. 24
Panoramic radiograph after 24 hours of surgery showing the placed dental implants and the prosthesis for immediate loading. Also the extraction socket of the lower right second molar that was treated with Endoret (PRGF) without any complication.

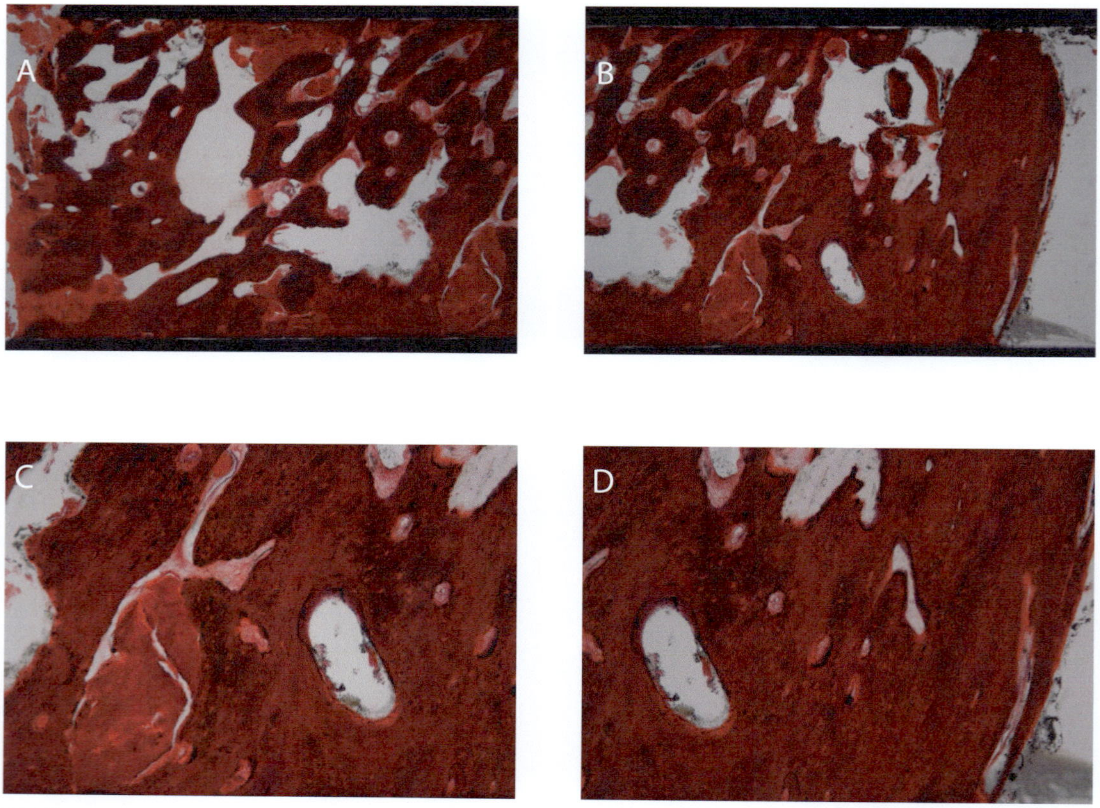

FIG. 25
Histological analysis of the two biopsies from regenerated bone at the area previously affected by BRONJ (C and D at 10x; A and B at 5x).

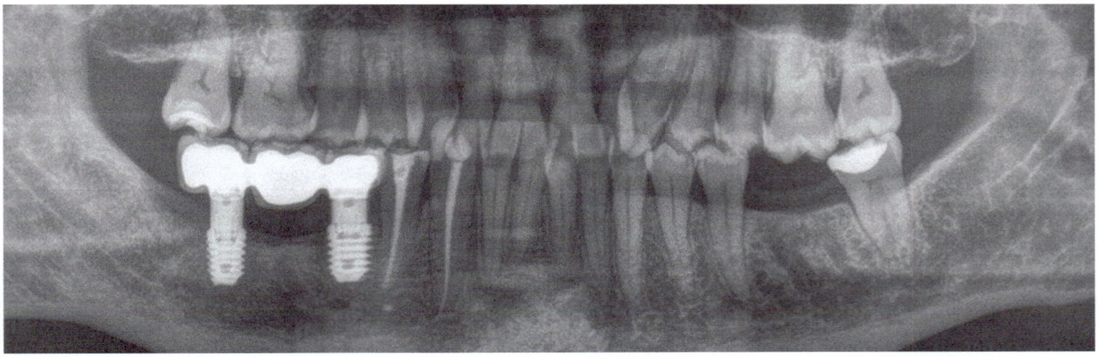

FIG. 26
Panoramic radiograph after 1 year of the placement of the prosthesis showing the proper healing of the extraction socket of the lower right second premolar and the well-osseointegration of the dental implants.

The efficacy of Endoret (PRGF) in the treatment of Medication-related osteonecrosis of the jaw from intravenous bisphosphonates has been evaluated in 32 patients[33]. All patients had received intravenous bisphosphonates for an average of 37 months when the BRONJ lesion had been diagnosed.

The treatment protocol included the surgical resection of the necrotic bone and the bio-stimulation of tissue regeneration with Endoret (PRGF)[33]. The patients had been followed for 48-50 months, confirming the efficacy of Endoret (PRGF) to stimulate the closure of the defect and the absence of intra- and post-operative complications[33].

Prevention and treatment of osteoradionecrosis

In a controlled split-mouth clinical trial[34], the capacity of Endoret (PRGF) in the prevention of osteoradionecrosis due to tooth extraction in patients who received radiotherpay.

In the study, 20 patients in need of bilateral paired dental extraction were treated as following: On the side directly impacted by radiation, the experimental side, extraction sockets were treated with Endoret (PRGF), whereas, on the other side (control), sockets were left to heal naturally (blood clot). To measure the effectiveness, the following variables were assesed: residual socket volume (RSV), healing index (HI), pain, and postsurgical complications. The study period was 30 days after surgery and included 4 evaluation sessions.

Endoret (PRGF) resulted in better values for RSV and HI at all checkups without any postoperative complications. However, in the control side, slower healing and 2 cases of bone exposure were observed. Interstingly, these two cases were then effectively treated with Endoret (PRGF) application. In this light, Endoret (PRGF) could be effective in the management of patients with a history of head and neck radiotherapy, accelerating and fostering mucosal healing and avoiding postextraction bone exposures.

In another study[35], osteoradionecrosis (ORN) defined as exposed necrotic bone, that not heal for at least 3 months. Ten patients with ORN were treated by debridement of necrotic bone using an ultrasound device followed by application of Endoret (PRGF) to improve and accelerate soft-tissue healing. Patients were followed up to 1 year clinically and radiographically. Visual analogue scale (VAS) was used to evaluate pain in the first week after surgery. A modified healing index assessed the clinical evolution of the cases.

Endoret (PRGF) was effective in the treatment of all patients with ORN without any intraoperative or postoperative complications. The authors have stated that the clinical and radiographic evaluations showed no signs of persistent infection or exposed bone up to 12 months of follow-up. The maturity and quality of the regenerated tissues was excellent, surgical wounds always achieving complete closure. VAS scores and trismus were very low in all patients, who did not require analgesics after the third day post-surgery.

These clinical findings recommend Endoret (PRGF) as effective tool not only for the treatment of osteoradionecrosis but also for its prevention.

7. CONCLUSIONS

The plasma rich in growth factors is an autologous, versatile, leukocyte-free platelet concentrate. The Endoret (PRGF) results in the formation of a fibrin scaffold and the release of growth factors that pave the way for tissue regeneration. More than 200 scientific papers evidence the safety and predictability of the Endoret (PRGF). Since its first intraosseous application in 1995, many randomized controlled clinical trials and observational studies have confirmed the properties of Endoret (PRGF) as antimicrobial and anti-inflammatory agent. Endoret (PRGF) improves the postoperative healing as patients experienced lesser pain, swelling, and hematoma than the control treatment (a blood clot). This has great impact on the patient's quality of life and the healing of medically-compromised patients. Clinical and histological evaluation of soft tissue healing indicates an accelerated defect closure by the formation of a thicker gingival tissue than the control treatment. Endoret (PRGF) alone or in combination with bone graft and/or bone substitutes has enhanced the bone tissue regeneration and results in a more mature bone tissue.

1. Mancuso JD, Bennion JW, Hull MJ, Winterholler BW. Platelet-rich plasma: a preliminary report in routine impacted mandibular third molar surgery and the prevention of alveolar osteitis. J Oral Maxillofac Surg. 2003;61 (8 suppl):40.

2. Rutkowski JL, Fennell JW, Kern JC, Madison DE, Johnson DA. Inhibition of Alveolar Osteitis In Mandibular Tooth Extraction Sites Using Platelet-Rich Plasma. J Oral Implantol. 2007;33:116-21.

3. Anitua E, Andia I, Ardanza B, Nurden P, Nudern AT. Autologous platelets as a source of proteins for healing and tissue regeneration. Thromb Haemost. 2004;91:4-15.

4. Anitua E. Plasma rich in growth factors: preliminary results of the use in the preparation of future sites for implants. In J Oral Maxillofacial Implants. 1999;14:57-63.

5. Anitua E, Orive G, Pla R, Román P, Serrano V, Andía I. The effects of PRGF on bone regeneration ando n titanium implant osseointegration in goats: a histologic and histomorphometric study. J Biomed Mat Res. 2009; 91º:158-65.

6. Anitua E, Orive G. Trattamento dei difetti post-estrattivi mediante la tecnologíaa PRGF: casi clinici. Italian Oral Surg. 2010;9:115-29.

7. Anitua E, Murias-Freijo A, Alkhraisat MH, Orive G. Clinical, radiographical, and histological outcomes of plasma rich in growth factors in extraction socket: a randomized controlled clinical trial. Clin Oral Investig. 2015;19:589-600.

8. Tatum H. Maxillary and sinus implant reconstructions. Dent Clin North Am. 1986; 30:1207–29.

9. Boyne PJ, James RA. Grafting of the maxillary sinus floor with autogenous marrow and bone. J Oral Surg. 1980; 38:613–16.

10. Anitua E. Atraumatic sinus elevation. In: Anitua E, ed. A new approach in surgery with implant-supported prosthesis. Vitoria: Puesta al día Publicaciones, 1996:75–99.

11. Anitua E, Prado R, Orive G. Bilateral sinus elevation evaluating plasma rich in growth factors technology: a report of five cases. Clin Implant Dent Relat Res. 2012;14:51-60.

12. Mountziaris PM, Kramer PR, Mikos AG. Emerging intra-articular drug delivery systems for the temporomandibular joint. Methods. 2009;47:134-40.

13. Sánchez M, Fiz N, Azofra J, Usabiaga J, Aduriz Recalde E, Garcia Gutierrez A, Albillos J, Gárate R, Aguirre JJ, Padilla S, Orive G, Anitua E. A randomized clinical trial evaluating plasma rich in growth factors (PRGF-Endoret) versus hyaluronic acid in the short-term treatment of symptomatic knee osteoarthritis. Arthroscopy. 2012;28:1070-8.

14. Vaquerizo V, Plasencia MÁ, Arribas I, Seijas R, Padilla S, Orive G, Anitua E. Comparison of intra-articular injections of plasma rich in growth factors(PRGF-Endoret) versus Durolane hyaluronic acid in the treatment of patients with symptomatic osteoarthritis: a randomized controlled trial. Arthroscopy. 2013;29:1635-43.

15. Anitua E, Sánchez M, Aguirre JJ, Prado R, Padilla S, Orive G. Efficacy and safety of plasma rich in growth factors intra-articular infiltrations in the treatment of knee osteoarthritis. Arthroscopy. 2014;30:1006-17.

16. Giacomello M, Giacomello A, Mortellaro C, Gallesio G, Mozzati M. Temporomandibular joint disorders treated with articular injection:the effectiveness of plasma rich in growth factors-endoret. J Craniofac Surg. 2015;26:709-13.

17. Fernández Sanromán J, Fernández Ferro M, Costas López A, Arenaz Bua J, López A. Does injection of plasma rich in growth factors after temporomandibular joint arthroscopy improve outcomes in patients with Wilkes stage IV internal derangement? A randomized prospective clinical study. Int J Oral Maxillofac Surg. 2016;45:828-35.

18. Fernández-Ferro M, Fernández-Sanromán J, Blanco-Carrión A, Costas-López A, López-Betancourt A, Arenaz-Bua J, et al. Comparison of intra-articular injection of plasma rich in growth factors versus hyaluronic acid following arthroscopy in the treatment of temporomandibular dysfunction: A randomised prospective study. Journal of Cranio-Maxillofacial Surgery. doi: 10.1016/j.jcms.2017.01.010

19. Cocero N, Pucci F, Messina M, Pollio B, Mozzati M, Bergamasco L. Autologous plasma rich in growth factors in the prevention of severe bleeding after teeth extractions in patients with bleeding disorders: a controlled comparison with fibrin glue. Blood Transfus. 2015;13:287-94.

20. Mozzati M, Gallesio G, di Romana S, Bergamasco L, Pol R. Efficacy of plasma-rich growth factor in the healing of postextraction sockets in patients affected by insulin-dependent diabetes mellitus. J Oral Maxillofac Surg. 2014;72:456-62.

21. Russell RG. Bisphosphonates: the first 40 years. Bone. 2011;49:2-19.

22. Allen MR, Burr DB. Bisphosphonate effects on bone turnover, microdamage, and mechanical properties: what we think we know and what we know that we don't know. Bone. 2011;49:56-65.

23. Marx RE. Pamidronate (Aredia) and zoledronate (Zometa) induced avascular necrosis of the jaws: a growing epidemic. J Oral Maxillofac Surg. 2003;61:1115-7.

24. Ruggiero SL, Mehrotra B, Rosenberg TJ, Engroff SL. Osteonecrosis of the jaws associated with the use of bisphosphonates: a review of 63 cases. J Oral Maxillofac Surg. 2004;62:527-34.

25. Advisory Task Force on Bisphosphonate-Related Osteonecrosis of the Jaws, American Association of Oral and Maxillofacial Surgeons: American Association of Oral and Maxillofacial Surgeons position paper on bisphosphonate-related osteonecrosis of the jaws. J Oral Maxillofac Surg. 2007;65:369.

26. Anitua E, Begoña L, Orive G. Treatment of hemimandibular paresthesia in a patient with bisphosphonate-related osteonecrosis of the jaw (BRONJ) by combining surgical resection and PRGF-Endoret. Br J Oral Maxillofac Surg. 2013;51:e272-4.

27. Ruggiero SL, Mehrotra B. Bisphosphonate-related osteonecrosis of the jaw: diagnosis, prevention, and management. Annu Rev Med. 2009;60:85-96.

28. Anitua E, Alonso R, Girbau C, Aguirre JJ, Muruzabal F, Orive G. Antibacterial effect of plasma rich in growth factors (PRGF-Endoret) against Staphylococcus aureus and Staphylococcus epidermidis strains. Clin Exp Dermatol 2012;37:652-7.

29. Drago L, Bortolin M, Vassena C, Taschieri S, Del Fabbro M. Antimicrobial activity of pure platelet-rich plasma against microorganisms isolated from oral cavity. BMC Microbiol. 2013;13:47.

30. Anitua E, Alkhraisat MH, Orive G. Perspectives and challenges in regenerative medicine using plasma rich in growth factors. J. Control Release. 2012;157: 29-38.

31. Mozzati M, Arata V, Gallesio G. Tooth extraction in patients on zoledronic acid therapy. Oral Oncol. 2012;48:817-21.

32. Scoletta M, Arata V, Arduino PG, Lerda E, Chiecchio A, Gallesio G, Scully C, Mozzati M. Tooth extractions in intravenous bisphosphonate-treated patients: a refined protocol. J Oral Maxillofac Surg. 2013;71:994-9.

33. Mozzati M, Gallesio G, Arata V, Pol R, Scoletta M. Platelet-rich therapies in the treatment of intravenous bisphosphonate-related osteonecrosis of the jaw: a report of 32 cases. Oral Oncol. 2012;48:469-74.

34. Mozzati M, Gallesio G, Gassino G, Palomba A, Bergamasco L. Can plasma rich in growth factors improve healing in patients who underwent radiotherapy for head and neck cancer? A split-mouth study. J Craniofac Surg. 2014;25:938-43.

35. Gallesio G, Del Fabbro M, Pol R, Mortellaro C, Mozzati M. Conservative treatment with plasma rich in growth factors-Endoret for osteoradionecrosis. J Craniofac Surg. 2015;26:731-6.

CHAPTER 7

The Scientific Rationale to Apply Plasma Rich in Growth Factors in Joint Tissue Pathologies: Knee Osteoarthritis

AUTHORS

Padilla S.[3,4,5], Anitua E.[3,4,5], Fiz N.[1], Pompei O.[1], Azofra J.[1], Sánchez M.[1,2]

[1] Arthroscopic Surgery Unit, Hospital Vithas San Jose, Vitoria-Gasteiz, Spain
[2] Advanced Biological therapy Unit, Hospital Vithas San José, Vitoria-Gasteiz, Spain
[3] BTI-Biotechnology Institute, Vitoria, Spain
[4] Eduardo Anitua Foundation for Biomedical Research. Vitoria-Gasteiz, Spain
[5] University Institute for Regenerative Medicine and Oral Implantology (UIRMI) from the University of Basque Country (UPV/EHU)

SUMMARY

Knee osteoarthritis (KOA) is a mechanically induced, cytokine and enzyme-mediated disorder with different biochemical, inflammatory, and genetic signatures undergoing distinct phases and phenotypes, and encompassing all joint tissues, with pain and inflammation as the clinical and biochemical hallmarks of the disease. In the daunting task of rebuilding a physiological-homeostatic network at the tissue level in synovial joint organ failure, as in severe KOA, a biologically inspired therapeutic approach consisting in intra-articular infiltrations of PRP has proven to substantially reduce pain in patients with KOA and to improve joint stiffness and physical function.

This chapter is an attempt to shed more light on the molecular and cellular data in joint homeostasis, pathophysiology, and to discuss some mechanistic aspects that have been proposed which provide the rationale for using PRP in KOA.

E. Anitua et al. (eds.), *Platelet Rich Plasma in Orthopaedics and Sports Medicine*,
https://doi.org/10.1007/978-3-319-63730-3_7

1. INTRODUCTION

The treatment of synovial joint injuries remains daunting despite advances in pharmacological management of the pain and inflammation, the refinement of surgical procedures and techniques, and the paramount contribution of the field of regenerative medicine. Synovial joint is a complex mechanical organ that includes articular cartilage (AC), an avascular hydrated tissue functionally sandwiched between two highly innervated and vascularized tissues, namely, synovial membrane (SM), which produces synovial fluid (SF), and subchondral bone (SB), ligaments, capsule, and periarticular muscles (PM)[1]. These tissues are highly specialized mechano-sensitive and/or load-bearing tissues whose homeostasis relies on the precise interaction between biomolecules and cells when the latter are subjected to physiological loading[2,3]. Intraarticular joint tissues are endowed with very distinct load-bearing cellular responses, which are responsible for the organization of their specific extracellular matrix (ECM), which account for the bulk mechanical properties of the tissues in order to transfer, absorb and dissipate the mechanical forces among them in a frictionless and pain-free movement[1,4]. Knee osteoarthritis (KOA) is a mechanically induced, cytokine and enzyme-mediated disorder with different biochemical, inflammatory, and genetic signatures undergoing distinct phases and phenotypes, and encompassing all joint tissues, with pain and inflammation as the clinical and biochemical hallmarks of the disease[5-7].

A biologically inspired therapeutic approach consisting in intra-articular infiltrations of PRP has proven to substantially reduce pain in patients with KOA[8-10] and to improve joint stiffness and physical function[11]. Unlike a single growth-factor-delivered therapeutic strategy in a bolus manner, PRP conveys many bioactive mediators within an autologous fibrin network released gradually, which have been shown to exert positive effects on reestablishing homeostasis of joint tissues through a breadth of actions such as antiinflammatory, immunomodulatory, and antioxidative effects[12-19], an analgesic effect[8,9,11,20], and finally chondroprotective and anabolic-trophic effects (figure 1)[21-24].

This chapter addresses current molecular and cellular data in joint homeostasis and pathophysiology, some mechanistic aspects that have been proposed, and provides the rationale for using PRP in KOA.

2. JOINT TISSUE RESPONSES TO MECHANICAL STIMULI: HOMEOSTASIS, ADAPTATION, AND INFLAMMATION

2.1. Joint homeostasis and mechanical stress

At a biomechanical level, knee components work as a network from which the joint´s functional property as an organ emerges, a property known as dynamic stability, whose equivalent at the tissular and cellular level is termed tissue and cell homeostasis. Such identities do not imply biological constancy but rather dynamic adaptability[25]. The phenotype of chondrocytes, synoviocytes, and osteoblasts is constantly adapting to its dependence on the biochemical, biophysical and mechanical loading features of their microenvironment[3,26-28]. Signals and ligands from extracellular matrix (ECM) drive cell responses and tightly fine tune the anabolic/catabolic balance in order to maintain or to adapt their ECM composition to the ongoing mechanical challenges[3], thereby protecting against the deleterious effect of some supraphysiological stimuli[29]. Abnormal mechanical stress and/or biochemical mediators variously stemming from trauma, obesity, lesion or disfunction of knee components, as well as from metabolic diseases, break knee dynamic stability and trigger biological responses that disrupt the homeostasis of cells and tissues of the joint in a local, sustained, low-grade inflammatory fashion leading to a matrix degradation (figure 2)[6,30,31].

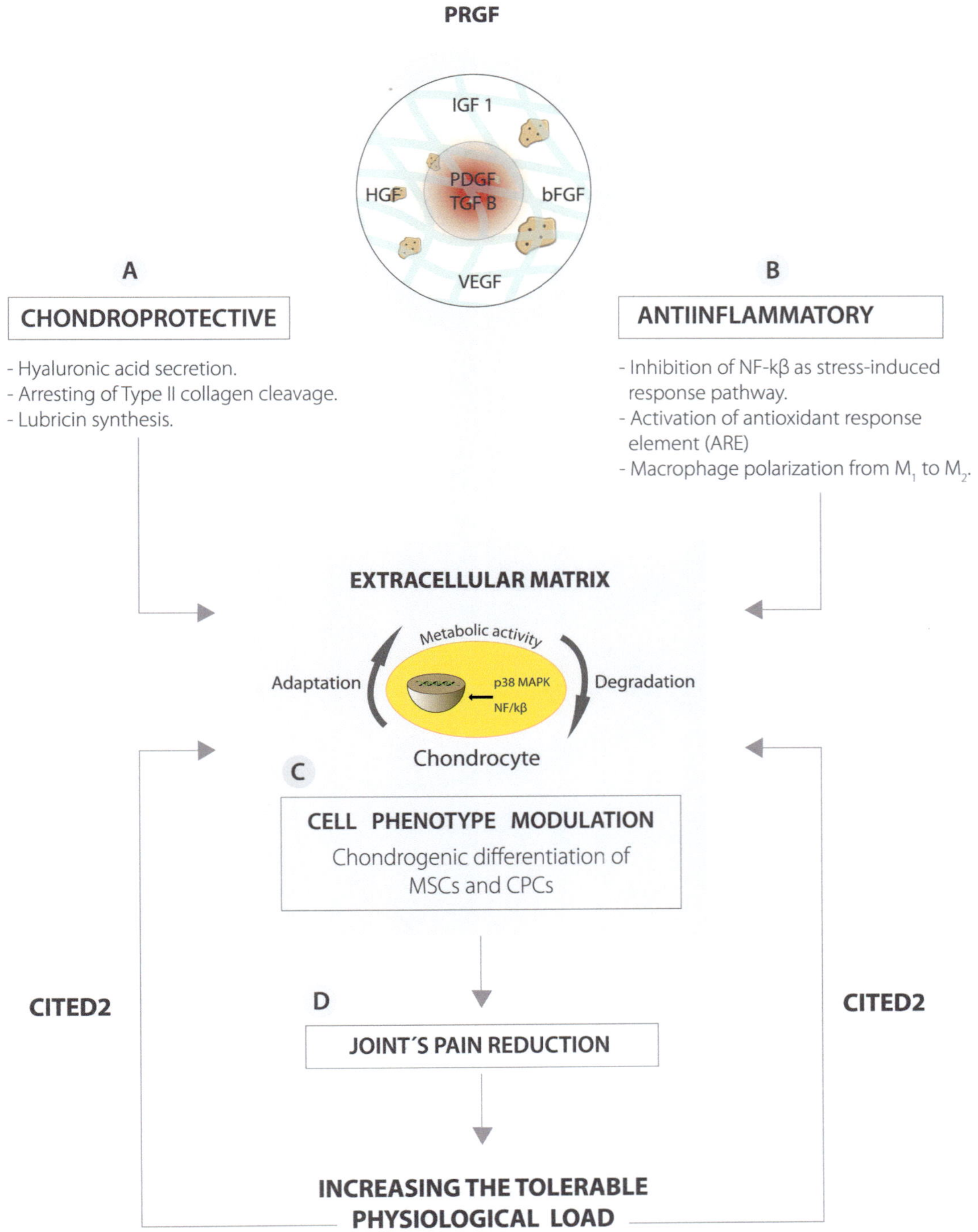

FIG. 1
The overall outcomes in basic science, preclinical, and clinical studies suggest four synergetic effects of PRGF application on the osteoarthritic joint. By modulating gene expression and gene products, PRGF may well influence cell behaviour which is conducive to maintaining the homeostatic state of the joint tissues, thereby reducing pain and improving joint function and motion[76]. (Reprinted with permission from Anitua et al.[76])

In the wake of this sterile matrix degradation of AC, there is a depletion of aggrecans and cleavage of collagen II, which leads to the erosion of cartilage, subsequently altering the nanostiffness of articular cartilage and weakening its load-bearing capacity[1,32]. Besides the release of matrix-degrading products, the ECM degradation deeply impacts the micromechanical environment of chondrocytes and changes the magnitude of dynamic compressive forces transferred from them to the underlying bone, and these aberrant new sustained (chronic) abnormal forces prompt chondrocytes and osteoblasts to respond with a pro-inflammatory gene expression through activation of the NFkB signalling pathway[26,33] and increased osteoclastogenesis, thereby increasing bone resorption and sclerosis[28,34] respectively (figure 2). Nevertheless, evidence is accumulating about

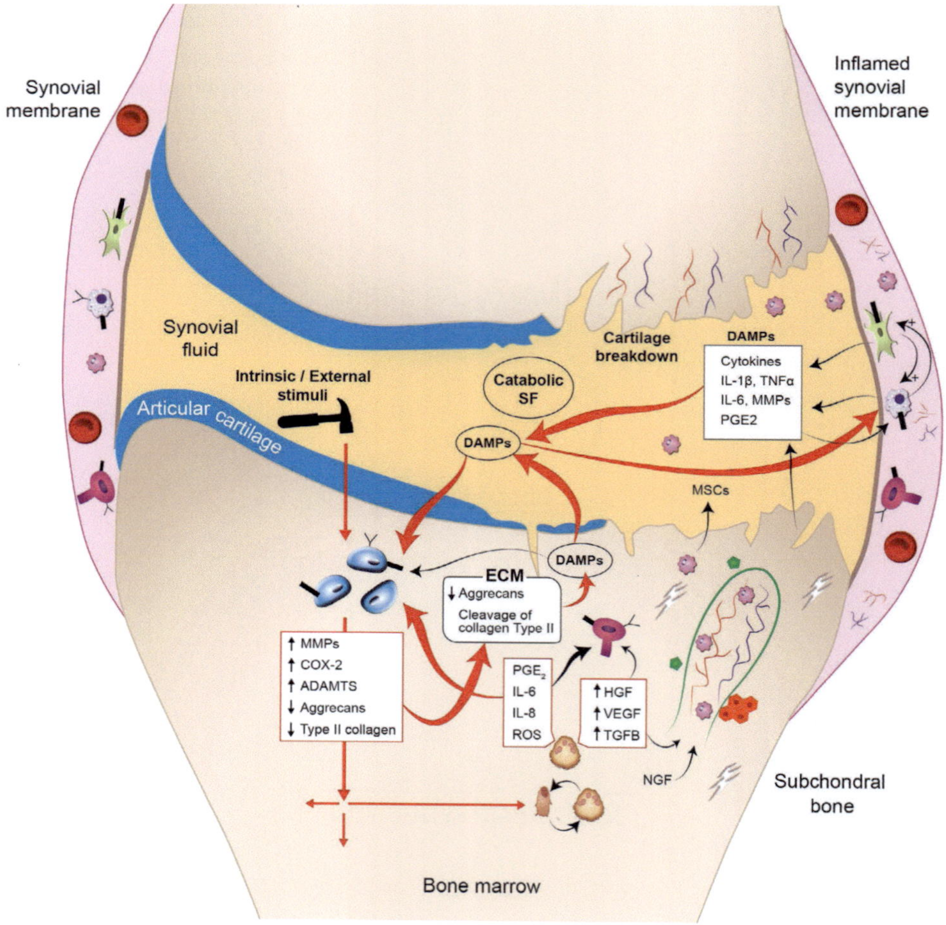

FIG. 2
Abnormal distribution of mechanical loading across joint cartilage breaks the homeostasis of articular cartilage and provokes adaptive or catabolic cell responses, which leads to an increased synthesis of matrix metalloproteinases (MMPs) and aggrecanases (ADAMTS), expression of proinflammatory cytokines and mediators such as interleukin-1B (IL-1B) and cyclooxygenase-2 (COX-2), high levels of reactive oxygen species (ROS), disruption of water tissue distribution, and matrix fragments[1,7,32,45]. Proinflammatory cytokines involved in OA, such as IL-1B and TNF-a, are major players in the destruction of AC by inhibiting the synthesis of aggrecans and collagen type II while at the same time stimulating the synthesis of MMPs in chondrocytes[41]. It has been reported that activation of TLRs of synovial macrophages and fibroblasts, and monocytes by DAMPs present in an inflammatory SF, is an important pathway in promoting synovitis in OA through the NFkB pathway[7], cells that respond with the production of MMP-1, MMP-3, and MMP13, IL-1B, TNFa, and IL-6, among other catabolic mediators, promoting synovitis in OA[7,41,42].
(Reprinted with permission from Sanchez, M. et al.[10])

how alterations of SB induced by mechanical or vascular stresses might be the start point in the catabolic loop of AC degradation and extend to SM (figure A)[5,35-37]. Cartilage is an avascular tissue whose cells rely on synovial fluid and subchondral plate to obtain oxygen and a supply of nutrients, having the subchondral bone account as source for at least 50% of articular cartilage requirements in oxygen and glucose[37,38]. Therefore, despite the fact that tracking down the "first pathogenic event" responsible for the initiation of KOA still proves an elusive quest, any induced mechanical or metabolic damage to joint tissues in combination with predetermined influences such as genetic, obesity, and aging, paves the way to initiating a harmful joint environment involving AC, SM, and SB, and then it is difficult to establish who was first[39].

2.2. Synovial membrane and subchondral bone in cartilage homeostasis and inflammation

In recent years, a great deal of evidence has been accumulating in favour of seeing as decisive the contribution of synovitis and SB on articular cartilage degradation and on the progression of KOA, where AC may after all be the victim, and not the culprit of catabolic inflammatory cytokines stemming from SM and SB, and triggered by abnormal mechanical stresses[1,7,40-42]. Hence, cartilage integrity is highly dependent on the underlying subchondral bed and vice versa, as well as on a healthy synovium and its product the SF[35,43].

Evidence in basic science, preclinical and clinical settings has been mounting for the role of synovium inflammation in the pathogenesis and progression of OA[6,7]. Matrix-degradation products such as fibronectin, tenascin C, high-mobility group protein B1 (HMGB1), and low molecular-weight hyaluronic acid (LWHA) among others in the SF[31,42] can act as Toll-like receptor (TLR) ligands or damage-associated molecular patterns (DAMPs) and activate TLR-2 and TLR 4 of synovial macrophages and fibroblasts, chondrocytes, and osteoblasts, leading to the activation of the intracellular signaling pathway nuclear factor kappa B (NFkB) (figure 2)[7,44]. The activation of the NFkB signaling pathway mediates the expression of several inflammatory genes and the synthesis of interleukin 1beta (IL-1B), interleukin 6 (IL-6), interleukin 10 (IL-10), nitric oxide (NO), prostaglandine E2 (PGE2), tumor necrosis factor alpha (TNF-a), interferon gama (IFN-j), and nerve growth factor (NGF) among other inflammatory cytokines (figure 2)[7,41,44-46]. Moreover, NFkB transcription factor has been postulated as a functional connection among the mechanobiological, developmental programming and stress-inflammatory responses of AC, SM, and SB, making the NFkB signaling pathway a potential multi-faceted target in KOA disease[26,44,47]. Another pathway involved in KOA synovitis is the activation of complement as it has been shown by Wang et al.[48] who reported that the expression and activation of complement is abnormally high in the human OA joint, where the presence of some products of dysregulated cartilage remodelling such as fibromodulin, cartilage oligomeric matrix protein (COMP), and osteoadherin in SF and SM might account for this activation[7].

Important clinical features of the inflamed synovium (synovitis) are pain, swelling, and stiffness[42], whereas histopathological changes are characterized by an uneven, abnormal cell infiltration and an aberrant proliferation of macrophages, fibroblasts, and blood and lymphatic endothelial cells that lead to a neofibroangiogenesis[42]. SM and SB are highly vascularized and innervated tissues endowed with heat receptors, chemoreceptors, and mechanoreceptors from where nociceptive stimuli, coming from a microenvironment undergoing non-physiological mechanical loading and/or pro-inflammatory cytokines and damage-associated molecular patterns (DAMPs), might initially lead to peripheral and eventually both peripheral and neuropathic pain by mechanisms yet to be fully identified[7,49]. In addition, proinflammatory cytokines may contribute to pain by stimulating hyperalgesia and sensitizing joint nociceptors to other stimuli[7,42] thereby perpetuating a catabolic vicious circle among SM, AC, and SB.

2.3. Joint Inflammation and Mesenchymal stem cells

Aggression and inflammation to AC, SM, menisci, and ligaments has been reported to bring about an increase of mesenchymal stem cells (MSCs) in SF[50,51], which is commonly interpreted as a tissue response to injury[52,53], equivalent to the response of migratory chondrogenic progenitor cells from SB to injured cartilage[54,55]. Moreover, several studies have reported that the accumulation of synovial fluid MSCs increases with the severity of osteoarthritis, joint damage and the disease duration[51,56,57]. Healthy human and osteoarthritic cartilage and SF contain a population of cells with characteristics of mesenchymal progenitor cells[52,58] with migratory and chondrogenic potential[52,54]. According to these observations, endogenous mesenchymal stem cells have been postulated as a reservoir of repair cells and immunomodulatory drugstore cells to dampen inflammation[59]. Although the source of MSC increase has yet to be determined, the most likely origin may be the SM[51,52], the breakdown zone of superficial AC[58], and the SB[54,55,60,61]. However, the SB origin of SF MSCs is less likely to occur for as some authors have suggested, the marrow of patients with severe OA is almost depleted in MSCs and the remaining MSCs are functionally deficient (figure 2)[56].

Bone, like cartilage, responds to mechanical stress in an intensity-dependent manner and a tight regulation between the sequential processes of deposition and resorption at the same site. These processes are carried out by the coupling of osteoblast and osteoclast metabolic activities[33] and unlike cartilage, when damaged, regenerates spontaneously due mainly to its highly elevated vascular and cellular network. Evidence is gathering not only about the involvement of bone, and more particularly SB in the development and progression in OA but also about how these SB changes might even precede changes in AC of OA joints[27,35,39,61,62].

2.4. The role of SB in the pathophysiology of osteoarthritis

Subchondral bone is the layer of bone which lies immediately below the calcified cartilage (figure 2)[63], and consists of two different anatomical entities, one called subchondral or cortical plate which is nonporous and poorly vascularized cortical bone, and the SB which contains bone marrow (fatty) and trabecular bone[38,64]. Together with the AC, it forms the osteochondral functional unit, which undergoes mechanical stresses that trigger adaptive cell responses and establish a crosstalk among them to adjust their architecture to ongoing physical and biochemical challenges[61,65]. The osteochondral unit in an OA joint undergoes several structural changes including loss of articular cartilage, development of inflamed synovium, calcified cartilage thickening and tidemark duplication, undermineralization of bone, sclerosis and stiffness of SB, bone marrow lesions (BMLs), cysts, osteophyte, and a localized bone marrow replacement by fibroneurovascular tissue[27,60,61,66].

There is now good evidence that even in a non-diseased joint, naturally occurring pores and holes enable communication between SB and AC via diffusion of small molecules[66-68]. This communication may be exacerbated by structural changes seen early in the osteochondral unit in KOA (figure 2) (Chapter 11 delves into this topic).

3. PLASMA RICH IN GROWTH FACTORS (PRGF) AS AN EFFECTIVE AND SAFE THERAPEUTIC APPROACH TO TREAT SYNOVIAL JOINT OSTEOARTHRITIS

Plasma rich in growth factors (PRGF) consists of a pool of autologous growth factors (GFs) and other bioactive mediators stemmed from platelets and plasma. Once PRP is activated, plasma fibrinogen polymerizes into a three-dimensional transient fibrin scaffold, which contains heparan sulfate binding domains for growth factors (PDGF, FGF, HGF, BDGF, VEGF, IGF, TGF-B), cytokines (TNF-a, IL-2,3,4,5), chemokines (PF4), ECM components (fibronectin, thrombospondin, tenascin), cell adhesion (L-selectin, N-CAM), acute phase proteins, and proteins related to lipid metabolism[69,70]. By sequestering several growth factors, microparticles, and other biomolecules released from the degranulation of platelets and plasma[70-72], this biocompatible and biodegradable scaffold provides plastic-elastic stiffness and generates growth factor gradients that are essential cues for cell proliferation, differentiation, migration and correct orientation in the nascent tissue[73]. Once infiltrated into the joint and subchondral bone, this liquid-to-gel ·3D injectable scaffold is converted into a matrix-like viscous and malleable structure, which adheres to SM, AC and SB, and covers them (see chapter 11, figure 3) 74. When fibrinolysis begins, a gradual, sustained release of GFs and other biomolecules occurs, in contrast to a bolus delivery modality[71,75]. Such a gradual yet sustained release of GF influence on cells, mimics the biological repair process[71,72,75], which is the topic of a review published by Anitua et al. 2013[76].

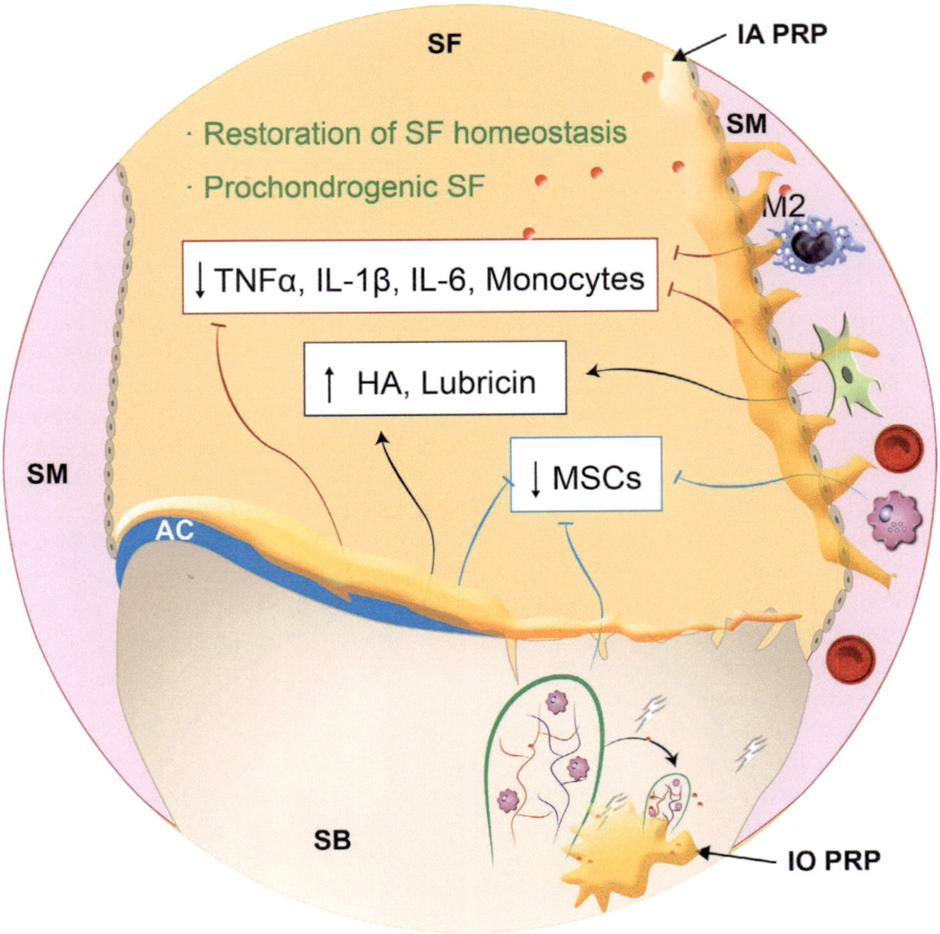

FIG. 3
Intraarticular infiltration of PRGF helps restore SF homeostasis by stimulating the synthesis of hyaluronic acid and lubricin by synoviocytes and chondrocytes respectively[16, 22, 23], dampening inflammation and suppressing the concentration chemoattractan cytokines in SF, which might contribute to the inhibition of the MSC release and migration[7, 10, 80]. PRGF might favour a homing and chondrogenic-differentiation effect on MSCs of subchondral mesenchymal progenitor cells and SF-MSCs[93-96]. (Reprinted with permission from Sanchez, M. et al.[10])

3.1. Inflammation and oxidative stress

In vitro and in vivo studies (Table I) have reported that PRGF and GFs within it such as HGF, IGF-1, PDGF, and TGFB, and platelet microparticles have proven to exert an immunomodulatory effect and promote an antiinflammatory environment. HGF and platelet microparticles have been reported to polarize macrophages from M1 to M2 phenotype[15,77,78]. IGF-I, PDGF, HG, and PRGF releasate modify the inflammatory status of chondrocytes by suppressing the NF-kβ signaling pathway[12-14], which might lead to the decreased presence of IL-β, and TNF-α and other pro-inflammatory cytokines in synovial fluid[7,79,80] (figure 3 and 4). Reinforcing this interpretation, Anitua et al. reported that LPS-treated osteoblasts and fibroblasts which had been cultured in the presence of releasates obtained from PRP without leukocytes, showed an increased expression of Ikβα, an antiinflammatory protein that anchors the transcription factor NFkβ to the cytoplasma and inhibits its activation, whereas releasates obtained from leukocyte-rich PRP induced a NFkβ activation[81]. In one recent study, Xie et al.[82] reported that PRP attenuated the multiple-cyclic tensile strain mediated MMPs, NO, and PGE2 synthesis in chondrocytes, suggesting that PRGF may protect chondrocytes from mechanically induced injury. Connective tissue factor (CTGF), one of the most abundant growth factors released by platelet activation[83] was reported to protect chondrocytes from age-related degenerative changes and from cellular stress, the latter mediated through NFkβ[84]. On the other hand, synovial fibroblasts from osteoarthritic patients cultured in 20% PRP supernatant produced a significant amount of HGF, even in the presence of IL-1β, which is known to inhibit the NFkβ on macrophages 15 and to mediate the antiinflammatory effects of PRGF on fibroblasts[53]. In a recent work, Assirelli et al.[85] observed that L-PRGF (leukocyte-rich PRP)-treated human synoviocytes sustained a long-term upregulation of IL-β, IL-8 and FGF-2, together with a down-regulation of HGF and TIMP-4 expression, two anti-catabolic mediators in cartilage, the former indicating a proinflammatory and procatabolic response. These observations were not present when the culture medium was obtained by P-PRP (Pure PRP) or PPP (Poor PPP), a notable signal that suggests there is indeed an impact of leukocytes on the biologic effects of PRP. This repertoire of antiinflammatory responses induced by PRP may break the catabolic loop, and dampen inflammatory response in SM and AC when these cells are exposed to proinflammatory cytokines and to abnormal mechanical stress and DAMPS, which is the significant OA context (figs. 3 and 4)[31]. One cellular process that accentuates the catabolic state of the AC and SB is the oxidative stress resulting from the imbalance between levels of reactive oxygen species (ROS) relative to antioxidant, which is amplified by aging[29,86,87]. Osteoblasts cultured in the presence of PRP supernatant showed an up-regulation of NrF2-ARE pathway and subsequent activation of antioxidant response element (ARE), an important mechanism involved in detoxifying ROS and protecting chondrogenic and osteogenic precursor cells[17]. Moreover, intraosseous infiltrations of PRP in mice can revert the decreased expression of SIRT1 in bone-marrow derived stem cells from aged animals, making stem cells more resistant to oxidative stress and maintaining their stemness, suppressing adipogenesis within the bone marrow and improving osteogenesis and bone mineral density[18,19]. Hence, PRP might additionally play a role as an anti-aging factor by stabilizing AC and protecting SB against oxidative stress[17-19,84]. However, as aging is one physiological risk factor for developing OA[29,87], there are some age-related changes in the composition of PRP, such as the reduction of IGF-1 and PDGF in elderly people, two important chondrogenic mediators[88], that might account for some contradictory outcomes in the application of this therapy.

3.2. OA and Pain

Pain is considered the clinical hallmark of KOA, and several clinical trials have been conducted to assess the efficacy of intraarticular injections of PRP for both pain and function of the knee. There are several relevant studies using the same type of PRP product (PRGF) demonstrating a significant pain reduction and an improvement in knee joint physical function[11] in patients with KOA treated by 3 weekly infiltrations of PRP[8,9,11,89]. The mechanism/s causing osteoarthritis pain remain yet to be fully identified[49] as do the proposed mechanisms of PRP effectiveness. Two mechanisms might likely link the pain reduction to PRP treatment. The first is the suppression of NFkβ on intraarticular inflamed cells, which leads to the reduction of proinflammatory cytokines that otherwise might contribute to pain by stimulating hyperalgesia and sensitizing joint nociceptors to other stimuli[7,42]. The second is the reported significant amount of endogenous cannabinoids within PRP 20 that might act as ligands for cannabinoid receptor 1 (CB1) and 2 (CB2) of chondrocytes, synovium cells, and bone cells 90 of OA patients, thereby supporting both a pain and inflammation reduction by targeting the endogenous cannabinoid systems (Figure 3 and 4)[20,90].

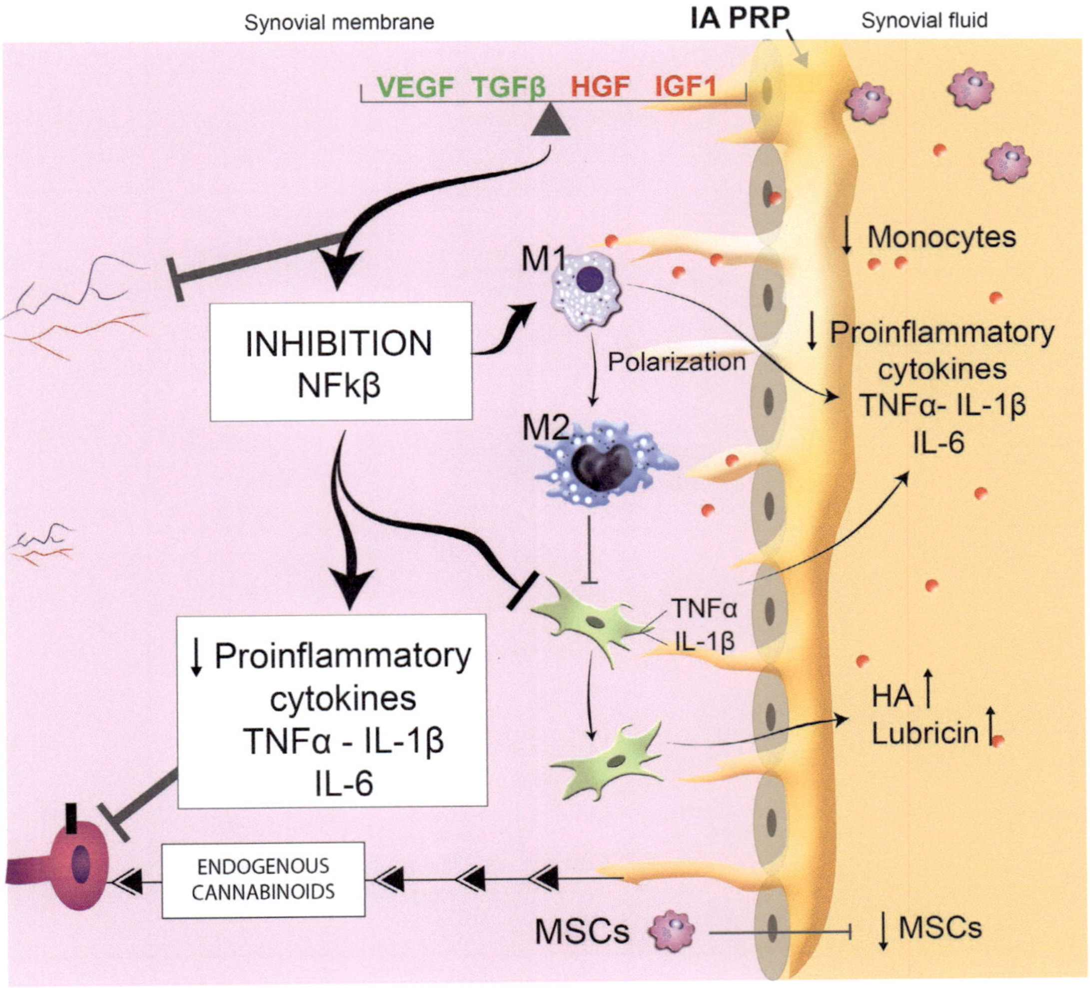

FIG. 4
This repertoire of antiinflammatory responses induced by PRP may break the catabolic loop, and dampen inflammatory response in SM and AC when these cells are exposed to proinflammatory cytokines and to abnormal mechanical stress and DAMPS, which is the significant OA context[5-7]. This sterile disruption of ECM homeostasis in osteoarthitic joint and an early inflammatory response has been suggested to resemble a chronic injury[7]. (Reprinted with permission from Sanchez, M. et al.[10])

Cell type/Animal model	Intervention	Outcome	Reference
Immortalized human chondrocytes	PRP releseate after thrombin and CaCl2 activation and single centrifugation	Reduction of transactivating activity of NFκB, decreased COX-2 and CXCR4 expression	Bendinelli P. 2010
Human monocytic tumor cell line	PRP releseate after thrombin and CaCl2 activation and single centrifugation	Decreased chemotaxis	Bendinelli P. 2010
Human osteoarthritic chondrocytes	10% PRP releseate after CaCl2 activation	Decreased IL-1β-related inflammation, inhibition of NFκB activation	Van Buul GM. 2011
Primary canine chondrocytes	Medium supplemented with HGF and IGF-1	Inhibition of IL-1β-mediated activation of NFκB, decreased apoptosis in chondrocytes	Montaseri A. 2011
Mouse bone marrow derived macrophages	Medium supplemented with HGF	Decreased IL-6 production, increased IL-10 production, reduction of transactivating activity of NFκB	Coudriet GM. 2010
Human osteoarthritic synoviocytes	Autologous conditioned plasma	Decreased TNF-α concentration, decreased MMP-13 expression, increased HAS-2 expression	Sundman EA. 2014
Human osteoarthritic chondrocytes	Autologous conditioned plasma	Decreases TNF-α concentration, increased cartilage synthetic activity	Sundman EA. 2014
Primary human osteoblast and osteoblast-like cell line	5% and 10% PRP releseate after activation and single centrifugation	Increased antioxidant response element activity, increased Nrf2 accumulation, increases VEGF gene expression	Tohidnezhad M. 2014
Human adipose-derived stromal cells	PRP releseate after thrombin activation	Increased cell proliferation, ALP activity and mineralization	Liu HY. 2011
Aged mouse bone marrow stem cells and adipose derived stem cells	PRP activated with bovine thrombin and single centrifugation	Increased cell proliferation, colony formation and osteogenesis, decreased adipogenesis, restoration cell senescence markers, resistance oxidative stress	Liu HY. 2014
Young-senescence-accelerated prone mouse strain (SAMP38) mice	PRP activated with bovine thrombin and single spin; injection into the tibia bone marrow	Delayed mice aging, improved survival and body weight, recovered cellular potential of stem cells	Liu HY. 2014
Human keratinocyte cell line	PRP releseate after freeze-thaw cycle activation and single centrifugation	Increased endocannabinoids anandamide and 2-arachidonoylglycerol (2-AG) production	Descalzi F. 2013
Mouse model of acute inflammatory pain induced	PRP releseate after freeze-thaw cycle activation and single centrifugation	Reduced nociceptive behavior	Descalzi F. 2013
Immortalized human chondrocytes cultured in a collagen scaffold	PRP activated with bovine thrombin and single centrifugation	Decreased IL-1β and TNF-α production, restored collagen type II and chondrogenesis	Wu CC. 2011
Human osteoarthritic chondrocytes	5% PRP releseate after double freeze-thaw cycle activation and single centrifugation	Increased cell proliferation, proteoglycan synthesis, Sox-9 and aggrecan expression, and chondrogenic differentiation proteins production	Spreafico A. 2009
Human osteoarthritic synoviocytes	20% PRP and 20% PRP releseate after CaCl2 activation	Increased hyaluronic secretion and HGF production	Anitua E. 2007 (Rheumatology)
Human synoviocytes, chondrocytes and anterior cruciate ligament-derived cells	Autologous conditioned plasma	Increased cell proliferation and superficial zone protein production	Sakata R. 2015
Mouse macrophages cell line	Different formulations of human and mouse PRP	Decreased nitric oxide, TNF-α and inducible NO synthase	Renn TY. 2015
Human acute monocytic leukemia THP-1 cells	Platelet-derived micropartilces	Promoted monocytes towards a resident phagocytic phenotype	Vasina EM. 2011

TABLE 1 (I)
Summary of in vitro and in vivo effects of Platelet-Rich Plasma and growth factors. (Reprinted with permission from Sanchez et al.[10])

Cell type/Animal model	Intervention	Outcome	Reference
Primary human gingival fibroblast and primary human alveolar fibroblast	Leukocyte-rich PRP	Increased NFκB activation, decreased cell proliferation, increased pro-inflammatory cytokines production	Anitua E. 2015
Bovine chondrocytes	PRP releseate after CaCl2 activation and single centrifugation	Increased type II collagen and aggrecan messenger RNA expression, decreased cyclic tensile strain-mediated catabolic and inflammatory response	Xie X. 2015
Huma osteoarthritic synovial fibroblasts	Leukocyte-rich PRP	Increased FGF-2, IL-1β and IL-8 production, decreased HGF and TIMP-4 production	Assirelli E. 2014
Human nasoseptal chondrogenic cells and human bone marrow mesenchymal stromal cells	PRP releseate after CaCl2 activation and single centrifugation	Promoted chondrogenic differentiation and their recommitment	do Amaral RJ. 107
Human cortico-cpongius progenitor cells	PRP releseate after freeze-thaw cycle activation and single centrifugation	Stimulated cell migration, increased cartilage matrix formation, promoted chondrogenic differentiation	Kruger JP. 2012
Human subchondral progenitor cells in polyglicol acid-hyaluronan scaffolds	PRP releseate after freeze-thaw cycle activation and single centrifugation	Induced collagen type II and IX, aggrecan and cartilage oligomeric matrix protein expression	Kruger JP. 2014
Human subchondral mesenchymal progenitor cells	Different PRP formulations	Modulated chondrogenic differentiation by PRP formulation	Kreuz PC. 2015
Human tenocytes	Different PRP releseate after CaCl2 activation supplemented with PDGF and TGF-β1	Modulated cell proliferation and collagen type I, HGF and VEGF production by TGF-β1 addition	Anitua E. 2007 (Plast Reconstr Surg)
Primary human keratocytes and conjunctival fibroblasts	PRP releseate after CaCl2 activation and single centrifugation	Stimulated cell proliferation and migration, inhibited TGF-β1-induced myofibroblast differentiation	
Anitua E. 2011			
Human tenocytes	PRP releseate after CaCl2 activation and single centrifugation	Stimulated cell proliferation and HGF and VEGF production	Anitua E. 2005
Human tenocytes and synoviocytes	PRP releseate after CaCl2 activation and single centrifugation	Stimulated cell migration	Anitua E. 2012
Human type B fibroblast-like synoviocytes	Different PRP formulations	Increased cell death and IL-1 β, IL-6 and TNF-α production by formulations contained leukocytes and red blood cells	Braun HJ. 2014
Human osteoarthritic chondrocytes	Different PRP formulations	Stimulated cell proliferation and chondrocyte anabolism by PRP, stimulated catabolic pathway by leukocyte-rich PRP	Cavallo C. 2014
Rabbit chondrocytes	Pool of rabbit PRP loaded in hydrogel scaffold	Increased cell viability and cannabinoid receptor CB1 and CB2 expression	Lee H-R. 2012
Male 4-month-old New Zeland white rabbits with induced articular cartilage defect in the groove of femur	Pool of rabbit PRP loaded in hydrogel scaffold	Enhanced cell proliferation and maturation of joint chondrocytes	Lee H-R. 2012

TABLE 1 (II)
(Reprinted with permission from Sanchez et al.[10])

3.3. Trophic and anabolic effects

PRP has been shown to have a consistent in vitro proliferative effect on cultured human chondrocytes in a dose-and time-dependent manner[22,24,91] and on rabbit chondrocyte when GFs are delivered in a sustained manner through the upregulation of CB1 and CB2 receptors[92]. Moreover, an in vitro and in vivo anabolic effect of PRP on chondrocytes has been reported by increasing the synthesis of proteoglycan and collagen type II[21] or decreasing catabolism by reducing MMP-13 expression and TNF-α concentration in synoviocyte and cartilage co-cultured systems with PRP media 16. Another chondroprotective effect is based on the visco-inducing effect of PRP, which stimulates the synthesis of hyaluronic acid and lubricin by synoviocytes and chondrocytes respectively[16,23,24], which help restore the SF homeostasis and function (figure 3), the latter preventing chondrocyte apoptosis, synovial cell overgrowth, cartilage breakdown, and inhibition of the MSC release and migration[24,80,93]. On the other hand, platelet rich plasma obtained by apheresis, and characterized by a low platelet concentration and very few leukocytes has been shown to exert positive effects on migration, proliferation and chondrogenic differentiation of cultured human subchondral mesenchymal progenitor cells[93-95]. Several soluble morphogens embedded in a fibrin network such as IGF-I and -II, PDGF, SDF-1, TGF-β, CCL5 and fibronectin, among other biomolecules, have been shown to be involved in the recruitment and homing, and in a chondrogenic-differentiation effect of PRP on chondroprogenitor or MSCs from subchondral mesenchymal progenitor cells[93,96]. Last but not least, dysregulated angiogenesis and fibroneurovascular tissue proliferation are two histological features of osteoarthritic SM and SB (figure 4). Despite the fact that PRP contains proangiogenic and profibrotic growth factors (VEGF, FGF, PDGF, and TGFβ) several in vitro and in vivo studies have reported no increase in the level of VEGF and TGFβ[97] nor were tissular fibrosis or an aberrant angiogenesis induced[97-100].

4. CONCLUSIONS

Intraarticular delivery is the conventional modality to deliver PRP in patients with KOA and it has been shown to be safe and efficacious in improving clinical symptoms. This route of drug delivery reaches the SM and the AC, which is sometimes inefficiently targeted by systemic drug delivery. Intraarticular delivery circumvents systemic toxicity and its side effects, offers an excellent bioavailability, and does not present molecular size limitation, in contrast to the systemically delivered molecules entering the joint via capillaries of the subsynovium. However this route does not target subchondral bone, and some mechanistic and dosage aspects remain to be elucidated in order to determine, harness, and optimize the therapeutic potential of platelet-rich plasma products. Some of these issues will be tackled in the ensuing chapters.

1. Brandt KD, Radin EL, Dieppe PA, van de Putte L. Yet more evidence that osteoarthritis is not a cartilage disease. Annals of the rheumatic diseases. 2006;65:1261-4.

2. Sun HB. Mechanical loading, cartilage degradation, and arthritis. Annals of the New York Academy of Sciences. 2010;1211:37-50.

3. Yokota H, Leong DJ, Sun HB. Mechanical loading: bone remodeling and cartilage maintenance. Current osteoporosis reports. 2011;9:237-42.

4. Hunziker EB, Lippuner K, Keel MJ, Shintani N. An educational review of cartilage repair: precepts & practice--myths & misconceptions--progress & prospects. Osteoarthritis and cartilage / OARS, Osteoarthritis Research Society. 2015;23:334-50.

5. Little CB, Hunter DJ. Post-traumatic osteoarthritis: from mouse models to clinical trials. Nature reviews. Rheumatology. 2013;9:485-97.

6. de Lange-Brokaar B, Ioan-Facsinay A, van Osch G, et al. Synovial inflammation, immune cells and their cytokines in osteoarthritis: a review. Osteoarthritis and Cartilage. 2012;20:1484-99.

7. Scanzello CR, Goldring SR. The role of synovitis in osteoarthritis pathogenesis. Bone. 2012;51:249-57.

8. Sanchez M, Fiz N, Azofra J, et al. A randomized clinical trial evaluating plasma rich in growth factors (PRGF-Endoret) versus hyaluronic acid in the short-term treatment of symptomatic knee osteoarthritis. Arthroscopy : the journal of arthroscopic & related surgery : official publication of the Arthroscopy Association of North America and the International Arthroscopy Association. 2012;28:1070-8.

9. Filardo G, Kon E, Pereira Ruiz MT, et al. Platelet-rich plasma intra-articular injections for cartilage degeneration and osteoarthritis: single- versus double-spinning approach. Knee surgery, sports traumatology, arthroscopy : official journal of the ESSKA. 2012;20:2082-91.

10. Sanchez M, Anitua E, Delgado D, et al. A new strategy to tackle severe knee osteoarthritis: Combination of intra-articular and intraosseous injections of Platelet Rich Plasma. Expert opinion on biological therapy. 2016;16:627-43.

11. Vaquerizo V, Plasencia MA, Arribas I, et al. Comparison of intra-articular injections of plasma rich in growth factors (PRGF-Endoret) versus Durolane hyaluronic acid in the treatment of patients with symptomatic osteoarthritis: a randomized controlled trial. Arthroscopy : the journal of arthroscopic & related surgery : official publication of the Arthroscopy Association of North America and the International Arthroscopy Association. 2013;29:1635-43.

12. Bendinelli P, Matteucci E, Dogliotti G, et al. Molecular basis of anti-inflammatory action of platelet-rich plasma on human chondrocytes: mechanisms of NF-kappaB inhibition via HGF. Journal of cellular physiology. 2010;225:757-66.

13. van Buul GM, Koevoet WL, Kops N, et al. Platelet-rich plasma releasate inhibits inflammatory processes in osteoarthritic chondrocytes. The American journal of sports medicine. 2011;39:2362-70.

14. Montaseri A, Busch F, Mobasheri A, et al. IGF-1 and PDGF-bb suppress IL-1beta-induced cartilage degradation through down-regulation of NF-kappaB signaling: involvement of Src/PI-3K/AKT pathway. PloS one. 2011;6:e28663.

15. Coudriet GM, He J, Trucco M, Mars WM, Piganelli JD. Hepatocyte growth factor modulates interleukin-6 production in bone marrow derived macrophages: implications for inflammatory mediated diseases. PloS one. 2010;5:e15384.

16. Sundman EA, Cole BJ, Karas V, et al. The anti-inflammatory and matrix restorative mechanisms of platelet-rich plasma in osteoarthritis. The American journal of sports medicine. 2014;42:35-41.

17. Tohidnezhad M, Wruck CJ, Slowik A, et al. Role of platelet-released growth factors in detoxification of reactive oxygen species in osteoblasts. Bone. 2014;65:9-17.

18. Liu HY, Wu AT, Tsai CY, et al. The balance between adipogenesis and osteogenesis in bone regeneration by platelet-rich plasma for age-related osteoporosis. Biomaterials. 2011;32:6773-80.

19. Liu HY, Huang CF, Lin TC, et al. Delayed animal aging through the recovery of stem cell senescence by platelet rich plasma. Biomaterials. 2014;35:9767-76.

20. Descalzi F, Ulivi V, Cancedda R, et al. Platelet-rich plasma exerts antinociceptive activity by a peripheral endocannabinoid-related mechanism. Tissue engineering. Part A. 2013;19:2120-9.

21. Wu CC, Chen WH, Zao B, et al. Regenerative potentials of platelet-rich plasma enhanced by collagen in retrieving pro-inflammatory cytokine-inhibited chondrogenesis. Biomaterials. 2011;32:5847-54.

22. Spreafico A, Chellini F, Frediani B, et al. Biochemical investigation of the effects of human platelet releasates on human articular chondrocytes. Journal of cellular biochemistry. 2009;108:1153-65.

23. Anitua E, Sanchez M, Nurden AT, et al. Platelet-released growth factors enhance the secretion of hyaluronic acid and induce hepatocyte growth factor production by synovial fibroblasts from arthritic patients. Rheumatology (Oxford). 2007;46:1769-72.

24. Sakata R, McNary SM, Miyatake K, et al. Stimulation of the superficial zone protein and lubrication in the articular cartilage by human platelet-rich plasma. The American journal of sports medicine. 2015;43:1467-73.

25. Buchman TG. The community of the self. Nature. 2002;420:246-51.

26. Nam J, Aguda BD, Rath B, Agarwal S. Biomechanical thresholds regulate inflammation through the NF-kappaB pathway: experiments and modeling. PloS one. 2009;4:e5262.

27. Karsdal MA, Bay-Jensen AC, Lories RJ, et al. The coupling of bone and cartilage turnover in osteoarthritis: opportunities for bone antiresorptives and anabolics as potential treatments? Annals of the rheumatic diseases. 2014;73:336-48.

28. Sanchez C, Pesesse L, Gabay O, et al. Regulation of subchondral bone osteoblast metabolism by cyclic compression. Arthritis and rheumatism. 2012;64:1193-203.

29. Liu-Bryan R, Terkeltaub R. Emerging regulators of the inflammatory process in osteoarthritis. Nature reviews. Rheumatology. 2015;11:35-44.

30. Berenbaum F. Osteoarthritis as an inflammatory disease (osteoarthritis is not osteoarthrosis!). Osteoarthritis and cartilage / OARS, Osteoarthritis Research Society. 2013;21:16-21.

31. Scanzello CR, Plaas A, Crow MK. Innate immune system activation in osteoarthritis: is osteoarthritis a chronic wound? Current opinion in rheumatology. 2008;20:565-72.

32. Stolz M, Gottardi R, Raiteri R, et al. Early detection of aging cartilage and osteoarthritis in mice and patient samples using atomic force microscopy. Nat Nanotechnol. 2009;4:186-92.

33. Henrotin Y, Pesesse L, Sanchez C. Subchondral bone and osteoarthritis: biological and cellular aspects. Osteoporosis international : a journal established as result of cooperation between the European Foundation for Osteoporosis and the National Osteoporosis Foundation of the USA. 2012;23 Suppl 8:S847-51.

34. Sanchez C, Deberg MA, Bellahcene A, et al. Phenotypic characterization of osteoblasts from the sclerotic zones of osteoarthritic subchondral bone. Arthritis and rheumatism. 2008;58:442-55.

35. Radin EL, Rose RM. Role of subchondral bone in the initiation and progression of cartilage damage. Clinical orthopaedics and related research. 1986:34-40.

36. Burr DB. The importance of subchondral bone in the progression of osteoarthritis. The Journal of rheumatology. Supplement. 2004;70:77-80.

37. Malinin T, Ouellette EA. Articular cartilage nutrition is mediated by subchondral bone: a long-term autograft study in baboons. Osteoarthritis and cartilage / OARS, Osteoarthritis Research Society. 2000;8:483-91.

38. Imhof H, Sulzbacher I, Grampp S, Czerny C, Youssefzadeh S, Kainberger F. Subchondral bone and cartilage disease: a rediscovered functional unit. Invest Radiol. 2000;35:581-8.

39. Lajeunesse D, Reboul P. Subchondral bone in osteoarthritis: a biologic link with articular cartilage leading to abnormal remodeling. Current opinion in rheumatology. 2003;15:628-33.

40. Radin EL, Burr DB, Caterson B, Fyhrie D, Brown TD, Boyd RD. Mechanical determinants of osteoarthrosis. Seminars in arthritis and rheumatism. 1991;21:12-21.

41. Kapoor M, Martel-Pelletier J, Lajeunesse D, Pelletier JP, Fahmi H. Role of proinflammatory cytokines in the pathophysiology of osteoarthritis. Nature reviews. Rheumatology. 2011;7:33-42.

42. Sellam J, Berenbaum F. The role of synovitis in pathophysiology and clinical symptoms of osteoarthritis. Nature reviews. Rheumatology. 2010;6:625-35.

43. Barr AJ, Campbell TM, Hopkinson D, Kingsbury SR, Bowes MA, Conaghan PG. A systematic review of the relationship between subchondral bone features, pain and structural pathology in peripheral joint osteoarthritis. Arthritis research & therapy. 2015;17:228.

44. Marcu KB, Otero M, Olivotto E, Borzi RM, Goldring MB. NF-kappaB signaling: multiple angles to target OA. Current drug targets. 2010;11:599-613.

45. [45] Goldring MB, Otero M, Plumb DA, et al. Roles of inflammatory and anabolic cytokines in cartilage metabolism: signals and multiple effectors converge upon MMP-13 regulation in osteoarthritis. European cells & materials. 2011;21:202-20.

46. Goldring MB, Marcu KB. Cartilage homeostasis in health and rheumatic diseases. Arthritis research & therapy. 2009;11:224.

47. Martel-Pelletier J, Wildi LM, Pelletier JP. Future therapeutics for osteoarthritis. Bone. 2012;51:297-311.

48. Wang Q, Rozelle AL, Lepus CM, et al. Identification of a central role for complement in osteoarthritis. Nature medicine. 2011;17:1674-9.

49. Malfait AM, Schnitzer TJ. Towards a mechanism-based approach to pain management in osteoarthritis. Nature reviews. Rheumatology. 2013;9:654-64.

50. Matsukura Y, Muneta T, Tsuji K, et al. Mouse synovial mesenchymal stem cells increase in yield with knee inflammation. Journal of orthopaedic research : official publication of the Orthopaedic Research Society. 2015;33:246-53.

51. Sekiya I, Ojima M, Suzuki S, et al. Human mesenchymal stem cells in synovial fluid increase in the knee with degenerated cartilage and osteoarthritis. Journal of orthopaedic research : official publication of the Orthopaedic Research Society. 2012;30:943-9.

52. Jones EA, Crawford A, English A, et al. Synovial fluid mesenchymal stem cells in health and early osteoarthritis: detection and functional evaluation at the single-cell level. Arthritis and rheumatism. 2008;58:1731-40.

53. Zhang J, Middleton KK, Fu FH, Im HJ, Wang JH. HGF mediates the anti-inflammatory effects of PRP on injured tendons. PloS one. 2013;8:e67303.

54. Koelling S, Kruegel J, Irmer M, et al. Migratory chondrogenic progenitor cells from repair tissue during the later stages of human osteoarthritis. Cell stem cell. 2009;4:324-35.

55. Seol D, McCabe DJ, Choe H, et al. Chondrogenic progenitor cells respond to cartilage injury. Arthritis and rheumatism. 2012;64:3626-37.

56. Barry F, Murphy M. Mesenchymal stem cells in joint disease and repair. Nature reviews. Rheumatology. 2013;9:584-94.

57. Lee DH, Sonn CH, Han SB, Oh Y, Lee KM, Lee SH. Synovial fluid CD34(-) CD44(+) CD90(+) mesenchymal stem cell levels are associated with the severity of primary knee osteoarthritis. Osteoarthritis and cartilage / OARS, Osteoarthritis Research Society. 2012;20:106-9.

58. Pretzel D, Linss S, Rochler S, et al. Relative percentage and zonal distribution of mesenchymal progenitor cells in human osteoarthritic and normal cartilage. Arthritis research & therapy. 2011;13:R64.

59. Singer NG, Caplan AI. Mesenchymal stem cells: mechanisms of inflammation. Annual review of pathology. 2011;6:457-78.

60. Lajeunesse D. Subchondral bone involvement in the pathophysiology of osteoarthritis. Understanding Osteoarthritis from Bench to Bedside. 2011:69-83.

61. Suri S, Walsh DA. Osteochondral alterations in osteoarthritis. Bone. 2012;51:204-11.

62. Zhao W, Wang T, Luo Q, et al. Cartilage degeneration and excessive subchondral bone formation in spontaneous osteoarthritis involves altered TGF-β signaling. Journal of Orthopaedic Research. 2015;DOI:10.1002/jor.23079.

63. Neuss S, Schneider RK, Tietze L, Knuchel R, Jahnen-Dechent W. Secretion of fibrinolytic enzymes facilitates human mesenchymal stem cell invasion into fibrin clots. Cells, tissues, organs. 2010;191:36-46.

64. Burr DB, Gallant MA. Bone remodelling in osteoarthritis. Nature reviews. Rheumatology. 2012;8:665-73.

65. Mapp PI, Walsh DA. Mechanisms and targets of angiogenesis and nerve growth in osteoarthritis. Nature reviews. Rheumatology. 2012;8:390-8.

66. Pan J, Wang B, Li W, et al. Elevated cross-talk between subchondral bone and cartilage in osteoarthritic joints. Bone. 2012;51:212-7.

67. Pan J, Zhou X, Li W, Novotny JE, Doty SB, Wang L. In situ measurement of transport between subchondral bone and articular cartilage. Journal of orthopaedic research : official publication of the Orthopaedic Research Society. 2009;27:1347-52.

68. Lyons TJ, McClure SF, Stoddart RW, McClure J. The normal human chondro-osseous junctional region: evidence for contact of uncalcified cartilage with subchondral bone and marrow spaces. BMC Musculoskelet Disord. 2006;7:52.

69. Anitua E, Prado R, Azkargorta M, et al. High-throughput proteomic characterization of plasma rich in growth factors (PRGF-Endoret)-derived fibrin clot interactome. Journal of tissue engineering and regenerative medicine. 2015;9:E1-E12.

70. Nurden AT. Platelets, inflammation and tissue regeneration. Thrombosis and haemostasis. 2011;105 Suppl 1:S13-33.

71. Martino MM, Briquez PS, Guc E, et al. Growth factors engineered for super-affinity to the extracellular matrix enhance tissue healing. Science. 2014;343:885-8.

72. Aird WC. Endothelial biomedicine. Cambridge university press; 2007. N.W.Shworak. Heparan sulfate.

73. Engler AJ, Sen S, Sweeney HL, Discher DE. Matrix elasticity directs stem cell lineage specification. Cell. 2006;126:677-89.

74. Sánchez M, Fiz N, Guadilla J, et al. Intraosseous Infiltration of Platelet-Rich Plasma for Severe Knee Osteoarthritis. Arthroscopy Techniques. 2014;DOI:http://dx.doi.org/10.1016/j.eats.2014.09.006.

75. Anitua E, Zalduendo MM, Prado R, Alkhraisat MH, Orive G. Morphogen and proinflammatory cytokine release kinetics from PRGF-Endoret fibrin scaffolds: evaluation of the effect of leukocyte inclusion. Journal of biomedical materials research. Part A. 2015;103:1011-20.

76. Anitua E, Sanchez M, Orive G, Padilla S. A biological therapy to osteoarthritis treatment using platelet-rich plasma. Expert opinion on biological therapy. 2013;13:1161-72.

77. Renn TY, Kao YH, Wang CC, Burnouf T. Anti-inflammatory effects of platelet biomaterials in a macrophage cellular model. Vox sanguinis. 2015.

78. Vasina EM, Cauwenberghs S, Feijge MA, Heemskerk JW, Weber C, Koenen RR. Microparticles from apoptotic platelets promote resident macrophage differentiation. Cell death & disease. 2011;2:e211.

79. Fahy N, de Vries-van Melle ML, Lehmann J, et al. Human osteoarthritic synovium impacts chondrogenic differentiation of mesenchymal stem cells via macrophage polarisation state. Osteoarthritis and cartilage / OARS, Osteoarthritis Research Society. 2014;22:1167-75.

80. Fahy N, Farrell E, Ritter T, Ryan AE, Murphy JM. Immune modulation to improve tissue engineering outcomes for cartilage repair in the osteoarthritic joint. Tissue engineering. Part B, Reviews. 2015;21:55-66.

81. Anitua E, Zalduendo M, Troya M, Padilla S, Orive G. Leukocyte inclusion within a platelet rich plasma-derived fibrin scaffold stimulates a more pro-inflammatory environment and alters fibrin properties. PloS one. 2015;10:e0121713.

82. Xie X, Ulici V, Alexander PG, Jiang Y, Zhang C, Tuan RS. Platelet-Rich Plasma Inhibits Mechanically Induced Injury in Chondrocytes. Arthroscopy : the journal of arthroscopic & related surgery : official publication of the Arthroscopy Association of North America and the International Arthroscopy Association. 2015;31:1142-50.

83. Kubota S, Kawata K, Yanagita T, Doi H, Kitoh T, Takigawa M. Abundant retention and release of connective tissue growth factor (CTGF/CCN2) by platelets. J Biochem. 2004;136:279-82.

84. Itoh S, Hattori T, Tomita N, et al. CCN family member 2/connective tissue growth factor (CCN2/CTGF) has anti-aging effects that protect articular cartilage from age-related degenerative changes. PloS one. 2013;8:e71156.

85. Assirelli E, Filardo G, Mariani E, et al. Effect of two different preparations of platelet-rich plasma on synoviocytes. Knee surgery, sports traumatology, arthroscopy : official journal of the ESSKA. 2014.

86. Goldring MB, Berenbaum F. Emerging targets in osteoarthritis therapy. Curr Opin Pharmacol. 2015;22:51-63.

87. Lotz M, Loeser RF. Effects of aging on articular cartilage homeostasis. Bone. 2012;51:241-8.

88. Dragoo JL, Korotkova T, Wasterlain AS, Pouliot MA, Kim HJ, Golish SR. Age-related changes of chondrogenic growth factors in platelet-rich plasma. Operative Techniques in Orthopaedics. 2012;22:49-55.

89. Sanchez M, Guadilla J, Fiz N, Andia I. Ultrasound-guided platelet-rich plasma injections for the treatment of osteoarthritis of the hip. Rheumatology (Oxford). 2012;51:144-50.

90. Richardson D, Pearson RG, Kurian N, et al. Characterisation of the cannabinoid receptor system in synovial tissue and fluid in patients with osteoarthritis and rheumatoid arthritis. Arthritis research & therapy. 2008;10:R43.

91. do Amaral RJ, Matsiko A, Tomazette MR, et al. Platelet-rich plasma releasate differently stimulates cellular commitment toward the chondrogenic lineage according to concentration. J Tissue Eng. 2015;6:2041731415594127.

92. Lee HR, Park KM, Joung YK, Park KD, Do SH. Platelet-rich plasma loaded hydrogel scaffold enhances chondrogenic differentiation and maturation with up-regulation of CB1 and CB2. Journal of controlled release : official journal of the Controlled Release Society. 2012;159:332-7.

93. Kruger JP, Hondke S, Endres M, Pruss A, Siclari A, Kaps C. Human platelet-rich plasma stimulates migration and chondrogenic differentiation of human subchondral progenitor cells. Journal of orthopaedic research : official publication of the Orthopaedic Research Society. 2012;30:845-52.

94. Kruger JP, Ketzmar AK, Endres M, Pruss A, Siclari A, Kaps C. Human platelet-rich plasma induces chondrogenic differentiation of subchondral progenitor cells in polyglycolic acid-hyaluronan scaffolds. Journal of biomedical materials research. Part B, Applied biomaterials. 2014;102:681-92.

95. Kreuz PC, Kruger JP, Metzlaff S, et al. Platelet-Rich Plasma Preparation Types Show Impact on Chondrogenic Differentiation, Migration, and Proliferation of Human Subchondral Mesenchymal Progenitor Cells. Arthroscopy : the journal of arthroscopic & related surgery : official publication of the Arthroscopy Association of North America and the International Arthroscopy Association. 2015;31:1951-61.

96. Kulawig R, Kruger JP, Klein O, et al. Identification of fibronectin as a major factor in human serum to recruit subchondral mesenchymal progenitor cells. The international journal of biochemistry & cell biology. 2013;45:1410-8.

97. Anitua E, Sanchez M, Nurden AT, et al. Reciprocal actions of platelet-secreted TGF-beta1 on the production of VEGF and HGF by human tendon cells. Plastic and reconstructive surgery. 2007;119:950-9.

98. Anitua E, Sanchez M, Nurden AT, et al. Autologous fibrin matrices: a potential source of biological mediators that modulate tendon cell activities. Journal of biomedical materials research. Part A. 2006;77:285-93.

99. Sanchez M, Anitua E, Azofra J, Prado R, Muruzabal F, Andia I. Ligamentization of tendon grafts treated with an endogenous preparation rich in growth factors: gross morphology and histology. Arthroscopy : the journal of arthroscopic & related surgery : official publication of the Arthroscopy Association of North America and the International Arthroscopy Association. 2010;26:470-80.

100. Anitua E, Sanchez M, Merayo-Lloves J, De la Fuente M, Muruzabal F, Orive G. Plasma rich in growth factors (PRGF-Endoret) stimulates proliferation and migration of primary keratocytes and conjunctival fibroblasts and inhibits and reverts TGF-beta1-Induced myodifferentiation. Investigative ophthalmology & visual science. 2011;52:6066-73

CHAPTER 8

A New Approach to Treat Joint Injuries: Combination of Intra-Articular and Intraosseous Injections of Platelet Rich Plasma

AUTHORS

Sánchez M.[1,2], Anitua E.[3,4,5], Delgado D.[2], Sanchez P.[2], Prado R.[3], Prosper F.[6,7], Fiz N.[1], Padilla S.[3,4,5]

[1] Arthroscopic Surgery Unit, Hospital Vithas San Jose, Vitoria-Gasteiz, Spain
[2] Advanced Biological therapy Unit, Hospital Vithas San José, Vitoria-Gasteiz, Spain
[3] BTI-Biotechnology Institute, Vitoria, Spain
[4] Eduardo Anitua Foundation for Biomedical Research. Vitoria-Gasteiz, Spain
[5] University Institute for Regenerative Medicine and Oral Implantology (UIRMI) from the University of Basque Country (UPV/EHU)
[6] Cell Therapy Program, Foundation for Applied Medical Research, University of Navarra, Spain.
[7] Hematology and Cell Therapy Department, Clínica Universidad de Navarra, University of Navarra, Spain.

SUMMARY

This chapter deals with the scientific rationale which underpins a new procedure for the treatment of severe knee osteoarthritis, namely, a combination of intra-articular and intraosseous injections of Platelet Rich Plasma. Intraarticular infiltration of platelet rich plasma is a promising treatment for knee osteoarthritis, but it still has some therapeutic limitations in severe osteoarthritis. Intraosseous infiltration delivers platelet rich plasma into the subchondral bone, acting on this tissue and consequently on cartilage-bone communication. Thus, this technique involves a new route of delivering platelet rich plasma that could be applied not only for severe osteoarthritis but also for other joint pathologies in which the subchondral bone is critical in its etiology such as osteonecrosis, osteochondral lesions, and bone marrow lesions.

This chapter explores some of the recent insights and observations concerning the involvement of subchondral bone in the pathophysiology of osteoarthritis and additionally we will describe a new technique of platelet rich plasma infiltration for the treatment of severe knee osteoarthritis.

E. Anitua et al. (eds.), *Platelet Rich Plasma in Orthopaedics and Sports Medicine*,
https://doi.org/10.1007/978-3-319-63730-3_8

1. INTRODUCTION

Subchondral bone has always been present in the equation of the cartilage repair process and OA[1-3] but it has suffered neglect for decades as an important player in the etiopathogenesis of OA[3,4]. There is an increasingly recognized communication between the subchondral bone and articular cartilage based on the changes that the subchondral bone undergoes in patients with severe OA, including microcracks and structural defects, vascularization of channels, nerve growth, and a progressive replacement of the subchondral marrow with fibroneurovascular mesenchymal tissue (figure 1)[5-8]. As it is yet to be established precisely which of the joint tissues or structures is the primary driver of knee osteoarthritis (KOA), and therapeutic strategies targeting solely one cell or tissue target may well prove to fail[9], it is advisable that approaches to severe KOA treatment should be aimed at reaching several joint tissues with the objective of reducing joint inflammation, controlling pain, improving joint functionality, and restoring the homeostasis of joint tissues.

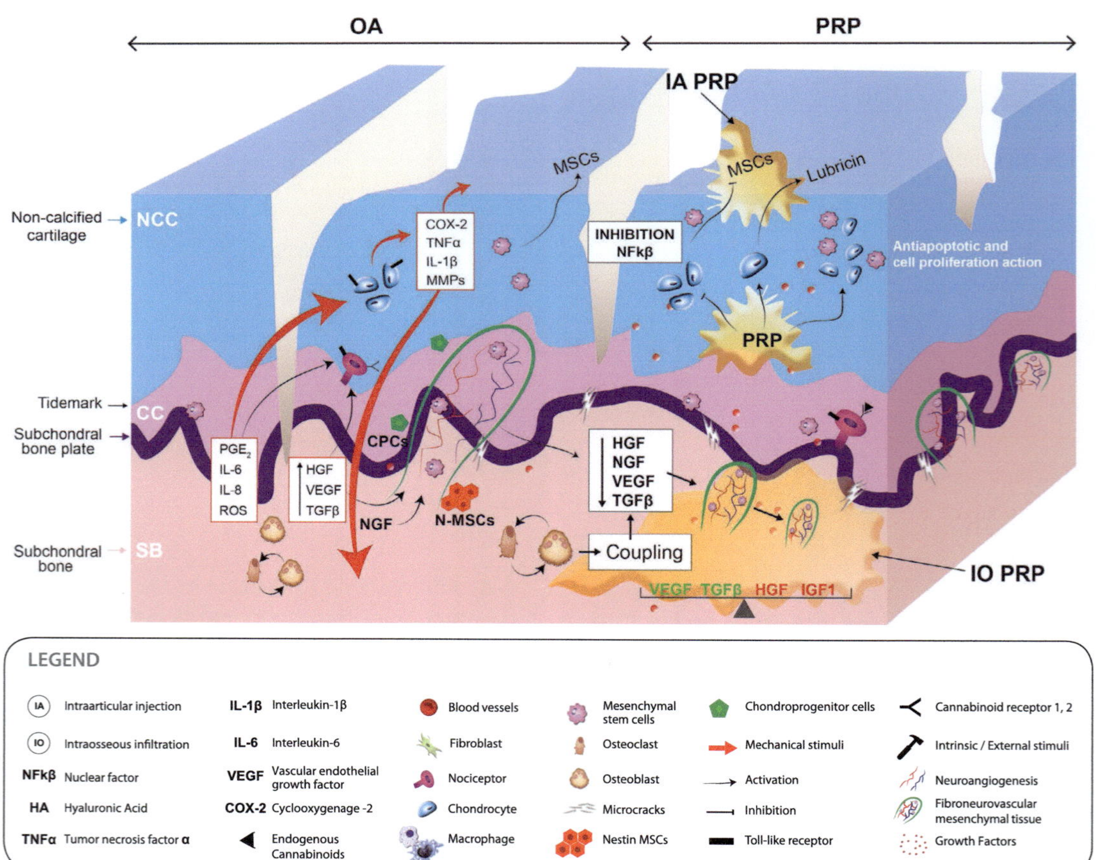

FIG. 1
Targeting the osteoarthritic subchondral bone with Intraosseous infiltration of PRP. This schematic drawing illustrates the outside-in (AC-SB) and inside-out (SB-AC) flow of mediators and cells. SB as a point of egress of morphogens and cells, through the channels and vessels breaching the osteochondral junction, partially recruited by the osteoarthritic synovial fluid 3,7. This cartilage cell invasion might be facilitated by the loss of aggrecans, collagen II cleavage, and disruption of water tissue distribution 8 of the articular cartilage as well as by the secretion by MSCs of fibrinolytic enzymes 22. The excessive presence of TGFB1 and VEGF in OA subchondral bone 3, 7 could be a driving factor for changes in osteoblast-osteoclast coupling thereby leading to a bone remodelling imbalance 28, 30, 38, NGF expression, and fibroneurovascular growth, changes that additionally might well contribute to overlying cartilage degradation, pain, and an osteoarthritic joint 25, 33, 47, 48, 49. (Reprinted with permission from Sánchez, M. et al.)[16]

In recent years, several clinical trials using intra-articular infiltrations of plasma rich in growth factors have shown promising results[10-14] ; however, there are still some concerns about whether this form of administration is able to reach the deeper layers of the cartilage and subchondral bone, thereby possibly limiting the growth factors therapeutic potential especially in severe osteoarthritis[11,15].

In light of recent studies reporting the importance of subchondral bone in the pathogenesis of osteoarthritis and cartilage-subchondral bone communication[16,17] we proposed a combination of intra-articular and intraosseous injections to treat severe osteoarthritis[18] In so doing, it is possible to expand the effective range of PRPs by not only acting on the subchondral bone and consequently on its cartilage communications, but also on mesenchymal stem cells, to modulate the affected tissue regeneration[19,20].

This chapter is based on two manuscripts published recently[16,18] an it will explore some of the recent insights and observations concerning the involvement of subchondral bone in the pathophysiology of osteoarthritis.

2. THE ROLE OF SUBCHONDRAL BONE (SB) IN PATHOPHYSIOLOGY AND CLINICAL SYMPTOMS OF OSTEOARTHRITIS

2.1. The subchondral bone-articular cartilage functional unit

Subchondral bone has always been present in the equation of OA pathogenesis, and more than 40 years ago, partially inspired by the 1827 proposal by surgeon Dr. P.P. Physick on the SB as an effective shock absorber, Radin et al[2,21] suggested a cause-effect connection among mechanical loading, subchondral bone sclerosis, and osteoarthritis. Subchondral bone is the layer of bone which lies immediately below the calcified cartilage (figure 1)[22], and consists of two different anatomical entities, one called subchondral or cortical plate which is nonporous and poorly vascularized cortical bone, and the SB which contains bone marrow (fatty) and trabecular bone[23,24]. Together with the articular cartilage (AC), it forms the osteochondral functional unit, which undergoes mechanical stresses that trigger adaptive cell responses and establish a crosstalk among them to adjust their architecture to ongoing physical and biochemical challenges[7,25]. In the functionality of the osteochondral unit, articular cartilage provides an elastic, gliding, smooth frictionless surface, while subchondral bone, a very low viscoelastic structure, together with periarticular muscles and ligaments, acts as shock absorber structures, accounting for 30% and 50% of the total absorbing energy and only 1-3% for the AC[23,26]. Besides the pivotal shock absorbing function, SB is a source of vessels whose perfusion rate enables an important nutritional route for AC but any damage to this microvasculature affects venous bony circulation thereby altering cartilage and chondrocyte function[5,23,27].

2.2. SB turnover and structural changes in OA

The osteochondral unit in an OA joint undergoes several structural changes including loss of articular cartilage, development of inflamed synovium, calcified cartilage thickening and tidemark duplication, undermineralization of bone, sclerosis and stiffness of SB, bone marrow lesions (BMLs), cysts, osteophyte, and a localized bone marrow replacement by fibroneurovascular tissue (figure 1)[5-7,28].

Despite the high turnover of SB in OA, an uncoupling between bone formation and resorption at the same site leads to an increase in bone volume without a concomitant increase in bone mineralization pattern[3,28,29]. This SB sclerosis is characterized by an increase of the osteoid volume, and a decrease of calcium bound to collagen fibre, and is associated with a gain of trabecular thickness, loss of trabecular number, and a trabecular network more separated and less interconnected[29,30]. It has been suggested that sclerotic subchondral bone, localized at subchondral plate, could decrease the load transfer to the underlying bone tissue leading to osteoporotic-like changes[5]. Moreover, SB can undergo microdamage, such as microcracks and clefts, that modify SB stiffness and reduce the shock-absorbing capacity of SB, thereby making chronic a microdamage context and perpetuating an accelerated bone remodelling, which impairs normal mineralization of bone once it has been deposited, most likely by a modified osteoblastic phenotype[5,24,31]. Magnetic resonance imaging (MRI) has helped to detect subchondral bone marrow edema-like lesions (BMLs), which have been found to be associated with pain and disease progression in KOA[32], and together with bone attrition, are strong indicators of a structural deterioration in knee and hip osteoarthritis[5,33].Several studies conducted in human knee and hip OA paralleling MRI bone marrow edema lesion (BMLs) studies with histological analysis of SB retrieved at the time of joint replacement, revealed microfractures and increased bone remodelling, subchondral ingrowth of fibrovascular tissue and increased vascularity, various types of bone marrow fibrosis[32,34,35] as well as numeric and topographic alterations in native mesenchymal stem cells (MSCs)[33]. These observations were confirmed in rodent models of OA[7,36].The increased activity of osteoclasts in OA cause channels to extend from SB to AC, passing across the calcified tissues into the noncalcified articular cartilage[25]. The neurovascular invasion of those new-formed channels is accompanied by a new fibroneurovascular mesenchymal tissue within the channel along with cells such as macrophages, osteoclasts, osteoblasts, and endothelial cells, which interact to stimulate angiogenesis and growth of sympathetic and sensory nerves[7] and reach the noncalcified cartilage (figure 1), a finding which has been supported by animal models of OA[7].

2.3. Cellular interactions and molecular crosstalk in osteochondral unit in OA

There is now good evidence that even in a non-diseased joint, naturally occurring pores and holes enable communication between SB and AC via diffusion of small molecules[6,37,38]. This communication may be exacerbated by structural changes seen early in the osteochondral unit in OA.The increased osteoclastic activity in the OA subchondral plate 28 may increase the permeability of bone-cartilage interface by inducing channel formation in the tidemark, in addition to the existent aberrant fibroneurovascular tissue and vasculature, and mechanical stress-induced microcracks[7,24,39]. Reinforcing this view, Pan et al.[37] have demonstrated the diffusion of small-size molecules between SB and AC by utilizing the FLIP method (Imaging method based on fluorescence loss, which quantifies diffusivity of small molecules) with sodium fluorescein in the distal femur of mice, and this communication is greatly increased in osteoarthritic joints of the mice model[6]. Therefore, the presence of these connections enables an elevated crosstalk among chondrocytes, osteoblasts, osteoclasts and MSCs through biological factors and signalling pathways (figure 1).

Several in vitro and in vivo studies have demonstrated that osteoblasts from sclerotic subchondral bone show an altered phenotype. In an in vitro study, Westacott et al 40 reported that osteoblasts in OA-affected bone exhibited a different phenotype, whose activity can degrade articular cartilage in vitro. Supporting this observation, Hilial et al.[41] reported that osteoblasts from OA subchondral bone have an abnormal metabolism with increased levels of PGE2 and TGFβ (figure 1). Using a co-culture model of OA subchondral bone osteoblasts with chondrocytes, Sanchez et al reported that osteoblasts induced a catabolic response of chondrocytes including a decrease in aggrecan, type II collagen and SOX-9, and an increase of MMP-3 and MMP-13 among other mediators[42,43]. Moreover, osteoblasts from scletoric subcondral bone have an elevated TGFβ expression[29] and under cyclical compression express proangiogenic factors such as VEGF,FGF, and IL-8[44]. Hepatocyte growth factor (HGF) is a pleiotropic morphogen present in articular cartilage but produced by osteoarthritic subchondral bone osteoblats, osteoclasts, and MSCs[45-47], with likely implications in both the chondrocyte anabolic state and the proliferation of an invasive fibroneurovascular tissue in SB[5,7,47], the latter when an uncoupling osteoclast-osteoblast activity may lead to an overexpression of HGF (figure 1)[45]. The excessive presence of TGFB1 and VEGF in OA subchondral bone likely stemmed from a dysregulated osteocyte[7,48] could be a driving factor for changes in osteoblast-osteoclast coupling thereby leading to a bone remodelling imbalance[5,30], NGF expression[49], and fibroneurovascular growth changes that additionally might well contribute to overlying cartilage degradation[30,48], pain[7,24,25] and an osteoarthritic joint[30,48]. In a recent study, Zhen et al. showed that by inhibiting TGF-β signalling in a specific population of MSCs present at the SB (Nestin positive MSCs), the severity of OA was reduced, a change associated with improvement of bone parameters, cartilage structure and joint function without affecting TGFB signalling in AC[48]. Moreover, in a recent study, Campbell et al (2016) reported functional and gene expression perturbations in native MSCs which could lead to further damage escalation[33]. These findings are in accordance with previous studies that have shown that the decrease of MSCs in the synovial fluid, in low degree OA, suggests clinical improvement[50]. MSCs from osteoarthritic bone marrow have been reported to be substantially reduced in yield and proliferative activity besides showing a weakened chondrogenic and adipogenic activity and increased osteogenic activity[51]. However, in vitro studies indicate that the inclusion of growth factors, as a supplementary culture medium, can be beneficial in reverting their chondrogenic activity[52].

2.4. Subchondral bone as a tissue target in OA treatment

The realization of the biological and mechanical connection between AC and SB has lead to numerous in vivo animal studies that have shown that targeting SB with some drugs can have protective structural effects on cartilage[4]. Blocking or limiting the bone remodelling with alendronate[53], zoledronic acid[54] or improving the microstructure and quality of subchondral bone in osteoarthritic and osteoporotic rabbits with parathyroid hormone[4], may prevent cartilage degradation and OA progression. Moreover, Sagar et al[55] reported a reduction in pain behaviour after a subcutaneous treatment with osteoprotegerin in a monosodium iodoacetate (MIA) rat model of OA pain, and Pelletier et al[56] demonstrated that an oral strontium ranelate treatment in an experimental osteoarthritic dog model reduced the progression of structural changes including the subchondral bone. Despite the fact that the translation of these promising observations in preclinical research to human clinical trials has often failed, as indicated by a recent metaanalysis of clinical trial with risedronate in knee osteoarthritis[57], recent clinical trials are raising expectations. For instance, using zoledronic in patients with clinical KOA associated with bone marrow lesions (BMLs) assessed by MRI, Laslett et al[58] reported a beneficial effect on pain and on BML evolution at 6 months. In participants from the osteoarthritis initiative, Laslett et al.[59] demonstrated significant pain reduction during the first 3 years of treatment with biphosphonates. Two more clinical trials have shown positive structural effects of strontium ranelate on KOA, one improving the joint space narrowing 60 and the other reducing the loss of cartilage volumes concurrent with the decrease of BMLs at 3 years of follow up[61].

Infiltrations of platelet rich plasma (PRP) into the bone marrow cavity of femur of young and old ovariectomized-SAMP8 age-related osteoporotic female mice have been reported to up-regulate osteogenesis and down-regulate adipogenesis[62]. The increase of fat tissue mass in BM is correlated with decreased bone mineralization in aged SAMPS8 mice[62,63], bone demineralization that occurs in osteoarthritic subchondral bone together with cysts[24]. Moreover, improvement of bone mineral density in PRP-treated osteoporotic mice concurred with both histological sections of the bone samples showing more trabecular bone areas and more intense calcium staining and a suppression of bone resorption process as evidenced by the decrease of RANKL transcript[62]. In a trial on 13 healthy volunteers, Philippart et al[64] reported fatigue on the first day as the only clinical adverse effect after a self-stimulation of BM of the iliac crest by injected autologous platelet rich plasma[64]. Supporting these findings, Figure 2 shows the histological analysis of cartilage and SB from a patient suffering from severe KOA who underwent intraosseous infiltrations of PRGF. Eight months later, the patient had not improved clinically and underwent a knee replacement. During the surgery, we took this sample of cartilage and subchondral bone from the femoral condyle in which 5cc of PRGF had been infiltrated intraosseously. Part of the biopsy showed a good gross appearance, with pearly areas similar to the original hyaline cartilage, though histological study revealed a fibrocartilage repair tissue. Another area showed nearly exposed bone.

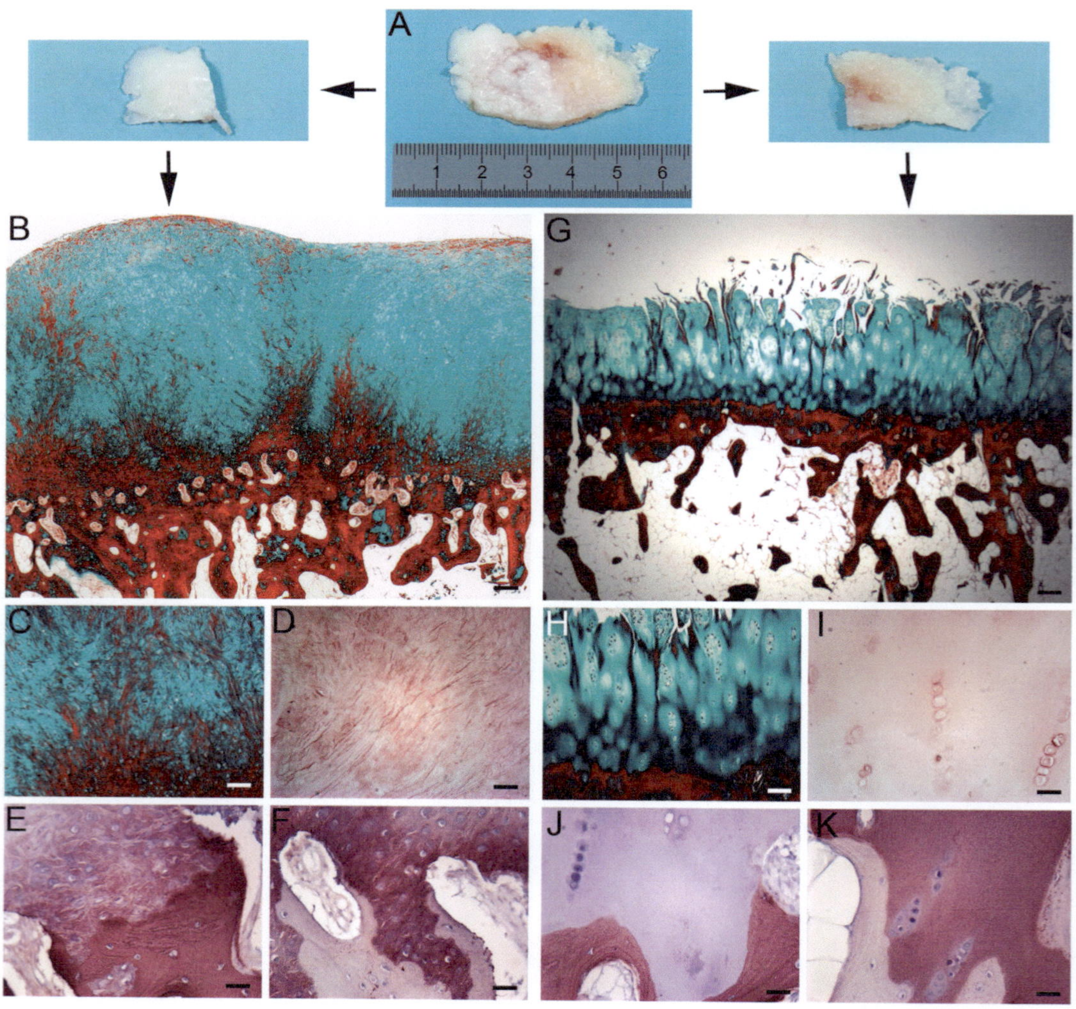

FIG. 2
Fibrocartilage repair tissue after intraosseus PRGF infiltrations in the treatment of human knee osteoarthritis: a histological study. (A) Macroscopic morphology of the sample. The sample was divided into two pieces. The fragment on the left corresponds to fibrocartilage repair tissue (B to F) while the right-hand fragment shows osteoarthritic cartilage (G to K). B and G show panoramic images of the sample (Masson's trichrome staining). In photomicrographs C and H, details of the structure of articular cartilage are observed (Masson's trichrome staining). The presence of elastic fibres is demonstrated by Orcein staining (D and I). These fibres can be seen in D, while they are absent in I. An immunohistochemical study was performed to detect the presence of type I (E and J) and type II (F and K) collagen. In all samples (E to K), both subchondral bone (always positive for type I and negative for type II collagens) and cartilage are observed. In fibrocartilage (E and F) both types of reactivity are observed, while in the degenerated cartilage, only type II collagen positivity is shown (K). Histologically, the pearly area (the left-hand side of the sample) is fibrocartilage repair tissue, while the right-hand side of the sample displays an osteoarthritic area with loss of cartilage surface integrity. (Reprinted with permission from Sánchez, M. et al.)[16]

3. INTRAOSSEOUS INFILTRATIONS OF PLASMA RICH IN GROWTH FACTORS

In light of the aforementioned research and others not mentioned here due to space limitation, and the significant clinical improvement obtained in some but not all patients with KOA treated with intraarticular infiltrations of PRP[11,13,14,65] our group arrived at the strategy of combining another drug delivery route, namely, the intraosseous infiltrations combined with intraarticular infiltrations of PRP[18-20,66,67]. (Figure 3)

The procedure is carried out in the operating room under a 4-5 degree of sedation of the patient. In addition, local anesthesia is conducted into the periosteum of condyle and tibial plateau by injecting 2mL of 2% mepivacaine. Intraosseous infiltrations are performed with a 13G trocar used

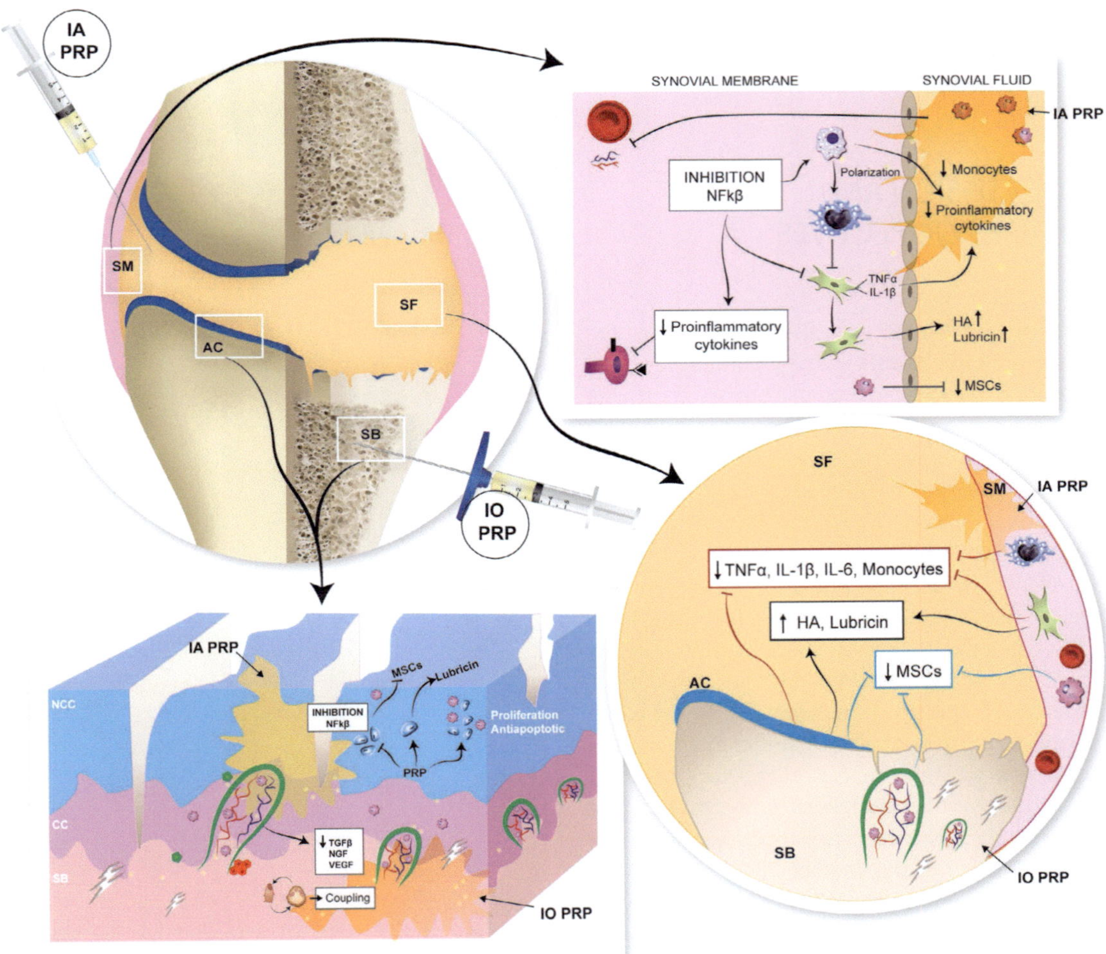

FIG. 3
Depiction of a new strategy to treat severe knee OA by targeting different knee joint structures such as synovial membrane (SM), synovial fluid (SF), articular cartilage (AC), noncalcified cartilage (NCC) and calcified cartilage (CC), and subchondral bone (SB) with intra-articular injections (IA) and intraosseous infiltrations (IO) of platelet rich plasma (PRP). This procedure reduces pain and mesenchymal stem cells (MSC) in SF, besides significantly improving knee joint function of patients with severe OA (Reprinted with permission from Sánchez, M. et al.)[19]

for bone biopsy, and the control of trocar placement is facilitated using a fluoroscope (Figure 4, 5, and 6)[18]. The first treatment includes one PRP intraarticular infiltration and two PRP intraosseous infiltrations (in femoral condyle and tibial plateau).Two more weekly intraarticular infiltrations are performed. The group of Sanchez et al. have found after a 6 month follow-up, a significant pain reduction and decrease of MSC and CFU-F in synovial fluid with no adverse effects[19,20,66]. We have been performing intraosseous infiltrations of PRGF since 2003 applying them regularly at the condyle and tibial tunnels in the arthroscopic reconstruction of anterior cruciate ligament, and in osteochondral injuries and osteonecrosis of the hip and knee[68].

4. DISCUSSION AND FUTURE PERSPECTIVES

Intraarticular delivery is an alternative modality to convey PRP in patients with KOA and it has been shown to be safe and efficacious in improving clinical symptoms[11,13,65]. This route of drug delivery reaches the synovial membrane (SM) and the AC, which is sometimes inefficiently targeted by systemic drug delivery. Intraarticular delivery circumvents systemic toxicity and its side effects, offers an excellent bioavailability, and does not present molecular size limitation, in contrast to the systemically delivered molecules entering the joint via capillaries of the subsynovium[69,70]. Nevertheless, intraarticular therapy faces other challenges when treating chronic nonsystemic sterile-inflammatory conditions as in the case of KOA. One significant challenge is a short joint dwell time of drugs, since the lymphatic drainage clears proteins in a few hours. This is not the case of PRGF, since it acts as a dynamic liquid scaffold with a fibrin network from where GFs are gradually released into the tissue[71,72]. Moreover, the increasingly recognized role of SB in the pathophysiology of OA[3,7,24,28] might make the intraarticular route insufficient to tackle all the joint tissues involved in KOA.

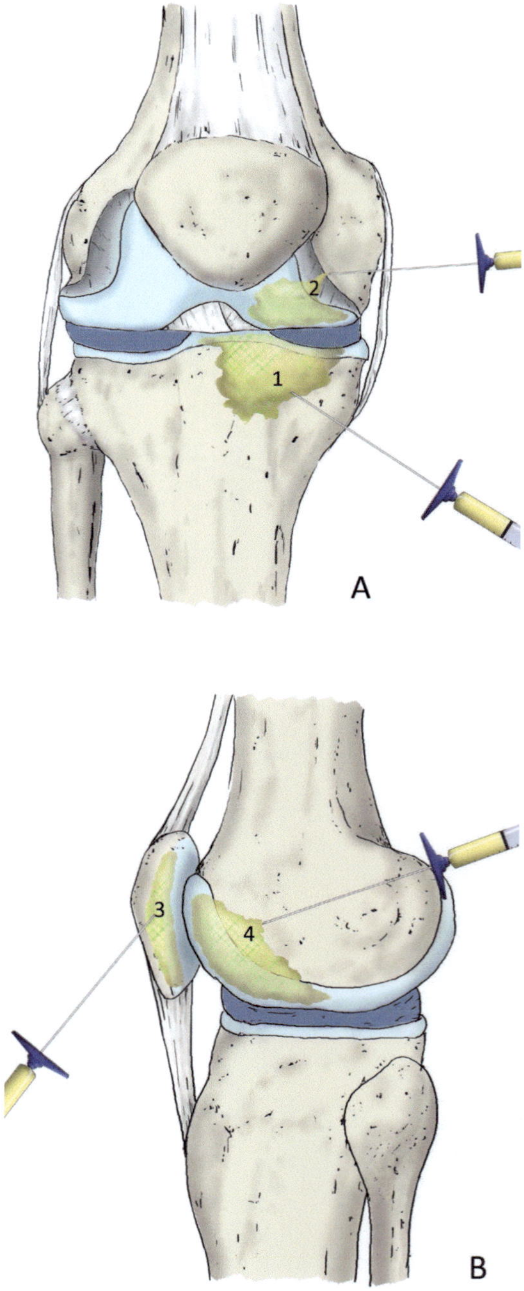

FIG. 4
(A) The platelet-rich plasma (PRP) intraosseous infiltration of a knee with severe femorotibial osteoarthritis is performed into the medial tibial plateau (1) and medial femoral condyle (2). (B) If the patient presents with femoropatellar osteoarthritis, the approach is external and the patella (3) and trochlea (4) are infiltrated. Before these intraosseous injections are performed, conventional knee intraarticular infiltration of PRP is conducted. (Reprinted with permission from Sánchez, M. et al.) [18]

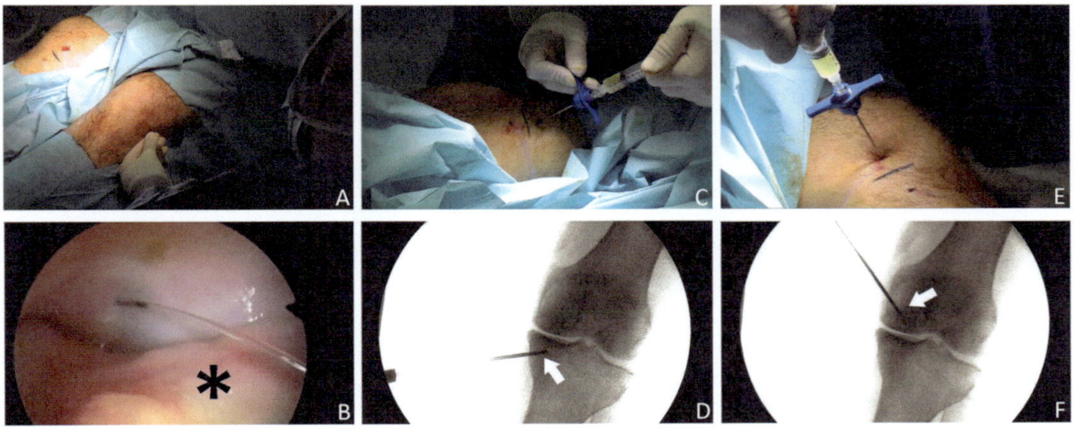

FIG. 5
After the patient is positioned supine on the operating room table, (A) intra-articular infiltration is performed into the joint through the external patellar wing, centred in the central region of the patella in the craniocaudal plane; (B) the infiltration is directed into the midpoint area of the femoropatellar region using an external approach and preventing infiltration into the synovial membrane, (asterisk). (C, D) Intraosseous tibial plateau infiltration is conducted into the medial tibial plateau, just to its middle area. The arrow indicates the trocar. (E, F). With respect to intraosseous femoral condyle infiltration, a trocar (arrow) is applied to the thickness of the medial femoral condyle, as far as the middle area of the medial condyle. (Reprinted with permission from Sánchez, M. et al.) [18]

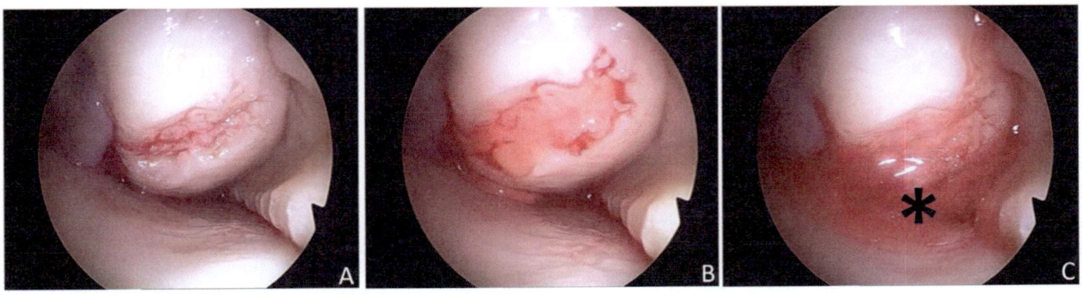

FIG. 6
(A) Communications between cartilage and subchondral bone are more pronounced in degenerated cartilage. (B) The platelet-rich plasma infiltrated into subchondral bone flows through the degenerated zones, and because of its viscous consistency, (C) it remains in the area, creating a matrix (asterisk). (Reprinted with permission from Sánchez, M. et al.) [18]

Intraosseous delivery strategy for local, prolonged, and sustainable release of GFs has been proven to be efficacious in some musculoskeletal pathology, non-union fractures, osteoporosis, and bone fracture healing among them[73,74]. Over the past 30 years, surgical experience in cartilage defect has revealed that only when the subchondral bone is involved through bone marrow stimulating procedures such as transcortical Pridie drilling and microfractures, is a temporary functional fibrocartilage tissue synthesized, with no serious adverse effect reported[75]. There is good in vitro and in vivo evidence that events in the subchondral bone concur with and have a direct effect on the overlying articular cartilage[4,27,29,76]. Moreover, although the titles and much of the text of Liu et al[63] and Philippart et al[64] papers are not focused on osteoarthitis, these studies shed important light on the role that intraosseous infiltrations of PRGF might play in subchondral bone homeostasis by targeting both osteoblast-osteoclast coupling and mesenchymal stem cell responses, as well as in its safety.

The combination of intra-articular and intraosseous injections of PRP is an in situ local biological "joint-centric" approach to treat severe KOA addresses the SM, SF and superficial zone of AC by intraarticular injections of PRGF, and deep zones of AC and SB through PRGF intraosseous infiltrations (figure 3)[18-20].These PRGF infiltrations convey a mimetic biomaterial embedded with a pool of growth factors acting as a smart scaffold[77] which might sustain a gradual delivery of growth factors at the dysfunctional and deregulated tissues as a niche therapy. Rebuilding a physiological-homeostatic network at knee organ failure tissue level, as is the case of severe knee OA, must be an orderly process, which entails a daunting therapeutic task. Our hypothesis is that the concurrent presence and a balanced ratio between platelet-secreted TGFB-1 and VEGF, and plasma growth factors such as IGF-1 and HGF[78-81], all conveyed by PRGF intraosseous infiltrations, might reduce or buffer the excess of TGFB in SB and restore HGF activity synthesized by subchondral bone cells. This modulatory effect of PRGF on TGFB-1 signaling pathway might shrink the fibroneurovascular tissue that replaces the bone marrow of OA subchondral bone, an explanation which parallels the antifibrotic mechanism already reported to be exerted by PRP on several cell phenotypes[79-81]. This new reestablished homeostatic balance between TGFB1 and HGF[39,48] would reduce the synthesis of NGF, VEGF and other inflammatory mediators thereby contributing as well to modulate the aberrant fibroneurovascular tissue and to alleviate pain and hyperalgesia[82].

In spite of a wealth of preclinical and clinical publications on PRP, many uncertainties remain regarding the ultimate molecular mechanism/s, the variability in its composition mainly due to the presence/absence of leukocytes, the platelet concentration, the donors age, and the manner in which PRPs are applied to the damaged tissues[83]. Moreover, we need to delve into the particular effect of PRP on MSCs in addition to the systemic effect that this procedure might entail since few human studies have been carried out regarding PRP treatments and systemic effects[84,85].

5. CONFLICT OF INTERESTS

The authors declare the following competing financial interest(s): One author is the Scientific Director of and two authors are scientists at BTI Biotechnology Institute, a dental implant company that investigates in the fields of oral implantology and PRGF-Endoret technology.

1. Pridie K, Gordon G. A method of resurfacing osteoarthritic knee joints. Paper presented at: Journal of Bone and Joint Surgery-British Volume1959.

2. Radin EL, Rose RM. Role of subchondral bone in the initiation and progression of cartilage damage. Clinical orthopaedics and related research. 1986:34-40.

3. Lajeunesse D, Reboul P. Subchondral bone in osteoarthritis: a biologic link with articular cartilage leading to abnormal remodeling. Current opinion in rheumatology. 2003;15:628-33.

4. Bellido M, Lugo L, Roman-Blas JA, et al. Improving subchondral bone integrity reduces progression of cartilage damage in experimental osteoarthritis preceded by osteoporosis. Osteoarthritis and cartilage / OARS, Osteoarthritis Research Society. 2011;19:1228-36.

5. Lajeunesse D. Subchondral bone involvement in the pathophysiology of osteoarthritis. Understanding Osteoarthritis from Bench to Bedside. 2011:69-83.

6. Pan J, Wang B, Li W, et al. Elevated cross-talk between subchondral bone and cartilage in osteoarthritic joints. Bone. 2012;51:212-7.

7. Suri S, Walsh DA. Osteochondral alterations in osteoarthritis. Bone. 2012;51:204-11.

8. Stolz M, Gottardi R, Raiteri R, et al. Early detection of aging cartilage and osteoarthritis in mice and patient samples using atomic force microscopy. Nat Nanotechnol. 2009;4:186-92.

9. Martel-Pelletier J, Wildi LM, Pelletier JP. Future therapeutics for osteoarthritis. Bone. 2012;51:297-311.

10. Sanchez M, Guadilla J, Fiz N, Andia I. Ultrasound-guided platelet-rich plasma injections for the treatment of osteoarthritis of the hip. Rheumatology (Oxford). 2012;51:144-50.

11. Sanchez M, Fiz N, Azofra J, et al. A randomized clinical trial evaluating plasma rich in growth factors (PRGF-Endoret) versus hyaluronic acid in the short-term treatment of symptomatic knee osteoarthritis. Arthroscopy : the journal of arthroscopic & related surgery : official publication of the Arthroscopy Association of North America and the International Arthroscopy Association. 2012;28:1070-8.

12. Kon E, Filardo G, Di Martino A, Marcacci M. Platelet-rich plasma (PRP) to treat sports injuries: evidence to support its use. Knee surgery, sports traumatology, arthroscopy : official journal of the ESSKA. 2011;19:516-27.

13. Vaquerizo V, Plasencia MA, Arribas I, et al. Comparison of intra-articular injections of plasma rich in growth factors (PRGF-Endoret) versus Durolane hyaluronic acid in the treatment of patients with symptomatic osteoarthritis: a randomized controlled trial. Arthroscopy : the journal of arthroscopic & related surgery : official publication of the Arthroscopy Association of North America and the International Arthroscopy Association. 2013;29:1635-43.

14. Wang-Saegusa A, Cugat R, Ares O, Seijas R, Cusco X, Garcia-Balletbo M. Infiltration of plasma rich in growth factors for osteoarthritis of the knee short-term effects on function and quality of life. Archives of orthopaedic and trauma surgery. 2011;131:311-7.

15. Khoshbin A, Leroux T, Wasserstein D, et al. The efficacy of platelet-rich plasma in the treatment of symptomatic knee osteoarthritis: a systematic review with quantitative synthesis. Arthroscopy : the journal of arthroscopic & related surgery : official publication of the Arthroscopy Association of North America and the International Arthroscopy Association. 2013;29:2037-48.

16. Sanchez M, Anitua E, Delgado D, et al. A new strategy to tackle severe knee osteoarthritis: Combination of intra-articular and intraosseous injections of Platelet Rich Plasma. Expert opinion on biological therapy. 2016;16:627-43.

17. Zhen G, Cao X. Targeting TGFbeta signaling in subchondral bone and articular cartilage homeostasis. Trends in pharmacological sciences. 2014;35:227-36.

18. Sanchez M, Fiz N, Guadilla J, et al. Intraosseous infiltration of platelet-rich plasma for severe knee osteoarthritis. Arthrosc Tech. 2014;3:e713-7.

19. Sánchez M, Delgado D, Sánchez P, et al. Combination of Intra-Articular and Intraosseous Injections of Platelet Rich Plasma for Severe Knee Osteoarthritis: A Pilot Study. BioMed research international. 2016;2016.

20. Muinos-Lopez E, Delgado D, Sanchez P, et al. Modulation of Synovial Fluid-Derived Mesenchymal Stem Cells by Intra-Articular and Intraosseous Platelet Rich Plasma Administration. Stem cells international. 2016;2016:1247950.

21. Radin EL, Paul IL, Rose RM. Role of mechanical factors in pathogenesis of primary osteoarthritis. Lancet. 1972;1:519-22.

22. Neuss S, Schneider RK, Tietze L, Knuchel R, Jahnen-Dechent W. Secretion of fibrinolytic enzymes facilitates human mesenchymal stem cell invasion into fibrin clots. Cells, tissues, organs. 2010;191:36-46.

23. Imhof H, Sulzbacher I, Grampp S, Czerny C, Youssefzadeh S, Kainberger F. Subchondral bone and cartilage disease: a rediscovered functional unit. Invest Radiol. 2000;35:581-8.

24. Burr DB, Gallant MA. Bone remodelling in osteoarthritis. Nature reviews. Rheumatology. 2012;8:665-73.

25. Mapp PI, Walsh DA. Mechanisms and targets of angiogenesis and nerve growth in osteoarthritis. Nature reviews. Rheumatology. 2012;8:390-8.

26. Brandt KD, Radin EL, Dieppe PA, van de Putte L. Yet more evidence that osteoarthritis is not a cartilage disease. Annals of the rheumatic diseases. 2006;65:1261-4.

27. Malinin T, Ouellette EA. Articular cartilage nutrition is mediated by subchondral bone: a long-term autograft study in baboons. Osteoarthritis and cartilage / OARS, Osteoarthritis Research Society. 2000;8:483-91.

28. Karsdal MA, Bay-Jensen AC, Lories RJ, et al. The coupling of bone and cartilage turnover in osteoarthritis: opportunities for bone antiresorptives and anabolics as potential treatments? Annals of the rheumatic diseases. 2014;73:336-48.

29. Henrotin Y, Pesesse L, Sanchez C. Subchondral bone and osteoarthritis: biological and cellular aspects. Osteoporosis international : a journal established as result of cooperation between the European Foundation for Osteoporosis and the National Osteoporosis Foundation of the USA. 2012;23 Suppl 8:S847-51.

30. Zhao W, Wang T, Luo Q, et al. Cartilage degeneration and excessive subchondral bone formation in spontaneous osteoarthritis involves altered TGF-β signaling. Journal of Orthopaedic Research. 2015;DOI:10.1002/jor.23079.

31. Burr DB, Radin EL. Microfractures and microcracks in subchondral bone: are they relevant to osteoarthrosis? Rheum Dis Clin North Am. 2003;29:675-85.

32. Felson DT, Chaisson CE, Hill CL, et al. The association of bone marrow lesions with pain in knee osteoarthritis. Annals of internal medicine. 2001;134:541-9.

33. Campbell TM, Churchman SM, Gomez A, et al. Mesenchymal Stem Cell Alterations in Bone Marrow Lesions in Patients With Hip Osteoarthritis. Arthritis Rheumatol. 2016;68:1648-59.

34. Taljanovic MS, Graham AR, Benjamin JB, et al. Bone marrow edema pattern in advanced hip osteoarthritis: quantitative assessment with magnetic resonance imaging and correlation with clinical examination, radiographic findings, and histopathology. Skeletal Radiol. 2008;37:423-31.

35. Hunter DJ, Gerstenfeld L, Bishop G, et al. Bone marrow lesions from osteoarthritis knees are characterized by sclerotic bone that is less well mineralized. Arthritis research & therapy. 2009;11:R11.

36. Mapp PI, Avery PS, McWilliams DF, et al. Angiogenesis in two animal models of osteoarthritis. Osteoarthritis and cartilage / OARS, Osteoarthritis Research Society. 2008;16:61-9.

37. Pan J, Zhou X, Li W, Novotny JE, Doty SB, Wang L. In situ measurement of transport between subchondral bone and articular cartilage. Journal of orthopaedic research : official publication of the Orthopaedic Research Society. 2009;27:1347-52.

38. Lyons TJ, McClure SF, Stoddart RW, McClure J. The normal human chondro-osseous junctional region: evidence for contact of uncalcified cartilage with subchondral bone and marrow spaces. BMC Musculoskelet Disord. 2006;7:52.

39. Tat SK, Lajeunesse D, Pelletier J-P, Martel-Pelletier J. Targeting subchondral bone for treating osteoarthritis: what is the evidence? Best Practice & Research Clinical Rheumatology. 2010;24:51-70.

40. Westacott CI, Webb GR, Warnock MG, Sims JV, Elson CJ. Alteration of cartilage metabolism by cells from osteoarthritic bone. Arthritis and rheumatism. 1997;40:1282-91.

41. Hilal G, Martel-Pelletier J, Pelletier JP, Ranger P, Lajeunesse D. Osteoblast-like cells from human subchondral osteoarthritic bone demonstrate an altered phenotype in vitro: possible role in subchondral bone sclerosis. Arthritis and rheumatism. 1998;41:891-9.

42. Sanchez C, Deberg MA, Piccardi N, Msika P, Reginster JY, Henrotin YE. Osteoblasts from the sclerotic subchondral bone downregulate aggrecan but upregulate metalloproteinases expression by chondrocytes. This effect is mimicked by interleukin-6, -1beta and oncostatin M pre-treated non-sclerotic osteoblasts. Osteoarthritis and cartilage / OARS, Osteoarthritis Research Society. 2005;13:979-87.

43. Sanchez C, Deberg MA, Piccardi N, Msika P, Reginster JY, Henrotin YE. Subchondral bone osteoblasts induce phenotypic changes in human osteoarthritic chondrocytes. Osteoarthritis and cartilage / OARS, Osteoarthritis Research Society. 2005;13:988-97.

44. Sanchez C, Pesesse L, Gabay O, et al. Regulation of subchondral bone osteoblast metabolism by cyclic compression. Arthritis and rheumatism. 2012;64:1193-203.

45. Grano M, Galimi F, Zambonin G, et al. Hepatocyte growth factor is a coupling factor for osteoclasts and osteoblasts in vitro. Proceedings of the National Academy of Sciences of the United States of America. 1996;93:7644-8.

46. Stella MC, Comoglio PM. HGF: a multifunctional growth factor controlling cell scattering. The international journal of biochemistry & cell biology. 1999;31:1357-62.

47. Guevremont M, Martel-Pelletier J, Massicotte F, et al. Human adult chondrocytes express hepatocyte growth factor (HGF) isoforms but not HgF: potential implication of osteoblasts on the presence of HGF in cartilage. Journal of bone and mineral research : the official journal of the American Society for Bone and Mineral Research. 2003;18:1073-81.

48. Zhen G, Wen C, Jia X, et al. Inhibition of TGF-beta signaling in mesenchymal stem cells of subchondral bone attenuates osteoarthritis. Nature medicine. 2013;19:704-12.

49. Davidson EB, van Caam A, Vitters E, et al. TGF-β is a potent inducer of Nerve Growth Factor in articular cartilage via the ALK5-Smad2/3 pathway. Potential role in OA related pain? Osteoarthritis and Cartilage. 2015;23:478-86.

50. Sekiya I, Ojima M, Suzuki S, et al. Human mesenchymal stem cells in synovial fluid increase in the knee with degenerated cartilage and osteoarthritis. Journal of orthopaedic research : official publication of the Orthopaedic Research Society. 2012;30:943-9.

51. Barry F, Murphy M. Mesenchymal stem cells in joint disease and repair. Nature reviews. Rheumatology. 2013;9:584-94.

52. Scharstuhl A, Schewe B, Benz K, Gaissmaier C, Buhring HJ, Stoop R. Chondrogenic potential of human adult mesenchymal stem cells is independent of age or osteoarthritis etiology. Stem cells. 2007;25:3244-51.

53. Hayami T, Pickarski M, Wesolowski GA, et al. The role of subchondral bone remodeling in osteoarthritis: reduction of cartilage degeneration and prevention of osteophyte formation by alendronate in the rat anterior cruciate ligament transection model. Arthritis and rheumatism. 2004;50:1193-206.

54. Lampropoulou-Adamidou K, Dontas I, Stathopoulos IP, et al. Chondroprotective effect of high-dose zoledronic acid: An experimental study in a rabbit model of osteoarthritis. Journal of orthopaedic research : official publication of the Orthopaedic Research Society. 2014;32:1646-51.

55. Sagar DR, Ashraf S, Xu L, et al. Osteoprotegerin reduces the development of pain behaviour and joint pathology in a model of osteoarthritis. Annals of the rheumatic diseases. 2014;73:1558-65.

56. Pelletier JP, Kapoor M, Fahmi H, et al. Strontium ranelate reduces the progression of experimental dog osteoarthritis by inhibiting the expression of key proteases in cartilage and of IL-1beta in the synovium. Annals of the rheumatic diseases. 2013;72:250-7.

57. Davis AJ, Smith TO, Hing CB, Sofat N. Are bisphosphonates effective in the treatment of osteoarthritis pain? A meta-analysis and systematic review. PloS one. 2013;8:e72714.

58. Laslett LL, Dore DA, Quinn SJ, et al. Zoledronic acid reduces knee pain and bone marrow lesions over 1 year: a randomised controlled trial. Annals of the rheumatic diseases. 2012;71:1322-8.

59. Laslett LL, Kingsbury SR, Hensor EM, Bowes MA, Conaghan PG. Effect of bisphosphonate use in patients with symptomatic and radiographic knee osteoarthritis: data from the Osteoarthritis Initiative. Annals of the rheumatic diseases. 2014;73:824-30.

60. Reginster JY, Badurski J, Bellamy N, et al. Efficacy and safety of strontium ranelate in the treatment of knee osteoarthritis: results of a double-blind, randomised placebo-controlled trial. Annals of the rheumatic diseases. 2013;72:179-86.

61. Pelletier JP, Roubille C, Raynauld JP, et al. Disease-modifying effect of strontium ranelate in a subset of patients from the Phase III knee osteoarthritis study SEKOIA using quantitative MRI: reduction in bone marrow lesions protects against cartilage loss. Annals of the rheumatic diseases. 2015;74:422-9.

62. Liu HY, Wu AT, Tsai CY, et al. The balance between adipogenesis and osteogenesis in bone regeneration by platelet-rich plasma for age-related osteoporosis. Biomaterials. 2011;32:6773-80.

63. Liu HY, Huang CF, Lin TC, et al. Delayed animal aging through the recovery of stem cell senescence by platelet rich plasma. Biomaterials. 2014;35:9767-76.

64. Philippart P, Meuleman N, Stamatopoulos B, et al. In vivo production of mesenchymal stromal cells after injection of autologous platelet-rich plasma activated by recombinant human soluble tissue factor in the bone marrow of healthy volunteers. Tissue engineering. Part A. 2014;20:160-70.

65. Filardo G, Kon E, Pereira Ruiz MT, et al. Platelet-rich plasma intra-articular injections for cartilage degeneration and osteoarthritis: single- versus double-spinning approach. Knee surgery, sports traumatology, arthroscopy : official journal of the ESSKA. 2012;20:2082-91.

66. Diego Delgado PS, Emma Muiños, Bruno Paiva, Froilán Granero, Eduardo Anitua, Sabino Padilla, Felipe Prósper, Mikel Sánchez. Phase II Clinical trial of intraosseous platelet rich plasma infiltration for severe knee osteoarthritis: preliminary results at 2 months. 2015. ICRS 2015 Chicago

67. Sanchez M, Anitua E, Azofra J, Andia I, Padilla S, Mujika I. Comparison of surgically repaired Achilles tendon tears using platelet-rich fibrin matrices. The American journal of sports medicine. 2007;35:245-51.

68. Sánchez M, Delgado D, Sánchez P, et al. Platelet Rich Plasma and Knee Surgery. BioMed research international. 2014;2014.

69. Evans CH, Kraus VB, Setton LA. Progress in intra-articular therapy. Nature reviews. Rheumatology. 2014;10:11-22.

70. Kang ML, Im GI. Drug delivery systems for intra-articular treatment of osteoarthritis. Expert Opin Drug Deliv. 2014;11:269-82.

71. Anitua E, Zalduendo MM, Prado R, Alkhraisat MH, Orive G. Morphogen and proinflammatory cytokine release kinetics from PRGF-Endoret fibrin scaffolds: evaluation of the effect of leukocyte inclusion. Journal of biomedical materials research. Part A. 2015;103:1011-20.

72. Martino MM, Briquez PS, Guc E, et al. Growth factors engineered for super-affinity to the extracellular matrix enhance tissue healing. Science. 2014;343:885-8.

73. Sanchez M, Anitua E, Cugat R, et al. Nonunions treated with autologous preparation rich in growth factors. Journal of orthopaedic trauma. 2009;23:52-9.

74. Kyllonen L, D'Este M, Alini M, Eglin D. Local drug delivery for enhancing fracture healing in osteoporotic bone. Acta biomaterialia. 2015;11:412-34.

75. Hunziker EB, Lippuner K, Keel MJ, Shintani N. An educational review of cartilage repair: precepts & practice--myths & misconceptions--progress & prospects. Osteoarthritis and cartilage / OARS, Osteoarthritis Research Society. 2015;23:334-50.

76. Burr DB. The importance of subchondral bone in the progression of osteoarthritis. The Journal of rheumatology. Supplement. 2004;70:77-80.

77. Conboy I, Freimer J, Weisenstein L. 5.526 - Tissue Engineering of Muscle Tissue. In: Ducheyne P, ed. Comprehensive Biomaterials. Oxford: Elsevier; 2011:345-59.

78. Anitua E, Andia I, Sanchez M, et al. Autologous preparations rich in growth factors promote proliferation and induce VEGF and HGF production by human tendon cells in culture. Journal of orthopaedic research : official publication of the Orthopaedic Research Society. 2005;23:281-6.

79. Anitua E, Sanchez M, Merayo-Lloves J, De la Fuente M, Muruzabal F, Orive G. Plasma rich in growth factors (PRGF-Endoret) stimulates proliferation and migration of primary keratocytes and conjunctival fibroblasts and inhibits and reverts TGF-beta1-Induced myodifferentiation. Investigative ophthalmology & visual science. 2011;52:6066-73.

80. Anitua E, Sanchez M, De la Fuente M, Zalduendo MM, Orive G. Plasma rich in growth factors (PRGF-Endoret) stimulates tendon and synovial fibroblasts migration and improves the biological properties of hyaluronic acid. Knee surgery, sports traumatology, arthroscopy : official journal of the ESSKA. 2012;20:1657-65.

81. Assirelli E, Filardo G, Mariani E, et al. Effect of two different preparations of platelet-rich plasma on synoviocytes. Knee surgery, sports traumatology, arthroscopy : official journal of the ESSKA. 2014.

82. Seidel MF, Herguijuela M, Forkert R, Otten U. Nerve growth factor in rheumatic diseases. Seminars in arthritis and rheumatism. 2010;40:109-26.

83. Wasterlain AS, Braun HJ, Dragoo JL. Contents and formulations of platelet-rich plasma. Operative Techniques in Orthopaedics. 2012;22:33-42.

84. Schippinger G, Fankhauser F, Oettl K, Spirk S, Hofmann P. Does single intramuscular application of autologous conditioned plasma influence systemic circulating growth factors? J Sports Sci Med. 2012;11:551-6.

85. Wasterlain AS, Braun HJ, Harris AH, Kim HJ, Dragoo JL. The systemic effects of platelet-rich plasma injection. The American journal of sports medicine. 2013;41:186-93.

CHAPTER 9

Knee Osteoarthritis: One versus Two Cycles of PRGF Infiltrations Treatment

AUTHORS

Vaquerizo V.[1], Ruiz de Castañeda MM.[1]

[1] Department of Orthopaedic Surgery, Príncipe de Asturias University Hospital, Alcalá de Henares, Spain

SUMMARY

Knee Osteoarthritis is a degenerative disease that produces an inflammatory response of the synovial membrane, cartilage and subchondral bone, and consequently produces pain and functional disability. Despite the enormous effort made to seek an early therapeutic intervention aimed at preventing progressive destruction of joint tissues or reversing the initial articular cartilage and bone damage, there is still a lack of disease-modifying osteoarthritis therapy. The application of the biological therapy PRGF has allowed significant improvement in the quality of life of patients, delaying implantation of prosthesis. According to the results shown in the various published studies, there are approximately 20% of patients do not respond to treatment with platelet rich plasma or the response is significantly lower than in other patients. There are several factors that determine this worse response such as the variance of level of degeneration, age, and the presence of alterations in terms of both platelet concentration and function. There is no straightforward agreement on the treatment to be followed. One of the options for improving the response could be to increase the number of infiltrations to get an effective response. Of late, there are no studies that determine the standard for the frequency and number of cycles that must be performed for the treatment of OA. Treatment with two cycles of PRGF show improved of quality of life in patients with knee OA, with greater reduction in pain and stiffness compared with one cycle, although these results are not statistically significant. In those patients with poor response to treatment an option is the application of intraosseous PRGF.

E. Anitua et al. (eds.), *Platelet Rich Plasma in Orthopaedics and Sports Medicine*,
https://doi.org/10.1007/978-3-319-63730-3_9

1. INTRODUCTION

Knee osteoarthritis (OA) is one of the most frequent causes of pain and loss of function in patients over 65 years, with an increasing prevalence given the increase in the older population itself. Osteoarthritis (OA) is a mechanically induced, cytokine and enzyme mediated clinicopathological syndrome, and characterized by the involvement of inflammatory events in early stages of the joint condition[1]. Inflammation affects joint tissues with neurovascular structures such as menisci, synovial membrane (SM), subchondral bone (SB), joint capsule, and ligaments[2-4] and where synovial fluid (FS) plays an important role in perpetuating a vicious cycle among knee joint`s tissues by maintaining a detrimental pro-inflammatory microenvironment for cells from SM and superficial articular cartilage to deep layers of articular cartilage, and to SB as well[2,5,6]. SM and SB are endowed with heat receptors, chemoreceptors, and mechanoreceptors from which the nociceptive stimulus may lead to peripheral pain. Indeed, this is the case in approximately 60% to 80% of patients with knee OA[7]. At the early and mild stages of OA, the pain is triggered by physical activity and relieved by rest[8]. Also included in the clinical assessment of OA patients is joint stiffness, and in conjunction with pain may well contribute to knee disability, ultimately resulting in a drastic reduction in patient quality of life.

Despite the enormous effort made to seek an early therapeutic intervention aimed at preventing progressive destruction of joint tissues or reversing the initial articular cartilage and bone damage, there is still a lack of disease-modifying osteoarthritis therapy, making joint replacement the only solution for these patients[9]. Based on the biological theory of OA, various therapies to modify the disease have been developed in recent years. Among the different biological therapies, the application of platelet-rich plasma has been an advance in the treatment, becoming a safe and effective autologous therapy[10-13]. With this biological approach, there is an increasing interest in autologous growth factor treatment such as the use of PRP. Platelets contain growth factors, cytokines, chemokines and lysosomal granules. The release of these may play a special role in cartilage repair including modulating inflammatory processes, cell proliferation, chemotaxis, migration, differentiation and syntheses of matrix. It has been shown that platelet rich plasma, PRGF, has a chondroprotective effect from both the hyaluronic acid secretion by synoviocytes[14] and the arresting of type II collagen, cleavage by the combination of TGFß and FGF. PRGF has been revealed as a mighty anti-inflammatory response that might be mediated on the basis of the high concentration of HGF present in PRP, besides being secreted by several cells, thereby inhibiting the intracellular signaling regulator of the inflammatory and stress-induced response pathway NF-kß. Some growth factors present in platelets such as PDGF and TGFß have been shown to promote the proliferation of osteoblasts[15,16]. PRP preparations facilitate bone repair by expressing the pro-osteogenic and angiogenic functions of endothelial cells, recruiting osteoblast precursors, and promoting expression of adhesion molecules (osteoprotegerin)[17].

The current molecular interventions mainly target the clinical hallmark of OA, namely, pain and subsequent loss of knee function. In fact, current studies on the application of platelet-rich plasma point to the efficacy of this treatment in the improvement of pain, stiffness and functional capacity compared to other conservative treatments[10-13,18-23]. There are several possible mechanisms that might likely link the pain reduction to PRP treatment. PRP and growth factors within it such as HGF, IGF-1, and PDGF suppress macrophage and fibroblast, and modifying the inflammatory sate of chondrocytes activation by inhibiting the NFκB pathway, thereby dampening the synovial and articular cartilage inflammatory response, and this could lead to decreased IL-β, TNF-α concentration and other proinflammatory cytokines in synovial fluid[24-26]. Another mechanism that has been reported is the significant amount of endogenous cannabinoids within PRP that might act as ligands for cannabinoid receptor 1 (CB1) and 2 (CB2) of chondrocytes, synovial cells and bone cells of OA patients, thereby supporting both a pain and inflammation reduction by targeting the endogenous cannabinoid systems[27].

In recent years there are many published studies have assessed the effectiveness of PRGF in patients with knee OA[21-23]. The results obtained are encouraging showing an improvement of quality of life in patients after long-term application compared with other conservative treatments. It is, however, complex to perform a meta-analysis due to the considerable heterogeneity of the PRP applied and the demographic differences of the patients. Variability in the OA degree including in the different studies, the significant difference of age groups, scales used, and PRP preparation themselves, conspire to make it difficult for us to reach a consensus on the standardization of treatment with PRP. However, it is clear that the studies performed by authors such as Sánchez et al show how the intra-articular application of PRGF improves patients' quality of life compared to accepted conservative treatments such as hyaluronic acid[10,12,13,18]. All papers show a significant reduction of pain and other symptoms such as stiffness, functional capacity, and mobility as measured according to the results of the WOMAC scales (Western Ontario McMaster Universities Osteoarthritis Index &), KOOS or Lequesne. This improvement was statistically significant. In addition, according to the OMERACT-OARSI clinical evaluation criteria, more than 80% of the patients presented a favorable response with reductions of over 50% in the scores[12,18]. As an autologous product, PRP is a safe treatment. In this regard, treatment with PRGF had no higher rate of adverse events than other treatments, all of which were related to injection technique. One of the problems of OA treatment is the limited effect over time, sometimes deriving adverse effects from chronic administration. In this sense the application of PRGF has not only shown effectiveness during the first 6 months, a beneficial effect has persisted for at least 12 months. The level of knee degeneration in all studies was one of the inclusion criteria. On the basis of this level, some studies reported more promising results with the use of PRP in knees with a lower level of joint degeneration. Although the response in patients over 65 years as well as in severe degrees of OA has been less studied, the work of Vaquerizo et al[12] shows that this improvement is lower in these patients although the patients were satisfied with the results obtained. According to the results reported in the various published studies, there are approximately 20% of patients do not respond to treatment with platelet rich plasma or the response is significantly lower than in other patients. There are several factors that determine this poor response such as the variable levels of degeneration, age, the presence of functional alterations, and in terms of preparations of platelet concentrations. In addition to this, there is no clear standard in the treatment to be followed. One of the options for improving the response could be to increase the number of infiltrations to get an adequate response. At the present, there are no studies, which determine the frequency and number of cycles that must be performed for the treatment of OA. In the light of this terra incognita, it was worth considering increasing the number of cycles to improve the symptoms of osteoarthritis such as pain, stiffness and functional capacity. We aimed to evaluate the effectiveness of two cycles of PRGF in the treatment of OA. The goal of this study was to assess, the clinical efficacy and safety of one cycle (OC) versus two cycles (TC) of intra-articular injections of PRGF on patients with knee OA. As in other studies we used WOMAC and Lequesne scores as outcomes measures. Our hypothesis was that treatment with 2 cycles of PRGF might add a greater clinical efficacy than a single cycle of PRGF in patients with OA, thus TC therapeutic dosage to improve associated symptoms of knee OA, pain stiffness and functional capacity. This study was performed during a second therapeutic open phase of the same randomized clinical trial[12], in the same centre in accordance with current law and regulatory rules, and the international guidelines for Good Clinical Practice (International Conference on Harmonization, June 1996), Declaration of Helsinki in its latest revised version (Fortaleza, 2013) was also followed. The study protocol was previously reviewed and approved by the institutional review board. All patients signed the informed consent prior to inclusion in the RCT. In the first blind phase of the RCT, an experimental group treated with PRGF (3 injections on a weekly basis) was compared with a control group receiving Viscous-supplementation with a follow-up of 48 weeks. In this posterior open phase of the RCT, after a washout period of 6 months at the end follow-up period, patients of the control group received treatment with 2 sequential cycles of PRGF (6 months separately), while patients in the control group previously had received a single cycle of three intra-articular infiltrations of PRGF (OC group).

The objective of this second phase was to compare the efficacy of these two different therapeutic regimens (one cycle of treatment vs. two cycles) of treatment with Endoret (PRGF) in OA. The study selection criteria were: over 50 years, osteoarthritis of the knee confirmed by radiographic (Kellgren-Lawrence classification grade II-IV), no severe mechanical deformity, no systemic autoimmune rheumatic disease or blood disorders, values of body mass index < 35, and no viscous-supplementation treatment in the past 6 months. Each patient also received a booklet that contained detailed instructions for the study and the Western Ontario and McMaster Universities Osteoarthritis Index WOMAC questionnaire.

PRGF was prepared following the technique described by Sanchez et al[18]. At each visit blood volume from each patient ranged from 36 to 72 mL, depending on the knees to be treated. Blood was collected in sterile conditions with a Sodium Citrate buffer. The blood was centrifuged for 8 minutes at 580g in a BTI System centrifuge. After centrifugation the BTI Plasma Transfer Device® was used to aspirate fractions of plasma enriched in platelets immediately above the buffy coat, taking care to avoid disturbing the buffy coat. Following activation of the PRGF with 50 microliters of Cl_2Ca 10% for every mL of plasma, the PRGF was infiltrated intraarticularly.

Clinical and demographic variables were analyzed (gender, age, body mass index (BMI), OA degree with Kellgren-Lawrence score, laterality and complications were collected at the beginning of the study.

The efficacy outcome measures were a reduction in the global score of the WOMAC Index (Western Ontario and McMaster University Osteoarthritis Index), as well as in the different sub-scales for pain, stiffness and physical function of this score, as well as the reduction, and in global LEQUESNE Index and its pain, MWD and ADL sub-scales, from baseline and at 6 and 12 months (48 weeks) of follow-up after treatment. At the end of the clinical trial and as a secondary objective, according to the guideline for Good Clinical Practice, all complications and/or adverse events were recorded at each patient visits. Severity grade, received treatment and evolution of all adverse events were assessed and documented. The use of rescue medication was also recorded daily in the patient's diaries.

In order to avoid bias in the analysis, an intention to treat (ITT) statistical analysis was performed for all variables, including all patients who received one or two cycles of intra-articular injections of Endoret (PRGF), and with at least one efficacy or safety assessment. Qualitative variables were expressed as absolute or relative frequencies and quantitative variables by either the mean and standard deviation or alternatively the median and its interquartile range in cases where normal distribution was not met. All comparisons between OC and TC groups were performed using the Student t-test or alternatively, with the Mann-Whitney U non-parametric statistical test for distributions other than normal. All statistical analysis was performed using the statistical program SPSS version 16.0.

90 patients were included in the study. Forty-eight patients had received one cycle of PRGF (OC group), while 42 patients received two cycles of PRG separated by 6 months (TC group) in this open phase. The mean age in the OC group was 63.55 years, and the mean body-mass index was 30.12, whereas in the two-cycle group (TC) mean age was 67.95 years and the mean body-mass index was 30.77. Comparing baseline values in both groups, no significant differences were observed in Kellgren grade or body mass index between groups, whereas a significant higher age was re-

corded in TC group. Moreover, a significantly higher Lequesne index and all WOMAC scores (global, pain, stiffness and function) were observed in patients of TC group (Table 1).

At 6 months of follow-up, all patients had a significant reduction in both scales (P <0.001). In both groups there was a clinical improvement of more than 30% in all subscales. Patients presented the best results at pain level (45%) and mobility (37%).

Results after both treatments showed a significant reduction at the end of follow-up (48 weeks) compared with the baseline values (p<0.001) for both treatment OC and TC groups. Patients in the OC group had a clinical worsening compared with the results obtained at 6 months in WOMAC and Lequesne score (Figure 1 and 2). This clinical worsening was not significant. On the other hand, patients in the TC group continued to improve at the end of follow-up, exceeding the results obtained by the OC group.

WOMAC AND LEQUESNE SCORE				
		OC	TC	P value
Patients		48	42	
Gender	Male	21	15	0.23
	Female	27	27	0.007*
Age (years)		63.6 ± 6.7	68 ±8.3	0.65
Laterality	Left	13	11	
	Right	22	17	
	Bilateral	13	14	
Kellgren-Lawrence		2.9 ± 0.7	2.9 ± 0.8	0.86
Body mass Index (kg/m^2)		30.1 ± 4	30.8 ±4.4	0.46
WOMAC scale	Pain score	9.7 ±2.5	11.01 ±3.4	0.024*
	Stiffness score	3.7 ±1.7	4.6 ±2	0.04*
	Function score	32.7 ±9.9	39.7 ± 12.2	0.005*
	Global	46 ± 12.7	55.4 ± 16.7	0.004*
Lequesne global Index		12.8 ± 3.8	15 ± 2.4	0.001*
*Statistical significance (P<0.05).				

TABLE 1. Demographic parameters and baseline values.

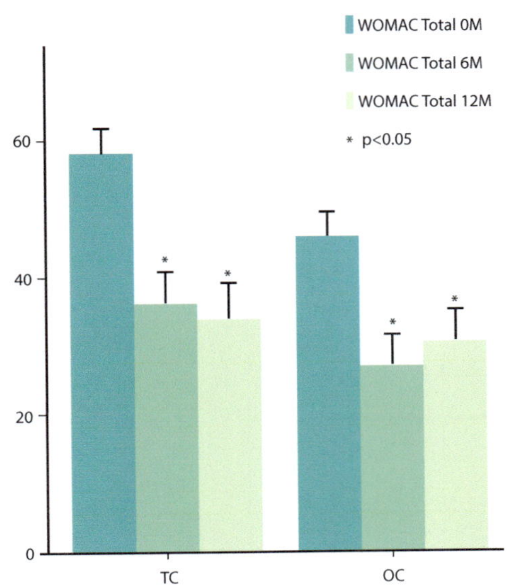

FIG. 1
Comparative Outcomes WOMAC score.

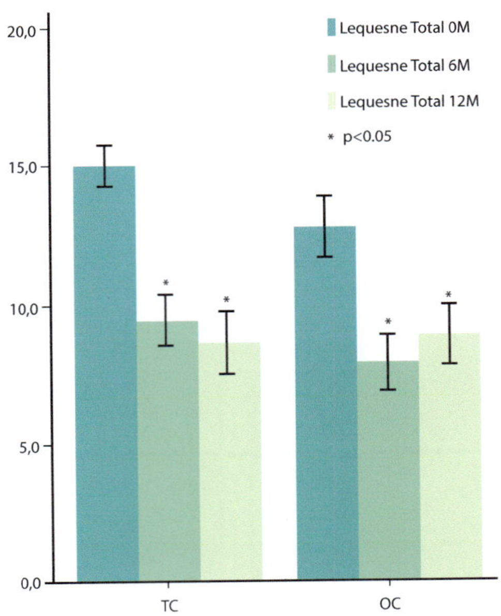

FIG. 2
Comparative Outcomes Lequesne score.

This reduction was observed for all WOMAC and Lequesne scales and sub-scales (Table 2). This substantial reduction from baseline was at least 24.6% (WOMAC stiffness score) for both groups and scores at the end of follow-up (48 weeks) as observed in Table 3.

Comparing the results in outcome measures in both OC/TCs treatment groups globally, the differences between groups were more relevant in the LEQUESNE score than in the WOMAC score as shown in Table 3. Regarding WOMAC score, patients of TC group showed a significantly higher reduction from baseline in WOMAC stiffness subscales compared with patients of OC group (P<0.05). In WOMAC global score and in pain and function sub-scales, despite a better response to treatment at the end of follow-up no significant differences between groups were detected. Regarding LEQUESNE index, a significantly higher

WOMAC AND LEQUESNE OUTCOMES					
		OC		TC	
		Mean ± SD	P value	Mean ± SD	P value
WOMAC Score	Pain score	9.7 ±2.5	<0.001	11.01 ± 3.4	<0.001
		6.3 ±3.3		6.7 ± 3.7	
	Stiffness score	3.7 ±1.7	<0.001	4.6 ±2	<0.001
		2.6 ± 1.4		2.7 ±1.6	
	Function score	32.7 ±9.9	<0.001	39.7 ± 12.2	<0.001
		21.9 ± 11.3		23.8 ± 12.8	
	Global	46 ± 12.7	<0.001	55.4 ± 16.7	<0.001
		30.8 ± 15.5		33.2 ± 17.5	
Lequesne Score	Pain score	5.6 ±1.4	<0.001	6.2 ± 1	<0.001
		4.1 ± 1.6		4.2 ± 1.9	
	MWD	2.8 ± 1.9	<0.001	3.3 ±1.6	<0.001
		1.5 ± 1.3		1.0 ± 0.9	
	ADL	4.5 ± 1.5	<0.001	5.6 ±0.9	<0.001
		3.3 ± 1.6		3.4 ± 1.7	
	Global	2.8 ± 3.8	<0.001	15 ± 2.4	<0.001
		8.9 ± 3.7		8.6 ± 3.7	

TABLE 2. WOMAC and Lequesne outcomes.

COMPARATIVE RESULTS				
		OC	TC	P value
WOMAC Score	Pain score	33.5 ± 30.9	33.5 ±30.9	0.96
	Stiffness score	24,7 ± 40.4	18.7 ±60.8	0.04*
	Function score	33.7 ± 28.7	37.1 ± 31.4	0.59
	Global	34 ± 27.6	36.5 ± 32.6	0.71
Lequesne Score	Pain score	25.3 ± 29	30.9 ±31.9	0.29
	MWD	29.7 ± 60.1	61.5 ± 53.6	0.006*
	ADL	25 ±30.7	39.7 ± 28.4	0.04*
	Global	30.2 ± 23	442 ± 24.7	0.02*

TABLE 3. Comparative results of outcome measures (%) between OC/TC groups. 48 weeks respect baseline.

reduction from baseline either in global score, in MWD sub-scale (maximum walking distance), in ADL (Activities of daily living) sub-scale, was observed. The improvement rate was 31.8 % higher for the TCs PRGF group compared with OC PRGF group (P<0.01) in MWD sub-scale. Specifically, in patients receiving two cycles of PRGF- (TC group), the improvement for the Lequesne global score was 11.84% higher than in the OC group (P<0.05), whereas in Lequesne MWD and ADL subscales the improvement compared to the OC group reached the 31.8% and 14.66% respectively (P<0.05). For pain assessment on the WOMAC scale, in Lequesne pain sub-scale patients in the TCs group had a greater pain reduction than patients in the OC group, although this difference was not significant.

Patients who have been treated with two cycles of PRGF (TC group) showed a higher pain reduction, compared with OC group, although this differ- ence was not significant. The reason might be related to the significant difference in baseline values observed for WOMAC and LEQUESNE pain score values between both groups (higher baseline values in TC group) among other reasons.

At the end of the study, there were no significant differences in rescue medication used in both groups. Only 7 patients in both groups presented pain during the first 24 hours. All of these events were related to post-injection pain. No new adverse events or complications in TC group were reported during this second therapeutic phase.

Biological therapies improve symptoms of OA, this is an obvious fact, but at present it is difficult to adopt a mechanism-based approach to pain management for several reasons, including the heterogeneity of the OA syndrome[28], the poor understanding of mechanisms underlying joint pain, the different tissue sources of pain, and the dual central and peripheral features of OA pain[2,28].

If we compare the results obtained in this clinical trial, assessed by both Lequesne and WOMAC scores in patients with severe knee OA treated with one or two cycles of intraarticular injections of PRGF, the significant improvement is consistent with the results reported previously by Sanchez et al[10,13,18] and Vaquerizo et al[12]. PRP has proven to significantly reduce pain and joint stiffness, and to improve physical function in patients with knee OA[21,23]. In the absence of pertinent studies, however, there is evidence that application of PRGF indirectly slows the progression of osteoarthritis, delaying surgery[11-13,18-23].

There are several potential mechanisms by which intraarticular injections of PRGF might reduce OA knee pain. Although pain is the clinical hallmark of OA, tissue inflammation and degeneration appear to underlie the molecular, cellular, and clinical phenomena characterizing the cluster of degenerative joint conditions known as OA[29]. In patients with severe knee OA, extracellular matrix fragments stemming from the degrading proteoglycans and cleaved collagen I may act as DAMPs (damage-associated molecular patterns)[30-32], and activate the intracellular signalling pathway known as nuclear factor kappa B (NFkB) on cells such as nociceptors, chondrocytes, synovial fibroblasts and macrophages[2,30-32]. This NFkB activation induces the gene expression of pro-inflammatory cytokines such as interleukin 1beta (IL-1B), interleukin 6 (IL-6), and tumor necrosis factor alpha (TNF-a). These are not only the major mediators of joint inflammation, they also contribute to generating and perpetuating inflammation-evoked pain by eliciting hyperalgesia and sensitizing joint tissue nociceptors for mechanical stimuli[24,25].

In vitro and in vivo studies have reported that PRP and growth factors within it such as HGF, IGF-1, and PDGF suppress macrophage, fibroblast, and chondrocyte activation by inhibiting the NFkB signaling pathway[15,16] and thereby breaking the catabolic loop, to dampen the synovial and articular cartilage inflammatory response when these cells are exposed to pro-inflammatory cytokines, abnormal mechanical stress and DAMPs, comprising the OA context[5]. In addition, the significant amount of endogenous cannabinoids within PRP might act as ligands for cannabinoid receptor 1 (CB1) and 2 (CB2) of chondrocyte and synovial cells of OA patients thereby supporting a pain reduction by targeting the endogenous cannabinoid system[5,7,9].

The greater degree of degeneration of structures may produce a lower initial response of patients to treatment. The fact that two cycles of PRGF treatment (TC group) did not add a significantly higher pain reduction in patients, compared with OC group treatment, might be related to the significant difference in baseline values observed for WOMAC and Lequesne pain score values between both groups (higher baseline values in TC group) among other reasons (Table 1).

However, patients treated with two cycles of Endoret (PRGF) underwent a significantly higher improvement in WOMAC stiffness, maximum walking distance, activities of daily living and both global sub-scales than patients receiving only one Endoret (PRGF) cycle (OC group) ($p<0.05$) at 6 months and at the end of follow-up. The sensation of knee stiffness is one of the six criteria evaluated in the WOMAC questionnaire, and although it is a symptom whose origin is complex, factors such as synovial fluid lubrication and composition, and periarticular muscle conditions play an important role in this symptom since these two joint elements are the most important shock absorbers at knee level. The anti-inflammatory effect of PRP on synovial membrane and articular cartilage of knee osteoarthritis patients may well reduce knee swelling which otherwise would trigger a spine reflex and inhibit the activation of periarticular muscle, thereby leading to muscle weakness and atrophy, and eventually contribute to knee stiffness. On the other hand, it has been shown by in vitro studies that PRP enhances the synthesis of hyaluronic acid by osteoarthritic synoviocytes even in the presence of IL-B 14. Moreover, another key component in knee lubrication and chondrocyte protection is lubricin, whose production by synovial cells and superficial zone chondrocytes decreased with age and after injury, and in knee OA is significantly enhanced by the application of PRP. Overall, the secretion of HA and lubricin together with a reduction in inflammatory synovial fluid, might well contribute to a reduction in knee stiffness.

In this study, patients undergoing two cycles of PRGF treatment showed a significantly higher improvement in efficacy outcomes such as maximum walking distance (MWD), activities of daily living (ADL) and Lequesne global sub-scale compared with patients of the OC group. This increase in tolerable physical load might entail a positive chondroprotective and anti-inflammatory effect since as several lines of evidence suggest, moderate mechanical loading of joints prevents cartilage degradation by suppressing the activation of NFkB 33. It is worth mentioning that the application of intraarticular infiltrations of PRGF does not entail any reduction in physical activity and patients resume their daily activities immediately after the procedure is performed. It can then be surmised that the increased physiological loading may well work in synergy with the anti-inflammatory effect of PRGF treatment, to reinforce as well as strengthen the periarticular muscles and contribute to a reduction in knee joint stiffness.

A limitation of this study includes the different WOMAC-Lequesne baseline values of both groups, which results are unfavorable for the TC group. Patients with worse degrees of osteoarthritis showed better results at the end of follow-up in TC group, although due to the initial differences these results were not significant. This fact was observed when comparing the results according to the patient age. However, in order to overcome this pitfall, the clinical improvement of WOMAC and Lequesne outcomes were shown in % relation from the baseline values for both treatment groups.

On the other hand, as with previous published studies, there are no biochemical data analyzing the synovial fluid composition. A more ideal study would entail a close examination of synovial fluid in terms of inflammatory mediators and lubricant components, as well as assessing peri-articular muscle to reveal the real impact on quality of life and improvement of knee stability.

This study indicates that although two cycles of PRGF treatment does not produce a measurable higher pain reduction compared with one cycle of PRGF treatment on patients, both modalities of treatment (OC and TCs groups) were safe and clinically effective, which significantly reduce all assessed variables with WOMAC and LEQUESNE scores at the end of the follow-up period (48 weeks) compared with baseline values. In addition, patients treated with two cycles of PRGF showed a significant improvement in stiffness, maximum walking distance and activities of daily living, clearly indicating an improvement in life quality. Despite the best results obtained there are still other lines of research that may improve patient symptoms, and for this purpose the application of intraosseous PRGF can be a clear advance for the treatment of refractory cases. The application of intraosseous PRGF is explained below.

1. Little CB, Hunter DJ. Post-traumatic osteoarthritis: from mouse models to clinical trials. Nature reviews. Rheumatology. 2013;9:485-97.

2. Malfait AM, Schnitzer TJ. Towards a mechanism-based approach to pain management in osteoarthritis. Nature reviews. Rheumatology. 2013;9:654-64.

3. Felson DT. Clinical practice. Osteoarthritis of the knee. The New England journal of medicine. 2006;354:841-8.

4. Pelletier JP, Martel-Pelletier J, Abramson SB. Osteoarthritis, an inflammatory disease: potential implication for the selection of new therapeutic targets. Arthritis and rheumatism. 2001;44:1237-47.

5. Joos H, Wildner A, Hogrefe C, Reichel H, Brenner RE. Interleukin-1 beta and tumor necrosis factor alpha inhibit migration activity of chondrogenic progenitor cells from non-fibrillated osteoarthritic cartilage. Arthritis research & therapy. 2013;15:R119.

6. Scanzello CR, Goldring SR. The role of synovitis in osteoarthritis pathogenesis. Bone. 2012;51:249-57.

7. Dray A, Read SJ. Arthritis and pain. Future targets to control osteoarthritis pain. Arthritis research & therapy. 2007;9:212.

8. Felson DT. Developments in the clinical understanding of osteoarthritis. Arthritis research & therapy. 2009;11:203.

9. Martel-Pelletier J, Wildi LM, Pelletier JP. Future therapeutics for osteoarthritis. Bone. 2012;51:297-311.

10. Sanchez M, Anitua E, Azofra J, Aguirre JJ, Andia I. Intra-articular injection of an autologous preparation rich in growth factors for the treatment of knee OA: a retrospective cohort study. Clinical and experimental rheumatology. 2008;26:910-3.

11. Filardo G, Kon E, Pereira Ruiz MT, et al. Platelet-rich plasma intra-articular injections for cartilage degeneration and osteoarthritis: single- versus double-spinning approach. Knee surgery, sports traumatology, arthroscopy : official journal of the ESSKA. 2012;20:2082-91.

12. Vaquerizo V, Plasencia MA, Arribas I, et al. Comparison of intra-articular injections of plasma rich in growth factors (Endoret (PRGF)) versus Durolane hyaluronic acid in the treatment of patients with symptomatic osteoarthritis: a randomized controlled trial. Arthroscopy : the journal of arthroscopic & related surgery : official publication of the Arthroscopy Association of North America and the International Arthroscopy Association. 2013;29:1635-43.

13. Wang-Saegusa A, Cugat R, Ares O, Seijas R, Cusco X, Garcia-Balletbo M. Infiltration of plasma rich in growth factors for osteoarthritis of the knee short-term effects on function and quality of life. Archives of orthopaedic and trauma surgery. 2011;131:311-7.

14. Anitua E, Sanchez M, Nurden AT, et al. Platelet-released growth factors enhance the secretion of hyaluronic acid and induce hepatocyte growth factor production by synovial fibroblasts from arthritic patients. Rheumatology (Oxford). 2007;46:1769-72.

15. Bendinelli P, Matteucci E, Dogliotti G, et al. Molecular basis of anti-inflammatory action of platelet-rich plasma on human chondrocytes: mechanisms of NF-kappaB inhibition via HGF. Journal of cellular physiology. 2010;225:757-66.

16. van Buul GM, Koevoet WL, Kops N, et al. Platelet-rich plasma releasate inhibits inflammatory processes in osteoarthritic chondrocytes. The American journal of sports medicine. 2011;39:2362-70.

17. Cenni E, Ciapetti G, Granchi D, et al. Endothelial cells incubated with platelet-rich plasma express PDGF-B and ICAM-1 and induce bone marrow stromal cell migration. Journal of orthopaedic research : official publication of the Orthopaedic Research Society. 2009;27:1493-8.

18. Sanchez M, Fiz N, Azofra J, et al. A randomized clinical trial evaluating plasma rich in growth factors (Endoret (PRGF)) versus hyaluronic acid in the short-term treatment of symptomatic knee osteoarthritis. Arthroscopy : the journal of arthroscopic & related surgery : official publication of the Arthroscopy Association of North America and the International Arthroscopy Association. 2012;28:1070-8.

19. Gobbi A, Lad D, Karnatzikos G. The effects of repeated intra-articular PRP injections on clinical outcomes of early osteoarthritis of the knee. Knee surgery, sports traumatology, arthroscopy : official journal of the ESSKA. 2015;23:2170-7.

20. Gormeli G, Gormeli CA, Ataoglu B, Colak C, Aslanturk O, Ertem K. Multiple PRP injections are more effective than single injections and hyaluronic acid in knees with early osteoarthritis: a randomized, double-blind, placebo-controlled trial. Knee surgery, sports traumatology, arthroscopy : official journal of the ESSKA. 2017;25:958-65.

21. Meheux CJ, McCulloch PC, Lintner DM, Varner KE, Harris JD. Efficacy of Intra-articular Platelet-Rich Plasma Injections in Knee Osteoarthritis: A Systematic Review. Arthroscopy : the journal of arthroscopic & related surgery : official publication of the Arthroscopy Association of North America and the International Arthroscopy Association. 2016;32:495-505.

22. Laudy AB, Bakker EW, Rekers M, Moen MH. Efficacy of platelet-rich plasma injections in osteoarthritis of the knee: a systematic review and meta-analysis. British journal of sports medicine. 2015;49:657-72.

23. Dai Wi, Zhou AG, Zhang H, Zhang J. Efficacy of Platelet-Rich Plasma in the Treatment of Knee Osteoarthritis: A Meta-analysis of Randomized Controlled Trials. Arthroscopy: The Journal of Arthroscopic & Related Surgery. 2017;33:659-70.e1.

24. Schaible HG, von Banchet GS, Boettger MK, et al. The role of proinflammatory cytokines in the generation and maintenance of joint pain. Annals of the New York Academy of Sciences. 2010;1193:60-9.

25. Sellam J, Berenbaum F. The role of synovitis in pathophysiology and clinical symptoms of osteoarthritis. Nature reviews. Rheumatology. 2010;6:625-35.

26. Kapoor M, Martel-Pelletier J, Lajeunesse D, Pelletier JP, Fahmi H. Role of proinflammatory cytokines in the pathophysiology of osteoarthritis. Nature reviews. Rheumatology. 2011;7:33-42.

27. Descalzi F, Ulivi V, Cancedda R, et al. Platelet-rich plasma exerts antinociceptive activity by a peripheral endocannabinoid-related mechanism. Tissue engineering. Part A. 2013;19:2120-9.

28. Thakur M, Dickenson AH, Baron R. Osteoarthritis pain: nociceptive or neuropathic? Nature reviews. Rheumatology. 2014;10:374-80.

29. Fernandez-Tajes J, Soto-Hermida A, Vazquez-Mosquera ME, et al. Genome-wide DNA methylation analysis of articular chondrocytes reveals a cluster of osteoarthritic patients. Annals of the rheumatic diseases. 2014;73:668-77.

30. Sillat T, Barreto G, Clarijs P, et al. Toll-like receptors in human chondrocytes and osteoarthritic cartilage. Acta orthopaedica. 2013;84:585-92.

31. Gomez R, Villalvilla A, Largo R, Gualillo O, Herrero-Beaumont G. TLR4 signalling in osteoarthritis--finding targets for candidate DMOADs. Nature reviews. Rheumatology. 2015;11:159-70.

32. Houard X, Goldring MB, Berenbaum F. Homeostatic mechanisms in articular cartilage and role of inflammation in osteoarthritis. Current rheumatology reports. 2013;15:375.

33. Sanchez-Adams J, Leddy HA, McNulty AL, O'Conor CJ, Guilak F. The mechanobiology of articular cartilage: bearing the burden of osteoarthritis. Current rheumatology reports. 2014;16:451.

CHAPTER 10
PRGF on Sports-Related Ligament Injuries

AUTHORS

Cugat R.[1,2,3], Cuscó X.[1,3], Seijas R.[1,3,4], Barastegui D.[1,2,3], Álvarez-Díaz P.[1,2,3,4], Alentorn-Geli E.[1,2,3], Rius M.[1,2,3], Steinbacher G.[2], Sala E.[2], Boffa JJ.[2,3], Grossi S.[2], García-Balletbó M.[1,3], Tizol S.[1,3], Laiz P.[1,3].
PHYSIOTHERAPISTS: Marín M.[1], Álvarez X.[1], Lama N.[1].

[1] Fundación García-Cugat, Universidad CEU-Cardenal Herrera, Spain.
[2] Mutualidad Catalana de Futbolistas – Delegación Cataluña, Barcelona, Spain.
[3] Artroscopia GC, Hospital Quirón, Barcelona, Spain.
[4] Universidad Internacional de Cataluña, Sant Cugat del Vallès, Spain.

SUMMARY

Ligament injuries have a high incidence among young athletes and they occur most often in contact sports. Treatment of these injuries has a profound impact not only for athletes but also for everyone who engages in recreational sports practice.

Knee injuries are common and potentially career ending in amateur and professional sports. There are two ligaments on the knee cavity, anterior cruciate ligament (ACL) and posterior cruciate ligament (PCL). PCL injuries happen far less often than ACL injuries, because PCL is stronger than ACL and most commonly occurs in combined knee ligament injuries. The other two ligaments in the knee are the lateral collateral ligament (LCL) and the medial collateral ligament (MCL) which are located on both sides of the knee.

Ankle ligament injuries are also very common amongst young athletes. The front and middle bands of the lateral ligament are the ligaments commonly injured in a sprain. Recent epidemiology studies have revealed that ankle sprains have a high incidence among athletes, and are particularly common in those who practice team sport.
The benefit of using PRFG in ligament injuries is widely studied, over knee and ankle. These studies have shown that the PRGF seems to play an important role during the regeneration of the low healing potential ligament tissue, when applied. It also helps to restore the biomechanical properties of the tissue. It is important to restore the anatomy, recover function and to have a good biological environment so as to avoid degenerative processes in the cartilage joint.

E. Anitua et al. (eds.), *Platelet Rich Plasma in Orthopaedics and Sports Medicine*,
https://doi.org/10.1007/978-3-319-63730-3_10

1. INTRODUCTION

Since the emergence of regenerative medicine, a range of studies has demonstrated the efficacy of new biological treatments. During the tissular healing process, angiogenesis, tissular proliferation and extracellular matrix formation occurs. These processes are based on biological events controlled by a series of growth factors and proteins.

Until the emergence of PRGF therapies, it has not been possible to initiate healing in the same therapeutic agent using the necessary cell scaffold and molecular signals.

To understand the complexity of PRGF therapies, knowledge about platelet biology is fundamental. The primary and best-known function of platelets is their contribution to hemostasis. However, more functional facets of the platelets have been identified, and we now know that they play an important role in inflammatory and proliferative events, and also a critical role in tissue remodelling and wound healing; and furthermore, we now recognize their angiogenic power to deliver proteins to areas where tissue is damaged.

For these reasons, PRGF is a good vehicle to deliver GFs to the injured site, where it can mimic the physiological process of tissue repair.

Platelet Rich Growth Factor, PRGF, is a source of autologous Growth factors obtained by different methods. Depending on the system, the products obtained have different chemical and cellular composition, which consequently lead to different results after application. For that reason, it is very important to know the composition of the product administered.

There are studies suggesting that leukocytes in PRGF contribute to inflammatory cytokine production. But even more significant than simply minimizing inflammation is the maximizing platelet role to decrease inflammation and enhance matrix gene synthesis.

Growth Factors are substances whose biochemical signals are capable of modulating the cellular response. These substances can be vitamins or hormones with the main function of stimulating cell growth and differentiation. They are involved in a large number of other very important biological functions such as cellular proliferation, cellular survival, migration and even apoptosis.

Growth factors are cellular mediators synthetized by many different types of cells. The connective tissues are known to contain many of the signalling proteins that play a very important role in the remodelling and repair of the different types of connective tissue.

Growth Factors carry out their function at very low concentration, in the region of pico or nanograms. They bind to a cellular receptor; this receptor is specific for a second messenger where a tyrosine-kinase protein acts. This activation starts the signalling cascade, ending in the nucleus where the transcription factors activate one or more genes. The most important Growth Factors acting in ligament healing are PDGF, TGF-β, IGF, FGF, EGF and VEGF, but also NGF and HGF in a smaller proportion.

The PDGF has mitogenic properties as a very strong mesenchymal cell activator[1], modulates important processes as endocytosis or cell migration[2], and also plays a very important role in reparation and regeneration processes. TFG-β has many different functions such as proliferation, migration and cell metabolism. It stimulates or inhibits cell differentiation and proliferation depending on its concentration, tissue environment and cell type[2]. The functions of IGF are cellular replication, synthesis of glycogen, proteins and glycosaminoglycan, and the transport of glucose and amino acids throughout the cell membrane[2]. IGF also plays an important role in increasing cartilage, bone formation, and decreasing extracellular matrix degradation[3]. The main FGF biological activity is the mitogenic, chemotactic and angiogenic capacity over many cells[2]. EGF stimulates mitogenesis, increasing DNA, RNA and protein production in fibroblasts and in endothelial cells. VEGF is fundamental in tissue reparation-regeneration processes, and it plays an important role in early migration and proliferation phases, but is more active after the inflammatory process as a determinant in proliferation and the remodelling phase, where it is a great stimulant of angiogenesis[4]. NGF contributes to accelerate the cicatrization processes by modulating inflammatory phases, migration, angiogenesis and tissue remodelling[5]. HGF is a protein with mitogenic properties in endothelial cells which stimulates cell migration, and has a powerful synergic activity with VEGF in endothelial cells[6].

2. KNEE

ANATOMY AND FUNCTION

The knee is a large and complex joint, formed by two units:

A. The tibiofemoral joint, constituted by the distal end of the femur with the proximal end of the tibia, belonging to the bi-condylar group.
B. The patellofemoral joint, a trochlear diarthrosis genre-type, formed by the femoral trochlea and the back of the patella.

The knee has four major ligaments that help it avoid luxation. There are two positioned on the extra-articular side, called the Medial Collateral Ligament (MCL) and Lateral Collateral Ligament (LCL). There are two intraarticular ligaments crossed and located in the centre of the tibiofemoral joint, called the Anterior Cruciate Ligament (ACL) and Posterior Cruciate Ligament (PCL).

The other ligaments or capsular reinforcements are the following:

On the extra-articular of the anterior side: The Patellar Ligament connecting the patella to the tibia. On the extra-articular of the posterior side: The Oblique Popliteal Ligament or Recurring Tendon connecting the tendon of the semimembranous muscle to the external condyle of the femur. The Arched Popliteal Ligament connects the external condyle of the femur with the margin of the head of the tibia.

On the extra-articular of the inner side is the Medial Patellar Femoral Ligament (MPFL), which connects the border of the patella to the internal femoral condyle. The MPFL connects the patella to the medial meniscus. The Medial Collateral Ligament (MCL) is an extracapsular band-like ligament located in the inner side of the knee. The proximal end is inserted into the tuberosity of the medial femoral condyle and the distal end is inserted into the inner side of the tibia.

MCL function is to prevent lateral movement of the knee avoiding excessive genu valgum deformity. It also collaborates with the ACL.

On the extra-articular of the outer side is the Lateral Patellar Femoral Ligament (LPFL), which connects the patella to the edge of the lateral femoral condyle. The LPFL connects the patella to the lateral meniscus. The Lateral Collateral Ligament (LCL) or Fibular Collateral Ligament is a cordoned extracapsular ligament which is located in the outside of the knee. The proximal end is inserted into the external femoral condyle and the distal end is inserted in the outer zone of the fibular head.

As well as the MCL, its function is to prevent lateral mobility of the knee, avoiding, if necessary, excessive genu valgum. It also collaborates with the PCL and to a lesser degree with the ACL.

The intraarticular ligaments are the following: The Yugal Ligament or Transverse Ligament that connects the front face of both menisci; the Meniscofemoral Posterior Ligament or Humphrey Ligament which goes from the periphery of the posterior horn of the lateral meniscus to the medial femoral condyle; the Posterior Meniscofemoral Ligament or Wrisberg Ligament which goes from the periphery of the posterior horn of the lateral meniscus to the medial femoral condyle, located behind the Anterior Meniscofemoral Ligament.

The ACL is an intraarticular ligament located in the central area of the knee. It consists of few fascicles. The proximal end is inserted into the intercondylar area, specifically, in the postero-medial area of the lateral femoral condyle, and the distal end is inserted between the tibial spines on the antero-inner area of the tibia, adjacent to the anterior root of the medial meniscus.

The function of the antero-medial bundle is to avoid anterior displacement of the tibia relative to femur. Its injury results in Lachman Test positive and Pivot Shift negative.

The function of the postero-lateral bundle is to avoid the antero-lateral rotatory subluxation of the tibia relative to femur. Its injury produces Lachman Test negative and positive Pivot Shift.

The PCL is an intraarticular ligament located in the central area of the knee. It consists of several fascicles. The proximal end is inserted into the front area of the lateral face of the medial femoral condyle and the distal end is inserted in a depression of the posterior intercondylar area of the tibia and in the peripheral area of the posterior third of the lateral meniscus.

Its function is to prevent rear sliding of the tibia relative to femur, and with the ACL controls rotational stability of the knee.

INJURIES

When a ligament is injured, three important areas are altered: the anatomy, function and biology. This is why it is important to act on each one to solve the problem.

Epidemiology of knee injuries.

Time reviewed	Season 2014-15
Medial Colateral Ligament (MCL)	573
Lateral Colateral Ligament (LCL)	280
Anterior Cruciate Ligament (ACL)	926
Posterior Cruciate Ligament (PCL)	42

The epidemiology of knee injuries in the Mutualitat Catalana de Futbolistes, MCF, may differ from epidemiology in the general population. Soccer players from the MCF are highly active athletes whose knees suffer higher stress than the non-athlete population.

Medial Collateral Ligament (MCL)

Conservative Treatment

In acute isolated grade II and III injuries, as well as in chronic injuries with mild or moderate grade of instability, conservative treatment is recommended:

1. Ultrasound-guided infiltration with Fraction 2 (Platelet Rich) of PRGF leukocyte-free, 4 - 7 cc in the ligament and its insertions.
2. Anti-valgus brace placed for 3 weeks with free movement, unblocked.
3. Physiotherapy.
4. Rehabilitation program.
5. Regular medical and ultrasound controls.

Repetition of infiltration should be performed, if needed, according to the recovery evolution. Usually, from one to three infiltrations administered with an interval of 7-10 days is sufficient for healing.

Normally, there is a return to sport at 4-6 weeks in Grade II but 8-10 weeks in Grade III. (Figs. 1-2)

Surgical Treatment with Biological Augmentation

Surgical treatment is performed in acute grade III injuries associated with other injuries such as ACL and chronic injuries that cause instability. In these cases, surgery corrects the defect of anatomy and then biological treatment is applied with Fraction 2 PRGF. Since PRGF improves the quality of repairing tissue, and helps to have a more comfortable postoperative experience, it shortens the recovery process. Return to sport is estimated to be 6 months. (Fig. 3)

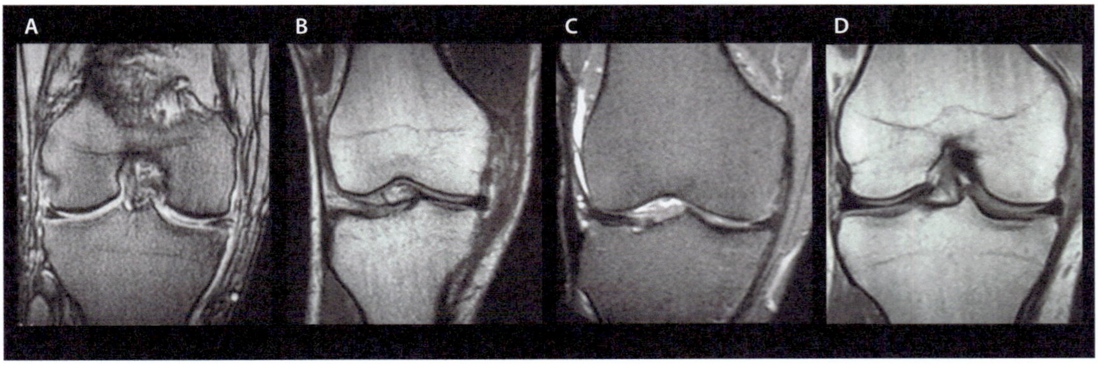

FIG. 1
MCL MRI. A) MCL rupture. Pre-treatment. B) Recovered MCL. Post- treatment with PRGF.

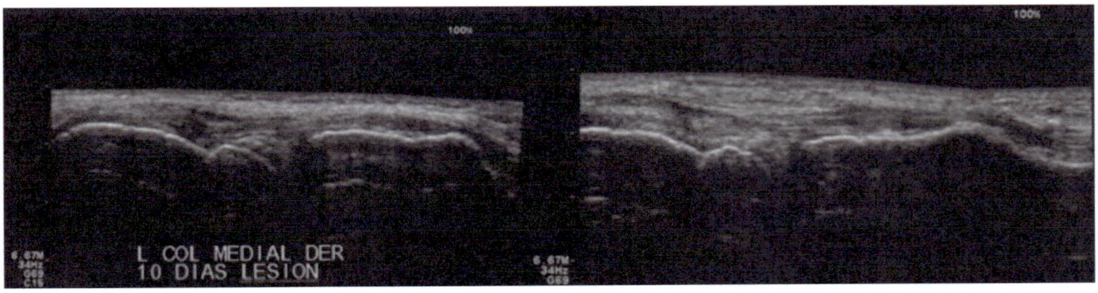

FIG. 2
Ultrasound follow-up in MCL injury with PRFG injection.

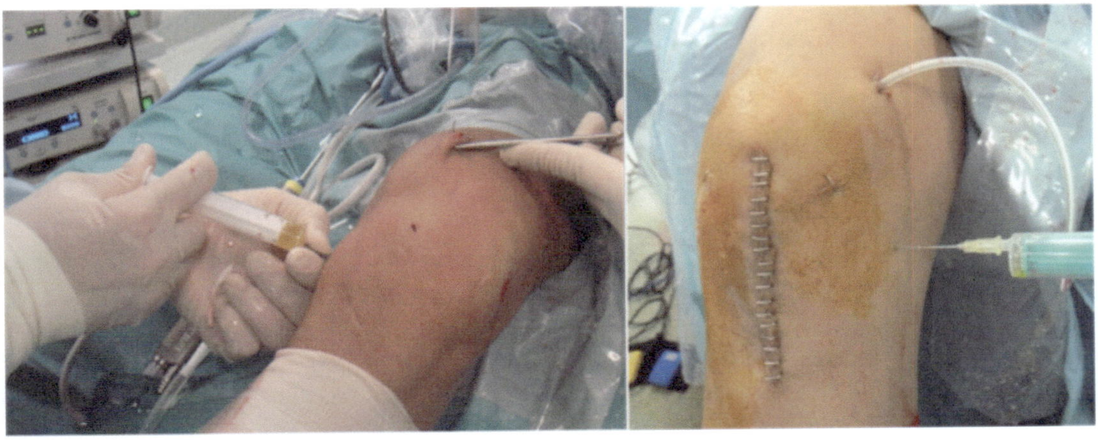

FIG. 3
Treatment of ACL and MCL ruptures: Arthroscopic ACL reconstruction with Bone- Patellar Tendon-Bone (BPTB), intraarticular injection and MCL infiltration of PRGF

In chronic injuries in which there is a major instability, reconstruction of the ligament by open surgery is mandatory. At the end of the procedure, infiltration of the new structure with Fraction 2 (Platelet Rich) of PRGF leukocyte-free, 4-6cc is recommended. After this, the Rehabilitation program is started and return to sport is estimated at between 12-16 weeks after the surgery. (Fig. 4)

Grade II Isolated Injury	• 4 – 6 cc PRGF: 1-2 Injections • Cryotherapy • Antivalgus Brace • Physiotherapy • Flexo-Extension Exercises immediately and without pain • Re-education Quadriceps & Hamstrings • Return to sport at 4-6 weeks
Grade III Isolated Injury	• 5 - 7 cc PRGF: 3 Injections • Cryotherapy • Antivalgus Brace • Physiotherapy • Flexo-Extension Exercises (without pain) • Re-education Quadriceps & Hamstrings • Return to sport 8-10 weeks

Grade II or III & ACL Injury	• ACL Arthroscopic reconstruction • 5 - 7 cc PRGF: 1 - 2 Injections • Perform Flexo-Extension with Antivalgus Brace • Re-education Quadriceps & Hamstrings • Return to sport starting at 6 months
Chronic Injury	• MCL Reconstruction • 4 - 6 cc PRGF: 1 - 2 Injections • Re-education Quadriceps & Hamstrings • Return to sport 12-16 weeks

Lateral collateral ligament (LCL)

The injury can be minimal and isolated or associated with a cascade of injuries after the LCL breakdown: avulsion of the Bicep Tendon, the Ilio-Tibial Tract and the Popliteus Tendon, traction of the internal popliteal sciatic nerve, lesion of the postero-lateral capsule and of the lateral meniscus, rupture of the ACL / PCL and internal popliteal sciatic nerve traction with or without popliteal vessel injury.

When the injury is partial, conservative treatment is recommended, as described previously for MCL:

1. Ultrasound-guided infiltration with Fraction 2 (Platelet Rich) of PRGF leukocyte-free, 4 - 7 cc on the ligament and its insertion.
2. Anti-varus brace placed for 4-7 weeks with free movement, unblocked.
3. Physiotherapy.
4. Rehabilitation program.
5. Regular medical and ultrasound controls.

Repetition of infiltration should be performed if needed, according to the evolution of healing. Usually, sufficiency comes from one to three infiltrations administered with an interval of 7-10 days.

Normally, the patient is back to sport at 8-10 weeks. (Fig. 5)

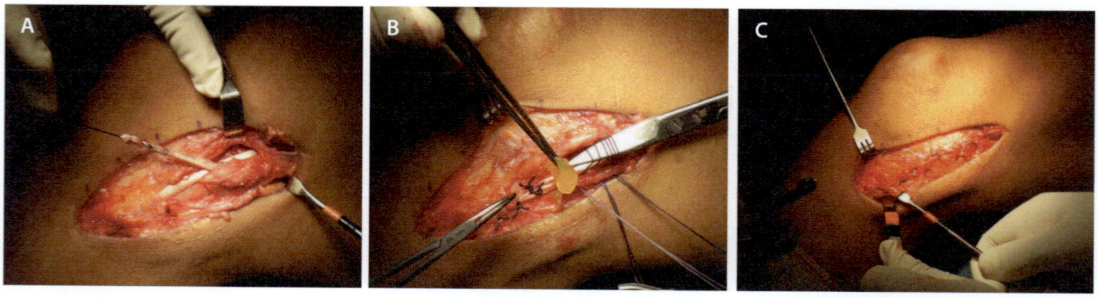

FIG. 4
MCL reconstruction surgery. A) Reconstruction with semitendinousus tendon (ST) and gracilis. B) PRGF clot after the the tendon suture. C) Articular capsule sutured.

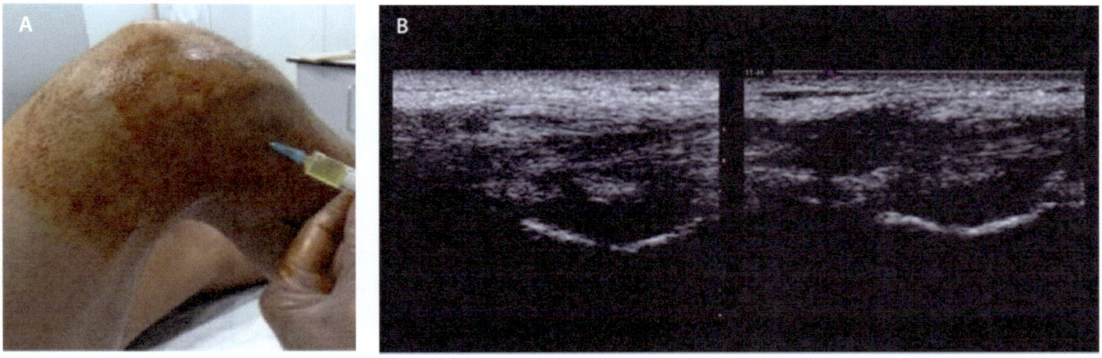

FIG. 5
A) LCL injury treated with PRGF. B) Ultrasound follow-up of the treated injury.

If the injury is complex, surgical treatment is advised. There are many surgical techniques that can be performed, and in all cases, after surgery infiltration into the repaired area with a Fraction 2 (Platelet Rich) of leukocyte-free PRGF, 4 to 7 cc. is recommended. (Fig. 6)

Isolated Injury	• 4 - 7 cc PRGF: 1 - 3 Injections • Cryotherapy • Antivarus Brace • Physiotherapy • Flexo-Extension Exercises (without pain) • Re-education Quadriceps & Hamstrings • Return to sport between 8-10 weeks
Complex Injury	• LCL reconstruction & other injured structures • 5 - 7 cc PRGF: 1 - 2 Injections • Physiotherapy • Rehabilitation program • Return to sport starting at 7-8 months

Anterior cruciate ligament (ACL)

Injuries causing only anteroposterior instability (Lachman Test + and Pivot Shift -) can be solved with a conservative therapy:

1. Infiltration should be performed under arthroscopic control of the Fraction 2 (Platelet Rich) of leukocyte-free PRGF, 3-4 cc, into the ligament and 5-6cc intraarticularly. Or alternatively, an intraarticular infiltration of the Fraction 2 (Platelet Rich) of the PRGF leukocyte-free, 7-8 cc. may be done.
2. Immobilization for 3-4 weeks.
3. Physiotherapy.
4. Rehabilitation program.
5. Regular medical controls between 8-12 weeks. (Fig. 7)

According to the recovery evolution, infiltration is repeated if needed. Usually, from one to three injections administered with an interval of 7-10 days is sufficient.

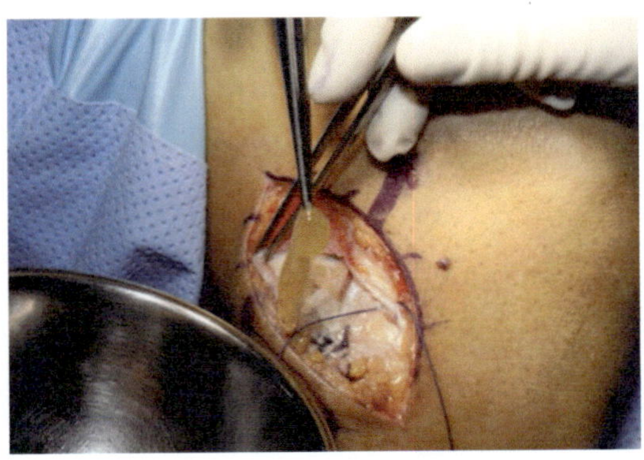

FIG. 6
Surgical Treatment of the LCL and Biological augmentation with PRGF clot.

However, injuries that cause rotational instability (Pivot Shift +), isolated or combined, the treatment performed is surgical with Biological augmentation with PRGF.

1. Arthroscopic ACL reconstruction and treatment of other structures if needed.
2. Intraarticular infiltration of Fraction 2 (Platelet Rich) of the PRGF leukocyte-free, 7 to 8 cc.
3. Physiotherapy.
4. Rehabilitation program and return to sport starting at 6 months. (Fig. 8)

Partial Rupture with Lachman Test +	• 3 – 4 cc PRGF ligament: 1 - 2 Injections • 5 – 6 cc PRGF intraarticular: 1 – 2 injections • Cryotherapy • Physiotherapy • Re-education Quadriceps & Hamstrings • Return to sport between 8-12 weeks
Injury with Pivot Shift +	• ACL arthroscopic reconstruction & surgical treatment to the other injured structures if it is necessary • 7 - 8 cc PRGF intraarticular • Physiotherapy • Rehabilitation program • Return to sport starting at 6 months

Posterior Cruciate Ligament (PCL)

In acute Grade I and II isolated injuries, a conservative treatment is recommended:

1. Infiltration under ultrasound control of the Fraction 2 (Platelet Rich) of the leukocyte-free PRGF, 3-4 cc, into the ligament and 5-6cc intraarticularly. If it is a grade II injury, more infiltrations may be needed.
2. 3-4 weeks (grade I) or 6-8 (grade II) of PCL brace placed, unblocked.
3. Physiotherapy.
4. Rehabilitation program.
5. Regular medical controls.

Depending on the recovery evolution of the patient, more infiltrations will be done. Usually, from one to three infiltrations administered with an interval of 7-10 days will suffice. (Figs. 9-10)

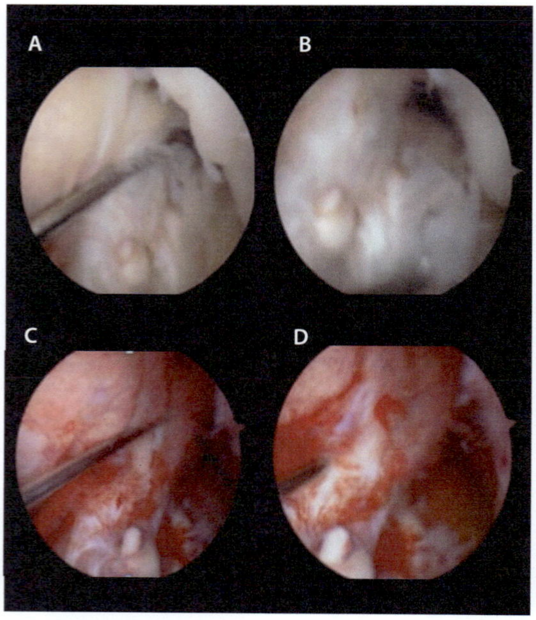

FIG. 7
A) ACL partial rupture. B) Infiltration with PRGF in the healthy posterolateral (PL) band of the ACL.

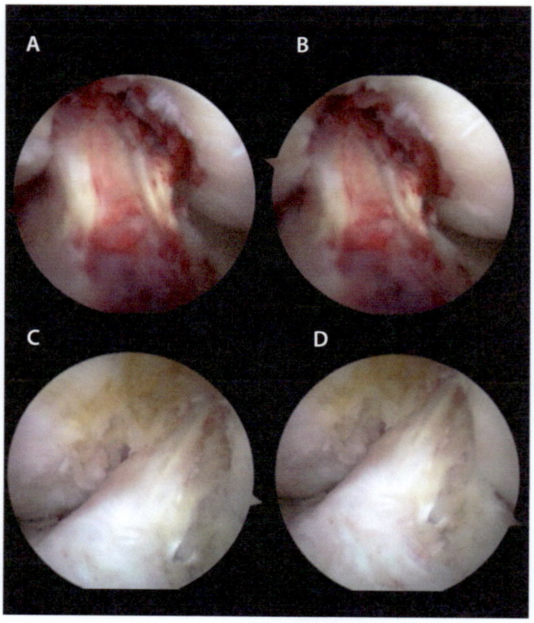

FIG. 8
A) Arthroscopic view, 7 weeks post ACL reconstruction and PRGF injection. B) Arthroscopic view, 14 weeks post ACL reconstruction and PRGF injection.

Grade I Isolated Injury	• 3 – 4 cc PRGF ligament: 1 - 2 Injections • 5 – 6 cc PRGF intraarticular: 1 – 2 injections • Cryotherapy • PCL Brace: 3 – 4 weeks • Physiotherapy • Re-education Quadriceps & Hamstrings • Return to sport 3-4 months after injury
Grade II Isolated Injury	• 3 - 4 cc PRGF ligament: 3 Injections • 5 – 6 cc PRGF intraarticular: 3 injections • Cryotherapy • PCL Brace: 6 – 8 weeks • Physiotherapy • Rehabilitation program • Return to sport 4-5 months after injury
Grade III Injury	• PCL arthroscopic reconstruction & surgical reconstruction to other injured structures if it is necessary • 3 - 4 cc PRGF intra-substance ligament & 5 - 6 cc PRGF intraarticular • 2 - 3 weeks postsurgery, PCL Brace: 3 – 4 months • Physiotherapy • Rehabilitation program • Return to sport 6-8 months after surgery
Complex Injury	• PCL arthroscopic reconstruction & surgical reconstruction to other injured structures if it is necessary • 3 - 4 cc PRGF intrasubstance ligament & 5 - 6 cc PRGF intraarticular • 2 - 3 weeks postsurgery, PCL Brace: 4 – 5 months • Physiotherapy • Rehabilitation program • Return to sport 8-10 months after surgery

Return to sport is at 3-4 months in the grade I isolated injury, and at 4-5 months in the grade II isolated injury.

In acute Grade III injuries and chronic injuries, a surgical treatment is recommended:

1. Arthroscopic PCL reconstruction and surgical reconstruction of other structures if necessary.
2. Infiltration of the Fraction 2 (Platelet Rich) of the leukocyte-free PRGF, 3-4 cc, in the ligament and 5-6cc intraarticularly.
3. 2-3 weeks after surgery, a PCL brace for 3-4 months, free and not blocked.
4. Physiotherapy.
5. Rehabilitation program

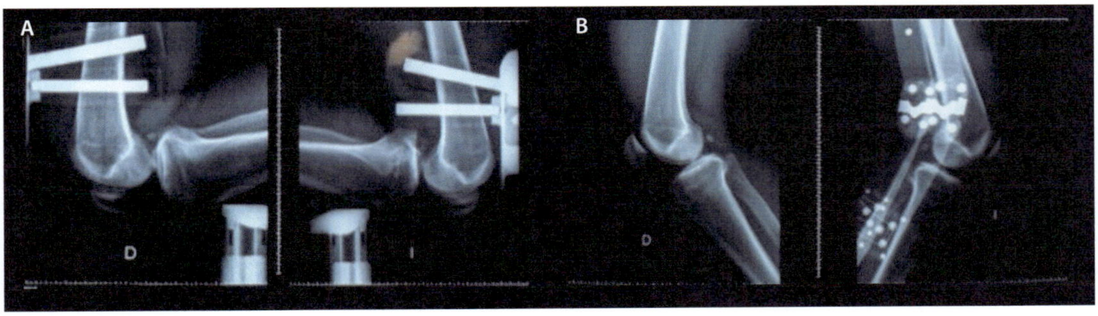

FIG. 9
A) Telos exam of both knees. D-Right (healthy knee) and I-Left (injured knee). B) X-ray profiles of both same knees. D-Right normal and I-Left with PCL brace which reduces the posterior tibial translation.

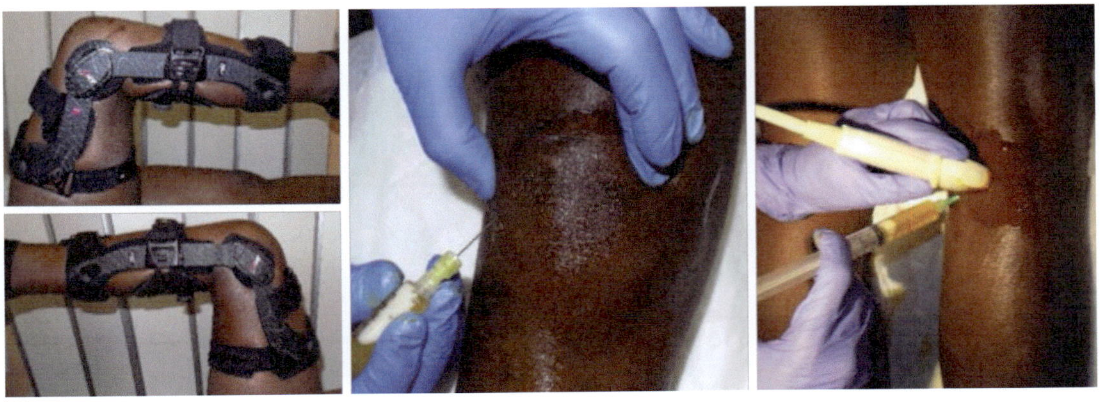

FIG. 10
PCL injury. Brace, PRGF intraarticular infiltration and PRGF ultrasound guided injection in the PCL.

3. ANKLE

ANATOMY AND FUNCTION

The ankle joint is made of three bones: Tibia and Fibula are the proximal while Talus is the distal bone.

The lower end of the tibia and fibula make an arch in which the trochlea of the talus is articulated. The peroneal malleolus, which is lateral, is bulkier than the tibial or medial malleolus.

This structure is surrounded by a fibrous capsule with ligaments, muscles and tendons. The muscles and tendons provide the movement.

Ligaments:
Internal Lateral Ligament or Deltoid Ligament is located in the medial part of the ankle joining the tibia with the talus and the calcaneus. It has two levels: deep and superficial. The deep one has two bands: anterior tibiotalus band and posterior tibiotalus band. The superficial one is larger with a triangular shape, connecting the tibia to the navicular in its lower edge and with the medial edge of the glenoid and the minor process of the calcaneus.

Lateral Collateral Ligament has three fascicles. The anterior bundle or the Anterior Talofibular Ligament joins the anterior edge of the peroneal malleolus to the talus. The medial band or Calcaneofibular Ligament (CFL) extends from the most prominent point of the peroneal malleolus to the lateral part of the calcaneus. The posterior band or Posterior Talofibular Ligament (PTFL) connects the medial side of the peroneal malleolus with posterioexternal tubercle of the talus.

The Anterior Ligament is a capsular thickening which is inserted into the talus.

The Posterior Ligament is a capsular thickening which is inserted into the talus.

The ligament of the anterior syndesmosis and the ligament of the posterior syndesmosis maintain the tibiofibular arch with the correct interosseous distance.

The movements of the tibiofibulotalar joint are plantar flexion or "flexion" and dorsal flexion or "extension".

INJURIES

Epidemiology of ligament injuries of the ankle.

Time reviewed	Season 2014-15
Anterior Talo-Fibular Ligament	1.355
Deltoid Ligament	233

The epidemiology of ankle injuries in the Mutualitat Catalana de Futbolistes, MCF, may well differ from general population epidemiology. Players from the MCF are highly active athletes in sports practise whose ankles suffer higher stress than normal.

Deltoid ligament

The injury diagnosis is confirmed with radiology (Stress Rx), MRI and static and functional ultrasound.

1. Infiltration of the Fraction 2 (Platelet Rich) of the leukocyte-free PRGF, 3-4 cc, in the ligament tissue and 5-6cc intraarticularly.
2. Placement of taping for 4-6 weeks.
3. Physical therapy.
4. Rehabilitation program.
5. Back to sport at 10-12 weeks. (Figs. 11-12)

Deltoid ligament Injury	• 3 - 4 cc PRGF intrasubstance ligament & 2 - 3 cc PRGF intraarticular • Taping for 4 – 6 weeks • Physiotherapy • Rehabilitation program • Return to sport 10-12 weeks

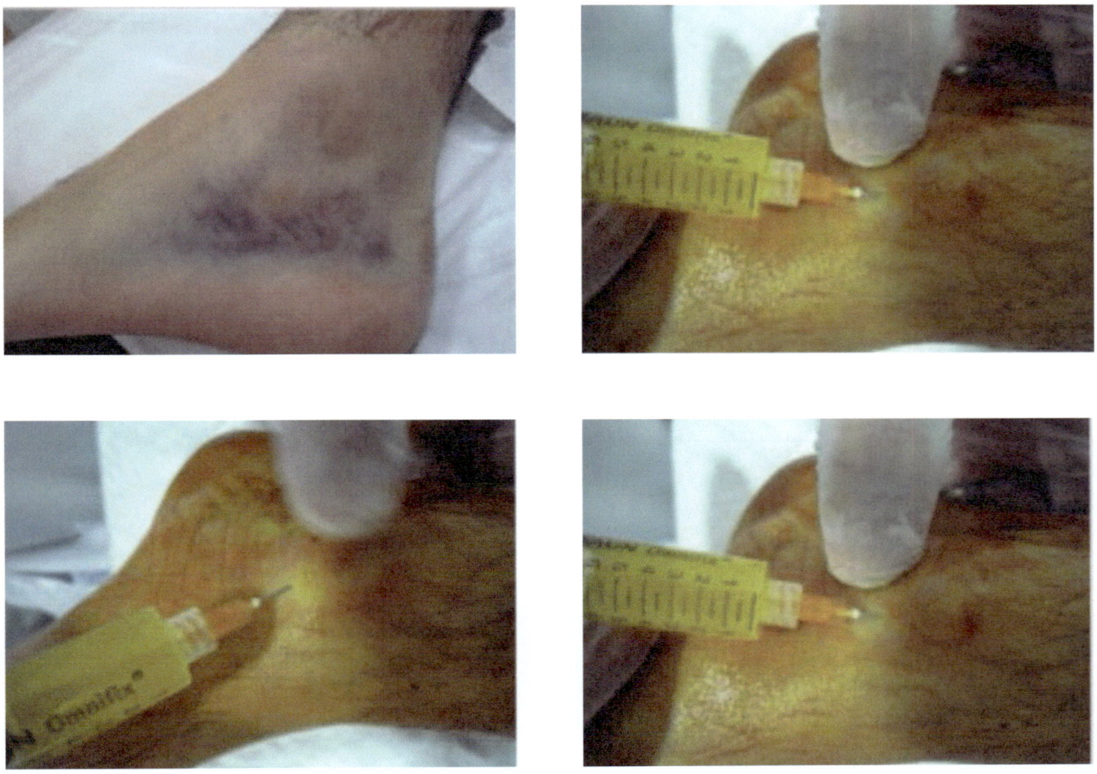

FIG. 11
Deltoid Ligament injury. Treatment with PRGF infiltration

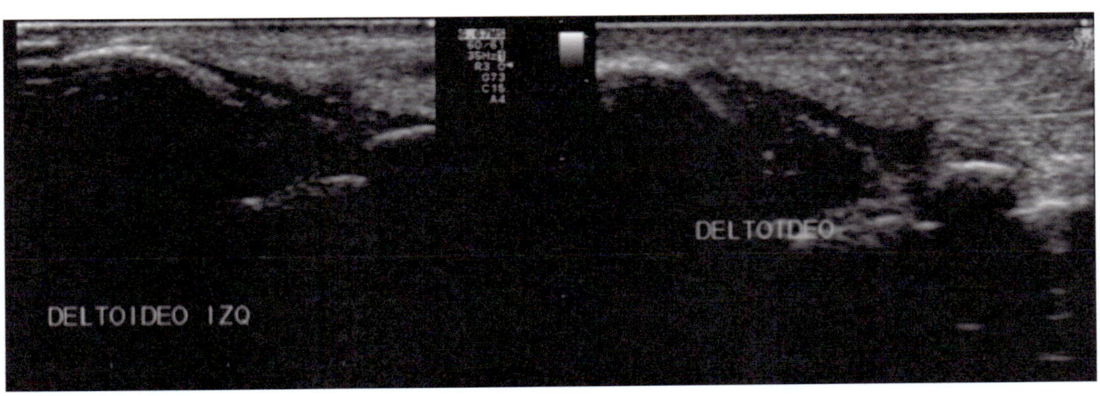

FIG. 12
Deltoid Ligament injury. Ultrasound follow-up control.

Anterior Talofibular ligament

The injury diagnosis is confirmed with radiology (Stress Rx), MRI and static and functional ultrasound.

1. Infiltration of the Fraction 2 (Platelet Rich) of leukocyte-free PRGF, 3-4 cc, in the ligament substance and 5-6cc intraarticularly.
2. Placement of taping for 4 weeks.
3. Physical therapy.
4. Rehabilitation program.
5. Back to sport at 4-7 weeks. (Figs. 13-14)

Anterior talofibular Injury	• 3 - 4 cc PRGF intrasubstance ligament & 2 - 3 cc PRGF intraarticular • Taping for 4 weeks • Physiotherapy • Rehabilitation program • Return to sport 4-7 weeks

4. REHABILITATION / RETURN TO SPORT

In ligament injuries the role of the physiotherapist is very Important. The main objective is to eliminate pain and decrease the swelling, then regain a good range of motion and finally re-establish the muscle mass.

The main objective of the first days is to diminish the swelling and pain, and next is to work with the physiotherapist on the range of motion to reestablish it, and then strength exercises must be conducted to maintain and restore good muscle tone.

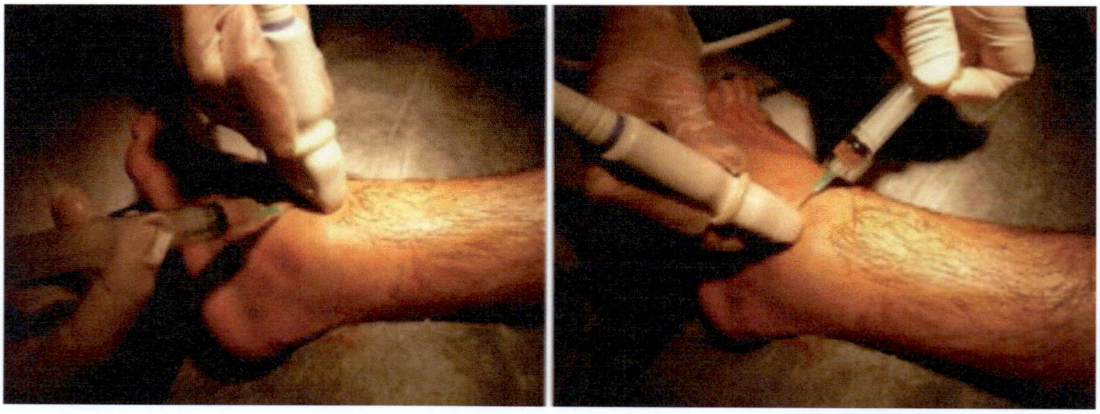

FIG. 13
Anterior Talo-Fibular Ligament injury. Treatment with PRGF injection.

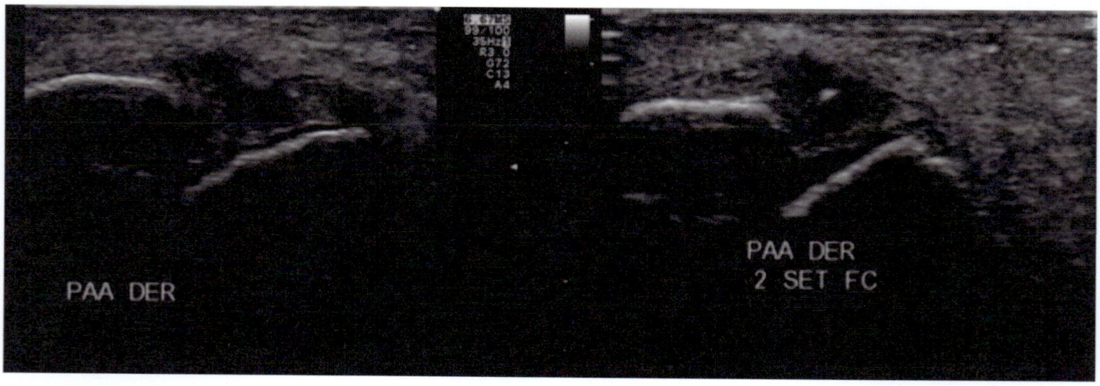

FIG. 14
Anterior Talo-Fibular Ligament injury. Follow-up control with Ultrasound.

When a brace is needed, the rehabilitation must be adapted to this circumstance.

If the injury requires surgical treatment, the recovery process could be longer and more delicate. (Fig. 15)

INJURIES IN EARLY AGE POPULATION – DEVELOPMENT IN ADVANCED AGE

Nowadays, increasing sports practise among children is a serious matter of concern. They practice sport as entertainment, training and taking part in championships, so the level of requirements has increased. It is very important to respect a young person's physical moment and age. The values, health and formative stage should be a priority. The physical formative stage is between 12 and 15 years. At that time, foundations must be created in mobility, strength, flexibility and endurance, in order to prevent a non-normal development during sports practice.

Severe injuries at an early age are becoming more common and the consequences are a subject of study. There are some studies that discuss this problem, and Dekker et al. conclude that early surgical treatment which is favoured to prevent concomitant articular injuries and an early return to play, can increase risk of re-injury and should be met with caution in this age group[7]. Conversely, Werner et al. demonstrated that paediatric and adolescent patients who underwent ACL reconstruction had significant increases in incidences of concomitant meniscal and cartilage procedures[8]. Similarly, the Vavken et al. study showed that more than half of the children and the adolescents treated for ACL tear have concurrent meniscal or chondral injury[9].

On the other side, the major problem years after the retirement of an elite athlete is osteoarthritis, OA, which he or she may develop in the injured joints. Therefore, a treatment to prevent a post-traumatic OA is fundamental to the normal behaviour of the injured joint after recovery.

PRGF treatment is not only positive and useful during an acute injury, it is also positive in the long term. PRGF injection avoids or diminishes the apparition of bone edema and early OA in ligament-injured joints. Some studies have concluded that not only are PRGF injections beneficial in treating injury, they are a good treatment to prevent OA.

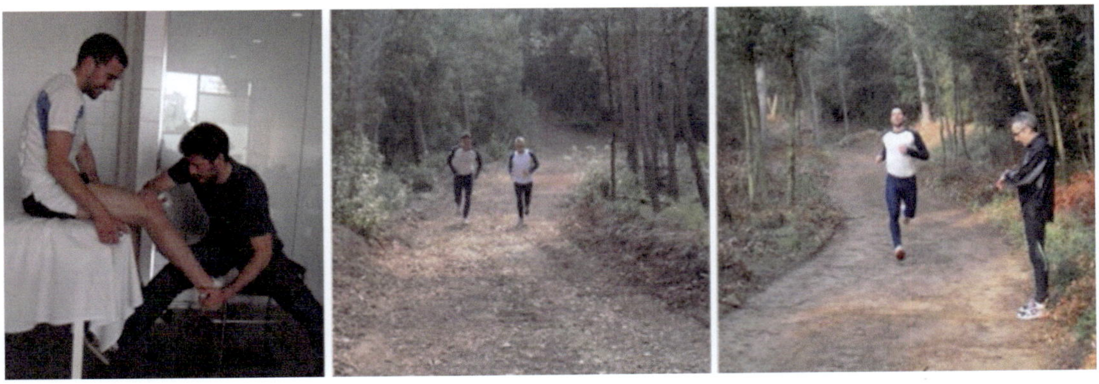

FIG. 15
Rehabilitation exercises in the gym and outdoor (in a more advanced stages of the recovery).

1. Pierce GF, Mustoe TA, Altrock BW, Deuel TF, Thomason A. Role of platelet-derived growth factor in wound healing. Journal of cellular biochemistry. 1991;45:319-26.

2. Kiritsy CP, Lynch AB, Lynch SE. Role of growth factors in cutaneous wound healing: a review. Critical reviews in oral biology and medicine : an official publication of the American Association of Oral Biologists. 1993;4:729-60.

3. Canalis E. Clinical review 35: Growth factors and their potential clinical value. The Journal of clinical endocrinology and metabolism. 1992;75:1-4.

4. Molloy T, Wang Y, Murrell G. The roles of growth factors in tendon and ligament healing. Sports Med. 2003;33:381-94.

5. Nico B, Mangieri D, Benagiano V, Crivellato E, Ribatti D. Nerve growth factor as an angiogenic factor. Microvascular research. 2008;75:135-41.

6. Anitua E, Andia I, Sanchez M, et al. Autologous preparations rich in growth factors promote proliferation and induce VEGF and HGF production by human tendon cells in culture. Journal of orthopaedic research : official publication of the Orthopaedic Research Society. 2005;23:281-6.

7. Dekker TJ, Rush JK, Schmitz MR. What's New in Pediatric and Adolescent Anterior Cruciate Ligament Injuries? Journal of pediatric orthopedics. 2016.

8. Werner BC, Yang S, Looney AM, Gwathmey FW, Jr. Trends in Pediatric and Adolescent Anterior Cruciate Ligament Injury and Reconstruction. Journal of pediatric orthopedics. 2016;36:447-52.

9. Vavken P, Tepolt FA, Kocher MS. Concurrent Meniscal and Chondral Injuries in Pediatric and Adolescent Patients Undergoing ACL Reconstruction. Journal of pediatric orthopedics. 2016.

CHAPTER 11

Tendinopathy and its Treatment: the Rationale and Pitfalls in the Clinical Application of PRP

AUTHORS

Wang J.[1], Zhou Y.[1,2], Nirmala X.[1]

[1,2]MechanoBiology Laboratory, Department of Orthopaedic Surgery, University of Pittsburgh School of Medicine, 210 Lothrop Street, BST, E1640, Pittsburgh, PA 15213, USA
[2]Joint Surgery and Sports Medicine Department, Shanghai Changzheng Hospital, Second Military Medical University, Shanghai 200003, China.

SUMMARY

Chronic tendon injuries or tendinopathy are prevalent among athletes and non-athletes worldwide. However, current treatment of tendinopathy in clinical settings is largely palliative. Platelet-rich plasma (PRP) is now a popular option to treat tendinopathy in orthopaedic surgery and sport medicine although some clinical studies cast doubt on the efficacy of PRP treatment for tendinopathy. Based on the findings from most basic science studies it seems clear that PRP can reduce pain and promote healing in tendinopathic tendons. However, the application of PRP treatment in clinics needs optimization. Currently, PRP treatments use a "one-size-fits-all" approach where a predetermined dose of a PRP preparation is used to treat tendon injuries in patients regardless of the conditions of tendon injury or patient's age, gender or treatment history. This "one-size-fits-all" approach would diminish the efficacy of PRP treatment and as a result, would create contradicting clinical outcomes. Thus, a "personalized approach" is necessary where PRP- and patient-related factors should be taken into account prior to PRP treatment. These may include selecting an appropriate PRP and also considering patients' age, gender, injury type, disease history, pre-injury activity level and post-treatment rehabilitation protocol. It is expected that such "personalized medicine" approach would enhance the efficacy of PRP treatment in clinics.

E. Anitua et al. (eds.), *Platelet Rich Plasma in Orthopaedics and Sports Medicine*,
https://doi.org/10.1007/978-3-319-63730-3_11

1. TENDINOPATHY

Tendons are connective tissues that link muscles to bones, and are mainly made of cells, collagen fibers and small amounts of proteoglycans that form the tendon extracellular matrix (ECM). The primary function of tendons is to transmit muscular forces to bones, enabling joint movements. Therefore, tendons like patellar and Achilles tendons are in general subject to large mechanical loads. Many studies have indicated that excess mechanical loading may induce chronic tendon injury or tendinopathy[1]. More recent studies have implicated tendon stem/progenitor cells (TSCs) in the mechanical loading-induced degenerative tendinopathy[2]. When exposed to mechanical overloading, TSCs were shown to differentiate not only into tenocytes, the dominant resident cells in the tendons, but also into non-tenocytes (adipocytes, chondrocytes and osteoblasts)[3] that may disrupt tendon structure and integrity.

Moreover, mechanical overloading is also implicated in inducing sterile tendon inflammation commonly observed in tendinopathic tendons[1]. Sterile inflammation is characterized by the presence of PGE2, an inflammatory mediator, in injured tendons. Studies have reported higher PGE2 levels in the Achilles tendons of humans subjected to mechanical loads in vivo[4] and in human tendon cells after mechanical loading in vitro[5]. Similar effects were also observed in animal models where intensive treadmill running increased PGE2 in the patellar and Achilles tendons of mice in vivo[6]. While low levels of PGE2 may increase tenocyte gene expression, high levels of PGE2 in the tendon may increase non-tenocyte gene expression and result in the formation of non-tendinous tissues by causing differentiation of TSCs into non-tenocytes[6] thus leading to tendinopathy (Fig. 1). The high levels of PGE2 production in injured tendons is the rationale behind using non-steroid anti-inflammatory drugs (NSAIDs) to treat tendinopathy; NSAIDs inhibit COX, which catalyze the conversion of arachidonic acids to PGE2[7]. Thus, inhibiting COX by NSAIDs reduces the levels of PGE2 in injured tissues like tendons thereby decreasing inflammation.

High levels of prostaglandin E2 (PGE2) may induce the development of tendinopathy

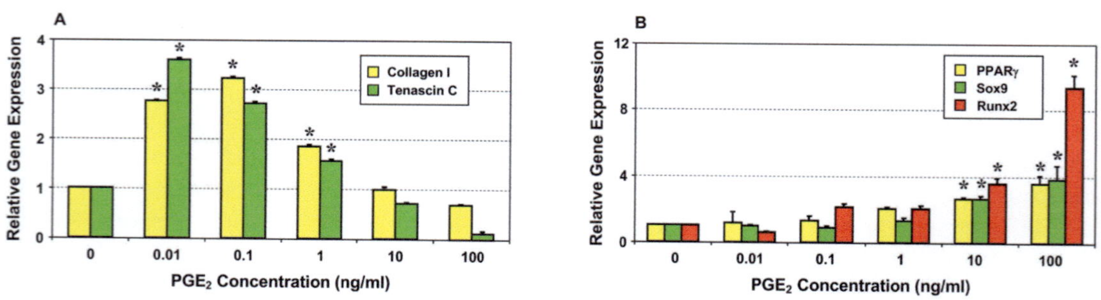

FIG. 1
(A) In tendon cells in vitro, PGE2 modulates the expression of tenocyte and non-tenocyte related genes in a dose-dependent manner. Specifically, at 0.01 ng/ml concentration, PGE2 induces a high level of expression of collagen type I (Collagen I) and Tenascin C, two tenocyte-related genes. (B) On the other hand, high concentrations of PGE2 increase non-tenocyte related genes, PPARγ (fat tissue marker, Sox9 (cartilage marker) and Runx2 (bone marker).

* $P < 0.05$ compared to 0ng/ml PGE2 concentration. For full description of the findings, refer to the paper[78].

Besides mechanical overloading, another common but less addressed causative factor of tendinopathy is aging, which affects a majority of the aging population. Typically, aging reduces the quality of human tendons by decreasing tendon cell numbers, protein synthesis and water content. Apart from these, non-tendinous tissues such as lipid deposition, proteoglycan accumulation, and calcification that are often observed in tendinopathic tendons[8] are also noticed in aging tendons. Using a mouse model, our study showed that tendons in aging mice (9 months old) had higher amount of lipids, proteoglycans and calcium deposits in comparison with young 2.5 months old mice[9]. TSCs isolated from aging mice also expressed higher amounts of non-tenocyte genes, LPL, Sox9 and Runx2[9] that have the potential to induce the development of lipids, proteoglycans and calcium, respectively. Moreover, the quality of TSCs in aging mice is evidently poor with lower proliferation rate and reduced expression of stem cell markers (Oct-4, Sca-1, and SEEA-1) (Fig. 2)[9], which may likely impair the healing of tendinopathic tendons because TSCs are necessary for the maintenance of intact tendons and repair of injured tendons by differentiating into tenocytes to replace cells and matrix proteins lost due to injury.

Aging causes tendinopathy by deteriorating tendon stem cells

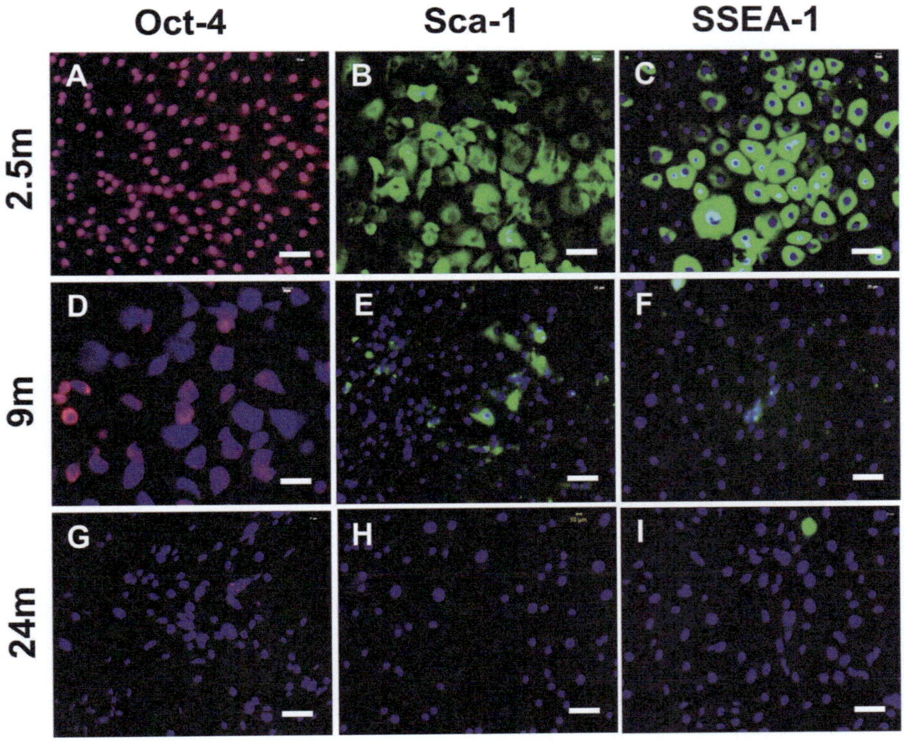

FIG. 2
Almost all tendon stem/progenitor cells (TSCs) from young, 2.5 months old mice express robust amounts of stem cell markers, Oct-4 (pink, A), Sca-1 (green, B) and SSEA-1 (green, C). But in 9 months old mice, fewer cells express these stem cell markers (D-F) and in 24 months old mice, none of the cells express these markers (G-I). Bar – 50μm. For full description of the results regarding the effects of aging on the quality and number of TSCs in mice, see the original paper [9].

2. TRADITIONAL TENDINOPATHY TREATMENT

Tendon and ligament injuries are one of the most prevalent musculoskeletal problems with millions of patients treated in orthopaedic clinics in the United States every year. Among the several tendons in a body, patellar, Achilles, and rotator cuff are the three tendon types that are more susceptible to injury than others due to mechanical overloading/overuse. Patients with tendinopathy experience inflammation and pain, and in many cases tendon rupture due to degenerative changes in the tendon. Currently, these patients receive only palliative care in clinics where pain and inflammation are treated mostly with NSAIDs, corticosteroids, physical therapy, shock wave therapy, or even rest with the last option being surgery. Although NSAIDs offer a short term pain relief, they have a negative impact on the structure of injured tendons, and are also reported to cause serious side effects such as abdominal discomfort, and gastrointestinal, cardiovascular and renal problems[7]. Besides, the use of corticosteroids itself may lead to tendon rupture by decreasing tendon cell proliferation and inducing degenerative changes in the tendon[10]. The other modalities often yield inconsistent results. Thus, alternative treatment options are in need for the safe and effective treatment of tendinopathy.

3. PLATELET-RICH PLASMA (PRP) TREATMENT OF TENDINOPATHY

Currently, PRP therapy is widely used as a promising option for tendinopathy treatment in orthopaedic/sports medicine across the United States and other countries[11]. Intuitively, the use of PRP for healing tendon injuries is reasonable, because in the event of an injury, platelets are indeed the "first responders" and thus PRP treatment may mimic the natural wound healing process. The primary benefits of PRP are a reduction in tendon pain and improvement in tendon function, which have been reported by patients treated for a variety of tendinopathy such as patellar tendinopathy[12], Achilles tendinopathy[13], elbow tendinopathy[14], and chronic plantar fasciitis[15].

In the PRP treatment of tendinopathy, the main factor to be considered is the PRP composition. The major PRP components are as follows.

Platelets

Platelets are present in large amounts because PRP is prepared with blood drawn from patients by centrifuging at low speed so they are re-suspended in a small volume of plasma. Platelets are anucleate cytoplasmic fragments produced in the bone marrow by megakaryocytes[16]. In the event of an injury, they are also the first responder cells that migrate to the wounded site and are well-known to play an important role in tissue healing[17,18].

It has been recognized that tissue wound healing is driven by growth factors, which are present in high amounts in PRP[17,18]. The main growth factors in PRP include platelet-derived growth factor (PDGF), transforming growth factor-β (TGF-β), vascular endothelial growth factor (VEGF), epidermal growth factor (EGF), insulin-like growth factor-I (IGF-I), fibroblast growth factor (FGF) and hepatocyte growth factor (HGF). These growth factors have been shown to enhance tendon healing[17,18]. Depending on the platelet concentration in PRP, the amount of growth factors released into a treated site may vary. While the rationale behind using PRP is to deliver concentrated amounts of growth factor-containing platelets to heal an injured tissue, studies have shown that very high levels of platelets may not be useful to treat tendon injuries[19] because they do not induce tendon cell proliferation[20]. In fact, the platelet concentration in most clinical and basic science studies is only 3-5-fold higher than in whole blood. At this concentration, PRP has been shown to increase the number of tendon cells[20,21], enhance collagen synthesis[20-22], improve fiber arrangement[23], and enhance tendon strength[24]. However, when the platelet concentration was more than 10-

fold higher than in whole blood, improvement in tendon function was not evident in patients with Achilles tendon ruptures[19]. Therefore, it is pertinent to regulate the platelet concentration in PRP, which are currently prepared using commercial kits in clinical settings.

Plasma

The majority of plasma is made of water (90%) and other components such as proteins. Plasma is necessary for the fluidity of the blood, and allows the flow of cells and other factors around the body.

Leukocytes

Another important component in PRP is the leukocyte, which has gained attention only recently in basic PRP research and clinical applications. Depending on the preparation method, PRP may contain a few or high amounts of leukocytes; PRP with no or only a few leukocytes are termed pure-PRP or P-PRP and those with high amounts of leukocytes are called leukocyte containing or leukocyte rich PRP both referred to as L-PRP.

Fibrinogen

PRP also contains abundant fibrinogen, which is a soluble plasma protein. When PRP is activated with thrombin or calcium chloride, fibrinogen is converted into polymeric fibrin, which forms a gel-like substance. In this gel form, PRP can act as a conducive bio-scaffold/matrix that facilitates the interaction between the components of PRP, tendon tissue and other migrating stem cells that are recruited to the healing site[25]. Because of this, PRP can also be used as an excellent carrier of cells or a bio-compound in wound repairs using tissue engineering approaches. For example, PRP was used as a carrier to deliver autologous adipose derived-stem cells (ASCs) to repair Achilles tendon defects in rabbits[26]. Our own studies have also used PRP as an effective carrier of kartogenin, a small bio-compound, to promote fibrocartilage formation in the tendon-bone interface[27].

Because PRP is a natural source and has a unique composition, it has a number of advantages that promote its use to treat tendon injuries.

1. PRP is safe because it is an autologous product derived from a patients' own blood and also contains physiological proportions of the growth factors;
2. PRP preparation in orthopaedic clinics is straightforward with many commercial kits available;
3. PRP can be easily applied via injections in clinical settings and therefore it is non-surgical and allows athletes to quickly return to sport activities;
4. PRP serves as a reservoir of numerous growth factors that can enhance tendon healing; and its fibrin gel can be used as a natural scaffold that is conducive to tendon healing; and
5. PRP can function as an anti-inflammatory "drug" to reduce tendon inflammation and hence pain. Such beneficial effects of PRP are better than the currently used steroid treatment that induces serious side effects.

4. CLINICAL STUDIES ON PRP

The findings of laboratory science become fruitful when validated by clinical studies such as randomized clinical trials (RCTs), which are considered as gold standards for clinical studies. Thus, a number of RCTs have been conducted to determine the efficacy of PRP to heal tendinopathic tendons with many reporting the beneficial effects of PRP in patients. For instance, significant pain reduction was observed in an RCT that included 14 patients with chronic lateral elbow epicondylitis 6 weeks after PRP treatment when compared to the 14 patients treated with autologous blood[28]. Similarly, pain reduction was realized 6 months after PRP treatment of patellar tendinopathy in an RCT with 12 patients[12]. In yet another larger double-blind, prospective, multicenter RCT, PRP treatment of chronic tennis elbow in 116 patients improved pain and function 6 months after treatment when compared to an active control group with 114 participants[29]. Furthermore, PRP also caused long-term pain-reduction effects. In a double-blind RCT that included 100 patients with chronic lateral epicondylitis, PRP treatment significantly reduced pain and improved elbow function in the 51 patients in this group in 1-year and 2-year follow-up studies when compared to corticosteroid injections given to 49 patients[14]. Besides, PRP has been used in conjunction with stem cells to improve PRP treatment efficacy. An animal RCT administered a combination of adipose derived mesenchymal stem cells and PRP, and found that the combination curtailed lesion progression, enhanced collagen fiber organization and decreased the presence of inflammatory cells[30]. Other clinical studies have also reported beneficial effects of PRP in patients with chronic plantar fasciitis[15], elbow tendinopathy[14,28,29], chronic Achilles tendinopathy[13] and patellar tendinopathy[12].

Despite the encouraging findings in these RCTs, others have reported the opposite results of PRP treatment; i.e. PRP did not produce beneficial effects when compared to the control. In fact, PRP did not significantly improve symptoms in patients ($n = 27$) with chronic Achilles tendinopathy when compared to the saline treated group up to 1 year after the treatment[19]. Similar results were also obtained in another RCT where PRP was used to treat rotator cuff tendinopathy in 20 patients; PRP treatment was similar to the saline treated group after a 1 year follow-up[31]. However, the study by Schepull et al.[19] used PRP with unusually high platelet concentration; 10-fold higher than in whole blood, while basic science studies use PRP with only 3-5 fold higher platelets level, which showed beneficial effects at the cellular and molecular levels[20,21]. Similarly, treatment of elbow tendinopathy with L-PRP or autologous whole blood yielded similar pain scores in 76 patients ($n=38$ per group) in a one year follow-up study[32]. Interestingly, using L-PRP to treat patellar tendinopathy in 10 patients in an RCT significantly improved pain and tendon function (VISA scores) in the PRP treated group when compared to the dry needling treatment group ($n = 13$) at 12 weeks[33]. However, at 26 weeks, the improved treatment effects of PRP were slightly lower than the dry needling treatment[33].

Thus, it is clear that while PRP appears to exert beneficial effects, such as reducing pain and improving tendon function, in some clinical trials, others reported no effects thus creating controversies in the efficacy of PRP to treat tendinopathy. Since RCTs are the gold standard for clinical studies, results from RCTs are considered highly relevant and important for judging the effectiveness of PRP treatment for tendinopathy. But it is important to note that while positive results from RCTs provide evidence for the efficacy of PRP among human participants, the negative results should be interpreted with caution taking into consideration the common factors that may lower PRP efficacy. A common weakness with RCTs is the small number of participants. In the RCTs mentioned above, except except for some with a few hundred participants the remaining had relatively small sample size ($n < 25$). Considering extreme variability among humans receiving the treatments, such a small sample size could reduce the statistical power such that the treatment effects of PRP may not be detected.

Another variable in the clinical trials of PRP treatment is the variations in PRP composition in the different preparations that may contribute to the controversy surrounding PRP efficacy. More importantly, the responses of study participants to PRP treatments may vary greatly and may not qualify to score as a positive effect. Conducting an RCT is highly complex where many factors such as age, gender, disease/treatment history and patient management protocols can affect the outcome. However, before evaluating these variables it is essential to understand whether there is any scientific basis for the use of PRP to treat tendinopathy. Below, we provide an analysis of basic science studies performed on cell (in vitro) and animal (in vivo) models under well-controlled conditions.

5. *IN VITRO* STUDIES OF PRP

Because in vitro studies are conducted in well-controlled experimental conditions it is possible to measure specific treatment effects of PRP. Below are some cellular events that are influenced by PRP.

Tendon cell proliferation
Studies have shown that PRP treatment of tendon cells in vitro increased their proliferation significantly in a dose-dependent manner[21,34]. However, a 10-fold higher platelet concentration in PRP did not benefit tendon healing[19] suggesting that a high concentration of platelets in PRP may not promote cell proliferation. Therefore, it is critical to use the optimal concentration of PRP (3-5-fold higher than in whole blood) to induce tendon cell proliferation[20,21]. Not only can PRP increase the proliferation of tendon cells it can also increase the proliferation of mesenchymal stem cells (MSCs), bone-marrow stem cells (BMSCs) and adipose derived stem cells (ADSCs) that may migrate into the injury site to promote tendon healing[24,34].

TSC differentiation into tenocytes
Like other adult stem cells, TSCs are also multipotent; i.e., they have the ability to differentiate into multiple cell types in the presence of appropriate induction factors. In the presence of PRP, rabbit TSCs differentiated into tenocytes but not non-tenocytes[20,21]. Moreover, PRP also increased the expression of tenocyte related genes, scleraxis and tenascin C[35], and matrix proteins, COMP, decorin and tenascin-C in tendon cells[36]. The newly formed tenocytes were also active because they upregulated total collagen production[21], specifically collagen I and III[20].

Anabolic and catabolic effects of PRP
Collagen is the most abundant protein in the tendon ECM and many studies have shown that PRP can significantly promote the expression of collagen type I[20,22]. Specifically, TGF-β increased collagen I synthesis in tendon cells in vitro[37]. So the anabolic effects caused by PRP treatment on cells may explain why PRP can promote healing of tendinopathic tendons. Moreover, our in vitro study showed that PRP increased collagen production and did not induce non-tenocyte differentiation of TSCs into chondrocytes, adipocytes, or osteocytes that may lead to degenerative changes in the tendon[21]. This finding suggests that PRP treatment does not increase the risk of non-tendinous tissue formation in tendons that may compromise tendon structure and function. The main components in PRP that cause catabolic effects are the leukocytes. While leukocytes can be beneficial because they can promote chemotaxis, cell proliferation and differentiation[38], they can also be detrimental because they release pro-inflammatory cytokines such as interleukin-1 β (IL-1β) and IL-6, tumor necrosis factor- α (TNF-α) and reactive oxygen species that can induce inflammation thereby exacerbating the tissue injury[20]. In rabbit TSCs cultured in vitro, L-PRP increased the levels of inflammatory and catabolic proteins, IL-1β, IL-6 and PGE2, and matrix metalloproteinase (MMP)-1, MMP-13 while P-PRP increased anabolic proteins including alpha-smooth muscle actin (α-SMA), and collagen types I and III[20]. Similar differential effects were also observed in chondrocytes; L-PRP induced catabolism while P-PRP induced anabolism by increasing collagen type II and aggrecan expression[39]. Interestingly, leukocytes in PRP did not decrease tendon cell proliferation in vitro[20]. While platelets increase collagen type I expression, leukocytes promote collagen type III expression[36]. This information is of high value because a high collagen type I/collagen type III ratio is expected in normal healthy tendons while the reverse with high collagen type III/collagen type I ratio indicates injured tendons or tendons with scar formation[40]. Besides, L-PRP also increased MMP-1 and MMP-3 in tendon cells[20,36] while PRP without leukocytes decreased these MMP levels[20,22]. In addition, platelets increase the tendon matrix proteins, COMP and decorin, while leukocytes exert the opposite effects[36]. Thus, leukocytes mostly induce catabolic effects on tendons and tendon cells. Considering the above, it may be appropriate to use P-PRP or PRP with a low level of leukocytes in the clinical treatments of tendinopathy.

Anti-inflammatory effects of PRP

The popularity of PRP is primarily due to its ability to reduce pain and inflammation in tendinopathy patients in clinical trials. However, the mechanisms of these effects were only recently discovered. In an in vitro study conducted in our laboratory, PRP reduced the levels of the pro-inflammatory mediators, COX-1, COX-2 and PGE2 in TSCs. Similar effects were obtained under the same conditions when the cells were treated with HGF. Moreover, in a series of in vivo experiments anti-HGF antibodies reversed these effects; i.e., COX-1, COX-2 and PGE2 levels were not lowered in the presence of anti-HGF antibodies indicating that HGF, in part, exerts the anti-inflammatory effects of PRP (Fig. 3)[41]. In a previous study, HGF treatment also decreased the production of the pro-inflammatory cytokine, IL-6, but increased the anti-inflammatory cytokine, IL-10[42].

Combining PRP with other approaches

As mentioned above, once activated, PRP forms a gel; therefore, PRP can be combined with other tissue engineering modalities by mixing stem cells with PRP gel to treat tendinopathy. Combining PRP with BMSCs or TSCs to treat tendon wound healing induced synergistic effects[43]. Moreover, adding PRP to dexamethasone (corticosteroid) or ciprofloxacin treatment of human TSCs suppressed the non-tenocyte differentiation of cells and also reversed the reduction in cell senescence and cell death, induced respectively by the two drugs[44]. Similarly, a decrease in human tenocyte viability induced by methylprednisolone (steroid) was reversed by the addition of PRP[45]. Thus, PRP can serve as a better alternative to steroid treatments for the treatment of tendinopathy and may improve clinical outcome when combined with drugs to treat tendinopathy.

HGF in PRP is an anti-inflammatory factor

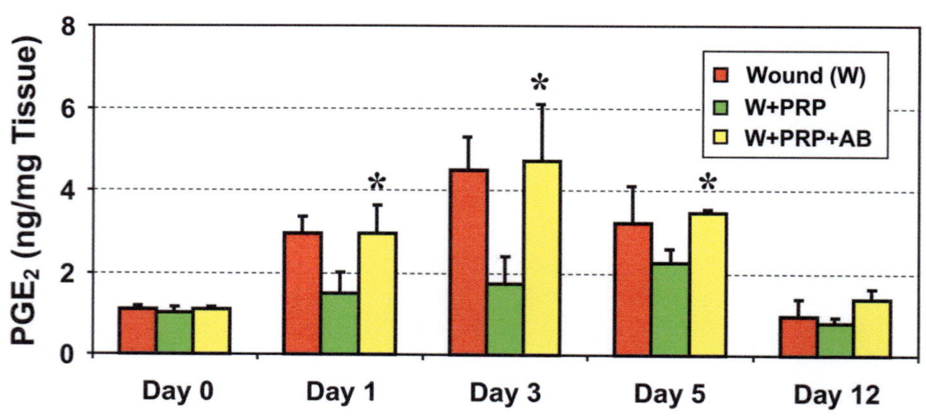

FIG. 3
In wounded mouse tendons, the concentration of PGE2, a tendon inflammation marker, increases on days 1-5 after wounding. However, treatment of the wounded area with PRP injection significantly reduces the levels of PGE2. In contrast, injecting HGF antibody along with PRP completely negates the PRP effects and as a result, PGE2 levels return to the levels in wounded tendons. AB, anti-HGF antibody.

* $P < 0.05$ when compared to the respective values on day 0. For complete results on the anti-inflammatory properties of PRP, see the original paper [41].

6. *IN VIVO* STUDIES OF PRP

In vivo studies have also shown the positive influence of PRP on tendon wound healing.

Intra-tendinous injections of PRP to treat tendinopathy in rat patellar and Achilles tendons increased joint mobilization and improved tendon fiber organization 25 days after treatment[46]. PRP gel injections into freshly ruptured patellar tendons also significantly increased the mechanical properties of tendons including stiffness, load at failure and ultimate stress over the saline treated control only 2 weeks after the treatment[47]. PRP also induced better cell orientation and tissue maturation in addition to increasing the expression of IGF-I in healed tendons[48]. Furthermore, individual growth factors including IGF-I[49], PDGF[50], FGF[51] or TGF-β[52] in PRP were demonstrated to increase cell proliferation and collagen production in tendon explants or when injected into horse, rabbit or rat tendons. Besides, combining platelet gel with a collagen implant effectively healed a rabbit Achilles tendon defect[53] and administering PRP with low-level laser therapy increased collagen type I and enhanced regeneration of the tendon tissue[54]. Thus, a number of in vivo studies have demonstrated that PRP treatment can enhance the healing of tendinopathic tendons. Lastly, our own studies in a wounded mouse Achilles tendon model established that PRP's anti-inflammatory function was mediated via HGF by suppressing the levels of COX-1, COX-2, and PGE2 production. The anti-inflammatory effects of PRP is of clinical relevance because high levels of PGE2 have been shown to increase pain[55], decrease cell proliferation and collagen production[56], and induce non-tenocyte differentiation of TSCs[21] that caused degenerative changes in rabbit tendons[57]. Therefore, PRP's ability to reduce PGE2 production is expected to benefit the healing of injured tendons.

7. FACTORS THAT MAY CONTRIBUTE TO THE PRP CONTROVERSY

As described above, findings from basic science studies provide support for the use of PRP to treat tendinopathy because PRP can increase cell proliferation, induce high expression of anabolic proteins, induce tenocyte differentiation, decrease inflammation and thus pain, which is of high clinical relevance. However, findings from some clinical trials do not align with basic science studies thus creating the well-known controversies in the PRP treatment efficacy for tendinopathy. We believe that the major factors that attribute to the inconsistent results observed in clinical trials are PRP-related factors, patient-related factors and insufficiencies of many clinical trials.

8. PRP-RELATED FACTORS

PRP treatment efficacy can be affected by a number of PRP associated factors including PRP composition, platelet concentration, activation, and application methods among others.

PRP composition

In current clinical practices, PRP is mostly prepared using various commercial kits, which do not yield "one-type" of PRP with the same composition. In contrast, PRP prepared from the kits vary in their composition. For example, PRP prepared from the same blood sample using three different kits (MTF Cascade, Arteriocyte Magellan and Biomet GPS III)[58] or three different preparation methods (apheresis-derived platelets, buffy coat-derived platelets and tube method-derived platelets)[59] had the same platelet concentration but had variable amounts of leukocytes. The potential negative effects of using L-PRP on tendon healing have been mentioned above. Therefore, it is suggested that PRP without leukocytes or with only small number of the leukocytes should be used to maximize anabolic effects of PRP on the healing of tendinopathic tendons thus enhancing treatment efficacy. Moreover, different commercial PRP preparation kits yield variable levels of growth factor. For instance, PRP prepared from MTF Cascade, Arteriocyte Magellan or Biomet GPS III PRP preparation systems varied widely in their PDGF and VEGF levels[58]. Therefore, optimization of PRP composition is critical to improve the PRP treatment efficacy in clinics.

Platelet concentration

The growth factors containing platelets vary considerably based on the type of kit used to prepare PRP. Platelet concentration could be 1- fold (Autolo Gel System, Secquire), 3-5-fold (Biomet GPS, Cell Saver Based Systems, Sorin Angel, Harvest Smart Pre BMC, Depuy Symphony, Arteriocyte Medical Magellan) or even 10-fold (GenesisCS) higher than in whole blood. Therefore, it is pertinent to choose the PRP preparation with optimal platelet levels because the presence of too many platelets may not benefit tendon wound healing. In at least one RCT, a 10-fold higher platelet concentration in PRP over that in whole blood did not improve treatment outcomes[19], and most clinical and basic science studies only use PRP with platelet concentrations 3-5-fold higher than in whole blood. At these levels, PRP has been shown to exert beneficial effects; decrease pain, increase tendon cell proliferation, and improve collagen synthesis and organization[20,21].

Activation of PRP

Regarding PRP activation there seems to be no consensus in the method used for activation, which is essential for the release of growth factors from the platelets[59]. Traditionally, both basic science studies and clinical trials have used thrombin or calcium chloride to activate PRP externally prior to treatment. However, non-activated PRP can also be used to treat tendinopathy because platelets can become activated when they come in contact with collagen in vivo[28]. Recently, platelets in PRP were shown to contain different components; specifically, pro- and anti-angiogenic components were shown to be released selectively after activation by using agonists to proteinase activated receptor-1 or -4 (PAR-1 or PAR-4)[60]. Further research on this topic is warranted.

These variations in PRP suggest the need for a universal PRP labeling system describing the PRP components present in the preparations used in clinical trials[18,61]. An example would be the use of PAW that includes Platelet concentration, Activation method and presence of White blood cells/ leukocytes on the label[18] or DEPA that describes the platelet Dose, Efficiency of production, PRP Purity and Activation on the label[61].

Lastly, the frequency of PRP treatment, and the mode of PRP application via injection or implantation of PRP gel should be studied more for optimization.

9. PATIENT-ASSOCIATED FACTORS

A number of variables related to patients also contribute to controversial PRP treatment outcomes. These may include patient's age, patient's gender, injury type, patient's disease and treatment history, and post-recovery plans.

Patient's age

Currently, there is no data from clinical trials that compared the efficacy of PRP treatment in young vs old patients. Almost all clinical trials conducted thus far (see above) have included patients both young and old with their ages ranging from 18 - 70 years. Thus, while PRP treatment for tendinopathy may work in young patients, it may not work in older patients. One biological reason for this is that with increased age, TSC number and quality decreases[9]. Specifically, it was also shown that aging decreased the numbers of human MSCs in the bone marrow[62]; moreover, the proliferation rate of some stem cells including ADSCs[63], BMSCs[63] and ACL-derived cells[64] were higher in young than in older animals. Furthermore, the differentiation potential of TSCs from older animals were found to be abnormal; i.e., TSCs from aging mice or rats could aberrantly differentiate into non-tendon cell types including adipocytes, chondrocytes and osteocytes[9,65] that develop into fat, cartilage-like and bone-like tissue in tendons and lead to tendon degeneration, which is a characteristic feature of degenerative tendinopathy[8]. In addition, some growth factors, for example in equine PDGF, had higher concentrations of PRP derived from younger horses than from older ones[66]. Thus, the increased number of TSCs, the higher TSC proliferation rate and higher amounts of growth factors in young individuals may result in a better PRP treatment efficacy than in older individuals. More importantly, the ability of aging TSCs to differentiate into non-tenocytes indicates how this stem cell characteristic could decrease the PRP treatment efficacy in older patients. Therefore, the PRP treatment efficacy in aging patients is expected to be low and if a clinical trial includes both young and old patients, it is expected that variations in clinical outcome of PRP treatment would be huge, which effectively reduces the statistical power to reveal the PRP treatment effects.

Patient's gender

Similar to age, clinical trials have not investigated the variations in PRP treatment efficacy based on patient's gender. Most clinical trials group males and females together and include more males than females. However, indirect evidence points to the likelihood of gender impacting PRP treatment efficacy in clinical trials. For instance, the levels of all human growth factors particularly EGF, HGF, IGF-1 and PDGF were found to be higher in females than males[67]. Besides, viscoelastic properties of tendons[68], and the incidences of Achilles tendon ruptures[69] and wound healing[70] are known to differ between genders. Moreover, among females PRP treatment efficacy can vary significantly between menopausal and post-menopausal women because estrogen impacts VEGF[71] and IGF-1[72] expression and lower estrogen levels decrease tensile strength[73] and diminish wound healing response of dermal fibroblasts[74].

Post-treatment recovery

Rehabilitation exercises after PRP treatment may benefit patients as shown in an RCT where patients were allowed eccentric exercise after PRP treatment of lateral elbow epicondylitis[28]. Besides, moderate mechanical loading can reduce inflammation[75] and excessive mechanical loading can increase inflammation by increasing PGE2 production[6]. Therefore, it is essential to understand the patient history to recommend the appropriate time and level of rehabilitation protocols that may be recommended after a PRP treatment. While some recommend rehabilitation along with any repair treatment[76] others suggest that resuming exercises a few days after any treatment may improve tendon's mechanical and biological parameters better than immediate loading or prolonged post-operative immobilization[77]. Currently, such recommendations in clinical trials are mostly subjective and are based on the practitioner. However, these recommendations should be based more on the patient and aim towards the "personalized medicine" approach.

Robustness of clinical trials

As mentioned earlier, in most current clinical trials investigating the efficacy of PRP treatment, the number of patients is relatively small (see above), which reflects the difficulties in recruiting a sufficient number of patients to participate in studies. A larger sample size in both control and treatment groups may likely increase the statistical power to detect the PRP treatment efficacy in clinical trials. These trials should take into consideration age, gender and other variables to minimize the inconsistent results obtained in PRP efficacy studies. Another variable that could affect PRP treatment efficacy is the measurement of PRP treatment outcome. Currently, various scoring systems are used as outcome measures; these include VAS (Visual Analog Scale), DASH (Disabilities of the Arm, Shoulder, and Hand), and VISA-A (Victorian Institute of Sport Assessment-Achilles) scale scores, which may be subjective because they are based on patients' assessment of pain intensity. Variations in these subjective scores can also be minimized by increasing the sample size in clinical trials and better yet, using objective measures such as ultrasound imaging technology to reveal tendon structure before and after PRP treatment. Lastly, guidelines should be established so that the results obtained from different studies that administered PRP are uniform and easier to compare.

Changing the PRP treatment approach

The controversies surrounding the use of PRP in clinical trials are well-known. This issue can be best addressed by optimizing the application of PRP treatment in clinics. Currently, clinical trials employ a "one size-fits-all" approach where "any" PRP preparation is used at a "pre-determined dose" to treat all types of tendon injuries in patients regardless of patient age, gender or history. This means that PRP containing higher amounts of leukocytes or too many platelets may also be used to treat tendinopathy in older patients. All these variables can individually decrease the PRP treatment efficacy and therefore should be avoided. Thus, a "tailored" approach is necessary. For example, PRP efficacy may be higher when leukocyte free PRP is used to treat younger patients particularly athletes who may have large number of "good-quality" TSCs that may proliferate at a higher rate and differentiate into tenocytes. This approach may also be effective when treating early stage tendinopathy, which is characterized mostly by inflammation and pain because PRP is known to have anti-inflammatory effects[41]. However, PRP may not effectively treat advanced stage tendinopathy, which is characterized by degenerative changes such as lipid deposition, proteoglycan accumulation and calcification in tendon lesions[8]. Besides, the number of TSCs in these degenerate tendons is also small and will not allow effective PRP treatment; i.e. PRP can promote the proliferation of only the few existing TSCs, which may not be sufficient for an effective healing and repair. Therefore, it is recommended that degenerate tissues be removed by wound debridement prior to PRP treatment; this procedure will eliminate the non-tenogenic environment in advanced stage tendinopathic tendon and allow TSCs to proliferate at a higher rate[17]. It should be noted that when PRP is used to treat injured tendon-bone interface, a fibrocartilage zone which is more complex than tendon alone[27], additional "materials," like a bio-compound, together with PRP may be required to improve treatment outcome (Fig. 4). Finally, selective release of pro- or anti-angiogenic components in PRP using specific activators may

PRP alone is not sufficient to promote the formation of fibrocartilage zone in the tendon-bone interface

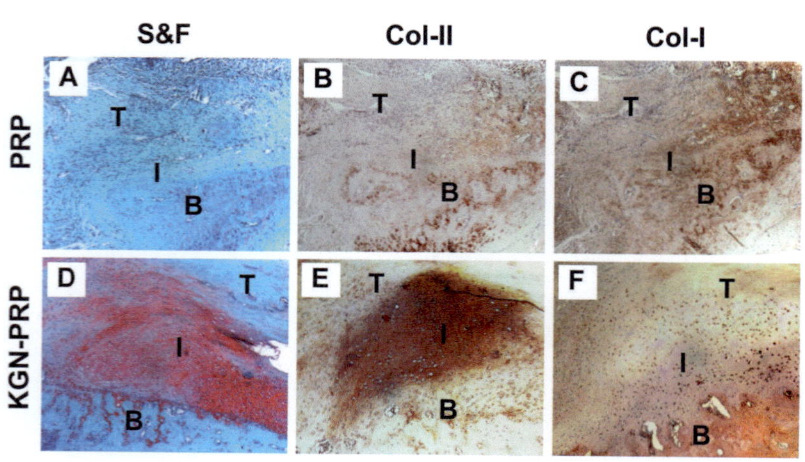

FIG. 4
Injection of PRP into the tendon-bone tunnel interface in a mouse model does not result in the formation of the fibrocartilage zone as evidenced by the lack of proteoglycan (A) and collagen type II (Col-II, B). In contrast, injection of KGN along with PRP induces robust formation of proteoglycan (pink, D), and abundant collagen type II (Col-II, brown, E). In both PRP and KGN+PRP groups, moderate amounts of collagen type I (Col-I, C, F) are formed. T - tendon; I – tendon-bone interface; B – bone.

For more detailed description of the results, see the original paper [27].

improve healing outcomes. All these converge on one point; i.e. if not monitored carefully, variations can occur easily during PRP treatment in clinical trials and may contribute to the reported inconsistent results.

10. CONCLUSION

PRP is an alternative option to traditional treatments of tendinopathy. PRP has a number of advantages; it is relatively safe and easy to use in clinics to treat tendinopathy. Findings from basic science studies have been consistent in demonstrating the beneficial effects of PRP including increased tendon cell proliferation, increased expression of anabolic genes and proteins, and reduced tendon inflammation among others. However, the efficacy of PRP in clinical trials is still controversial most likely driven by inconsistent protocols that use a "one-size-fits-all" approach. To obtain consistent results it is essential to use an individualized approach and optimize the variables related to PRP preparation and patients. Such efforts may improve the efficacy of PRP for the treatment of tendon injuries and may effectively address the controversies on PRP treatment efficacy in clinics.

Acknowledgements
This work was supported in part by the NIH under award numbers AR061395, AR065949, and AR070340.

1. 1Wang JH. Mechanobiology of tendon. Journal of biomechanics. 2006;39(9):1563-82. PubMed PMID: 16000201.

2. Zhang J, Wang JH. The Effects of Mechanical Loading on Tendons - An In Vivo and In Vitro Model Study. PloS one. 2013;8(8):e71740.

3. Zhang J, Wang JH. Characterization of differential properties of rabbit tendon stem cells and tenocytes. BMC Musculoskelet Disord. 2010;11(10):1471-2474.

4. Langberg H, Boushel R, Skovgaard D, Risum N, Kjaer M. Cyclo-oxygenase-2 mediated prostaglandin release regulates blood flow in connective tissue during mechanical loading in humans. J Physiol. 2003;551(Pt 2):683-9.

5. Wang JH, Jia F, Yang G, Yang S, Campbell BH, Stone D, et al. Cyclic mechanical stretching of human tendon fibroblasts increases the production of prostaglandin E2 and levels of cyclooxygenase expression: a novel in vitro model study. Connect Tissue Res. 2003;44(3-4):128-33. PubMed PMID: 14504032.

6. Zhang J JHW. Production of PGE(2) increases in tendons subjected to repetitive mechanical loading and induces differentiation of tendon stem cells into non-tenocytes. J Orthop Res. 2010;28(2):198-203.

7. Mehallo CJ, Drezner JA, Bytomski JR. Practical Management: Nonsteroidal Antiinflammatory Drug (NSAID) Use in Athletic Injuries. Clin J Sport Med. 2006;16(2):170-4.

8. Kannus P, Jozsa L. Histopathological changes preceding spontaneous rupture of a tendon. A controlled study of 891 patients. J Bone Joint Surg Am. 1991 Dec;73(10):1507-25. PubMed PMID: 1748700. Epub 1991/12/01. eng.

9. Zhang J, JH W. Moderate exercise mitigates the detrimental effects of aging on tendon stem cells. PloS one. 2015;10(6):e0130454.

10. Zhang J, Keenan C, Wang JH. The effects of dexamethasone on human patellar tendon stem cells: implications for dexamethasone treatment of tendon injury. J Orthop Res. 2013;31(1):105-10.

11. Andia I, Sánchez M, Maffulli N. Tendon healing and platelet rich plasma therapies. Expert opinion on biological therapy. 2010;10.

12. de Almeida AM, Demange MK, Sobrado MF, Rodrigues MB, Pedrinelli A, Hernandez AJ. Patellar tendon healing with platelet-rich plasma: a prospective randomized controlled trial. Am J Sports Med. 2012;40(6):1282-8.

13. Rabago D, Wilson J, Zgierska A. Platelet-rich plasma for treatment of Achilles tendinopathy. JAMA. 2010 May 5;303(17):1696-7; author reply 7-8. PubMed PMID: 20442382. Epub 2010/05/06. eng.

14. Peerbooms JC, Sluimer J, Bruijn DJ, Gosens T. Positive effect of an autologous platelet concentrate in lateral epicondylitis in a double-blind randomized controlled trial: platelet-rich plasma versus corticosteroid injection with a 1-year follow-up. Am J Sports Med. 2010;38.

15. Wilson JJ, Lee KS, Miller AT, Wang S. Platelet-rich plasma for the treatment of chronic plantar fasciopathy in adults: a case series. Foot & ankle specialist. 2014 Feb;7(1):61-7. PubMed PMID: 24287209.

16. Deutsch V, Tomer A. Megakaryocyte development and platelet production. Br J Haematol. 2006;134(5):453-66.

17. Anitua E, Sanchez M, Nurden AT, Nurden P, Orive G, Andia I. New insights into and novel applica-

tions for platelet-rich fibrin therapies. Trends Biotechnol. 2006;24(5):227-34.

18. DeLong JM, Russell RP, Mazzocca AD. Platelet-Rich Plasma: The PAW Classification System. Arthroscopy: The Journal of Arthroscopic & Related Surgery. 2012;28(7):998-1009.

19. Schepull T, Kvist J, Norrman H, Trinks M, Berlin G, Aspenberg P. Autologous platelets have no effect on the healing of human achilles tendon ruptures: a randomized single-blind study. Am J Sports Med. 2011 Jan;39(1):38-47. PubMed PMID: 21051425. Epub 2010/11/06. eng.

20. Zhou Y, Zhang J, Wu H, Hogan MV, Wang JHC. The differential effects of leukocyte-containing and pure platelet-rich plasma (PRP) on tendon stem/progenitor cells - implications of PRP application for the clinical treatment of tendon injuries. Stem Cell Research & Therapy. 2015;6(1):173. PubMed PMID: PMC4572462.

21. Zhang J, Wang JH. Platelet-rich plasma releasate promotes differentiation of tendon stem cells into active tenocytes. Am J Sports Med. 2010;38(12):2477-86.

22. Schnabel LV, Mohammed HO, Miller BJ. Platelet rich plasma (PRP) enhances anabolic gene expression patterns in flexor digitorum superficialis tendons. J Orthop Res. 2007;25.

23. Bosch G, Rene van Weeren P, Barneveld A, van Schie HT. Computerised analysis of standardised ultrasonographic images to monitor the repair of surgically created core lesions in equine superficial digital flexor tendons following treatment with intratendinous platelet rich plasma or placebo. Vet J. 2011;187(1):92-8.

24. Morizaki Y, Zhao C, An KN, Amadio PC. The effects of platelet-rich plasma on bone marrow stromal cell transplants for tendon healing in vitro. The Journal of hand surgery. 2010 Nov;35(11):1833-41. PubMed PMID: 20951509. Pubmed Central PMCID: Pmc2974778. Epub 2010/10/19. eng.

25. Xie X, Wang Y, Zhao C, Guo S, Liu S, Jia W, et al. Comparative evaluation of MSCs from bone marrow and adipose tissue seeded in PRP-derived scaffold for cartilage regeneration. Biomaterials. 2012 Oct;33(29):7008-18. PubMed PMID: 22818985.

26. Uysal CA, Tobita M, Hyakusoku H, Mizuno H. Adipose-derived stem cells enhance primary tendon repair: Biomechanical and immunohistochemical evaluation. Journal of Plastic, Reconstructive & Aesthetic Surgery. 2012;65(12):1712-9.

27. Zhou Y, Zhang J, Yang J, Narava M, Zhao G, Yuan T, et al. Kartogenin with PRP Promotes the Formation of Fibrocartilage Zone in the Tendon-Bone Interface Journal of Tissue Eng and Regenerative Medicine. 2016.

28. Thanasas C, Papadimitriou G, Charalambidis C, Paraskevopoulos I, Papanikolaou A. Platelet-rich plasma versus autologous whole blood for the treatment of chronic lateral elbow epicondylitis. Am J Sports Med. 2011;39.

29. Mishra AK, Skrepnik NV, Edwards SG, Jones GL, Sampson S, Vermillion DA, et al. Efficacy of platelet-rich plasma for chronic tennis elbow: a double-blind, prospective, multicenter, randomized controlled trial of 230 patients. Am J Sports Med. 2014 Feb;42(2):463-71. PubMed PMID: 23825183.

30. Carvalho Ade M, Badial PR, Alvarez LE, Yamada AL, Borges AS, Deffune E, et al. Equine tendonitis therapy using mesenchymal stem cells and platelet concentrates: a randomized controlled trial. Stem Cell Res Ther. 2013;4(4).

31. Kesikburun S, Tan AK, Yilmaz B, Yasar E, Yazicioglu K. Platelet-rich plasma injections in the treatment of chronic rotator cuff tendinopathy: a randomized controlled trial with 1-year follow-up. Am J Sports Med. 2013 Nov;41(11):2609-16. PubMed PMID: 23893418. Epub 2013/07/31. eng.

32. Raeissadat SA, Rayegani SM, Hassanabadi H, Rahimi R, Sedighipour L, Rostami K. Is Platelet-rich plasma superior to whole blood in the management of chronic tennis elbow: one year randomized clinical trial. BMC Sports Science, Medicine and Rehabilitation. 2014;6(1):1-10.

33. Dragoo JL, Wasterlain AS, Braun HJ, Nead KT. Platelet-rich plasma as a treatment for patellar tendinopathy: a double-blind, randomized controlled trial. Am J Sports Med. 2014;42(3):610-8. patellar tendon platelet-rich plasma randomized controlled trial symptoms tendinopathy tendon injuries.

34. Del Bue M, Ricco S, Conti V, Merli E, Ramoni R, Grolli S. Platelet lysate promotes in vitro proliferation of equine mesenchymal stem cells and tenocytes. Veterinary research communications. 2007 Aug;31 Suppl 1:289-92. PubMed PMID: 17682897. Epub 2007/10/10. eng.

35. Chen L, Liu JP, Tang KL, Wang Q, Wang GD, Cai XH, et al. Tendon derived stem cells promote platelet-rich plasma healing in collagenase-induced rat achilles tendinopathy. Cell Physiol Biochem. 2014;34(6):2153-68.

36. McCarrel T, Fortier L. Temporal growth factor release from platelet-rich plasma, trehalose lyophilized platelets, and bone marrow aspirate and their effect on tendon and ligament gene expression. J Orthop Res. 2009 Aug;27(8):1033-42. PubMed PMID: 19170097. Epub 2009/01/27. eng.

37. Klein MB, Yalamanchi N, Pham H, Longaker MT, Chan J. Flexor tendon healing in vitro: Effects of TGF-β on tendon cell collagen production. The Journal of hand surgery. 2002;27(4):615-20.

38. Wrotniak M, Bielecki T, Gazdzik TS. Current opinion about using the platelet-rich gel in orthopaedics and trauma surgery. Ortop Traumatol Rehabil. 2007;9(3):227-38.

39. Cavallo C, Filardo G, Mariani E, Kon E, Marcacci M, Pereira Ruiz MT, et al. Comparison of platelet-rich plasma formulations for cartilage healing: an in vitro study. J Bone Joint Surg Am. 2014;96(5):423-9.

40. Woo SL, Hildebrand K, Watanabe N, Fenwick JA, Papageorgiou CD, Wang JH. Tissue engineering of ligament and tendon healing. Clin Orthop Relat Res. 1999;367(23):S312-23.

41. Zhang J, Middleton KK, Fu FH, Im HJ, Wang JH. HGF Mediates the Anti-inflammatory Effects of PRP on Injured Tendons. PlosOne. 2013;8(6):e67303.

42. Coudriet GM, He J, Trucco M, Mars WM, Piganelli JD. Hepatocyte growth factor modulates interleukin-6 production in bone marrow derived macrophages: implications for inflammatory mediated diseases. PloS one. 2010;5(11):e15384. PubMed PMID: 21072211. Pubmed Central PMCID: 2970559.

43. Chen L, Dong S-W, Liu J-P, Tao X, Tang K-L, Xu J-Z. Synergy of tendon stem cells and platelet-rich plasma in tendon healing. Journal of Orthopaedic Research. 2012;30(6):991-7.

44. Zargar Baboldashti N, Poulsen RC, Franklin SL, Thompson MS, Hulley PA. Platelet-rich plasma protects tenocytes from adverse side effects of dexamethasone and ciprofloxacin. Am J Sports Med. 2011;39(9):1929-35.

45. Beitzel K, McCarthy MB, Cote MP, Apostolakos J, Russell RP, Bradley J, et al. The effect of ketorolac tromethamine, methylprednisolone, and platelet-rich plasma on human chondrocyte and tenocyte viability. Arthroscopy. 2013 Jul;29(7):1164-74. PubMed PMID: 23809450. Epub 2013/07/03. eng.

46. Dallaudiere B, Lempicki M, Pesquer L, Louedec L, Preux PM, Meyer P, et al. Efficacy of intra-tendinous injection of platelet-rich plasma in treating tendinosis: comprehensive assessment of a rat model. European radiology. 2013 Oct;23(10):2830-7. PubMed PMID: 23801419. Epub 2013/06/27. eng.

47. Lyras DN, Kazakos K, Verettas D, Polychronidis A, Tryfonidis M, Botaitis S, et al. The influence of platelet-rich plasma on angiogenesis during the early phase of tendon healing. Foot & ankle international. 2009 Nov;30(11):1101-6. PubMed PMID: 19912722. Epub 2009/11/17. eng.

48. Lyras DN, Kazakos K, Georgiadis G, Mazis G, Middleton R, Richards S, et al. Does a single application of PRP alter the expression of IGF-I in the early phase of tendon healing? J Foot Ankle Surg. 2011;50(3):276-82.

49. Dahlgren LA, van der Meulen MC, Bertram JE, Starrak GS, Nixon AJ. Insulin-like growth factor-I improves cellular and molecular aspects of healing in a collagenase-induced model of flexor tendinitis. J Orthop Res. 2002;20(5):910-9.

50. Yoshikawa Y, Abrahamsson SO. Dose-related cellular effects of platelet-derived growth factor-BB differ in various types of rabbit tendons in vitro. Acta Orthop Scand. 2001;72(3):287-92.

51. Chan BP, Fu S, Qin L, Lee K, Rolf CG, Chan K. Effects of basic fibroblast growth factor (bFGF) on early stages of tendon healing: a rat patellar tendon model. Acta Orthop Scand. 2000;71(5):513-8.

52. Kashiwagi K, Mochizuki Y, Yasunaga Y, Ishida O, Deie M, Ochi M. Effects of transforming growth factor-beta 1 on the early stages of healing of the Achilles tendon in a rat model. Scand J Plast Reconstr Surg Hand Surg. 2004;38(4):193-7.

53. Moshiri A, Oryan A, Meimandi-Parizi A, Koohi-Hosseinabadi O. Effectiveness of xenogenous-based bovine-derived platelet gel embedded within a three-dimensional collagen implant on the healing and regeneration of the Achilles tendon defect in rabbits. Expert opinion on biological therapy. 2014 Aug;14(8):1065-89. PubMed PMID: 24840092. Epub 2014/05/21. eng.

54. Barbosa D, de Souza RA, de Carvalho WR, Xavier M, de Carvalho PK, Cunha TC, et al. Low-level laser therapy combined with platelet-rich plasma on the healing calcaneal tendon: a histological study in a rat model. Lasers in medical science. 2013 Nov;28(6):1489-94. PubMed PMID: 23307438. Epub 2013/01/12. eng.

55. Fiorucci S, Mencarelli A, Palazzetti B, Distrutti E, Vergnolle N, Hollenberg MD, et al. Proteinase-activated receptor 2 is an anti-inflammatory signal for colonic lamina propria lymphocytes in a mouse model of colitis. Proc Natl Acad Sci U S A. 2001 Nov 20;98(24):13936-41. PubMed PMID: 11717450. Pubmed Central PMCID: 61145. Epub 2001/11/22. eng.

56. Cilli F, Khan M, Fu F, Wang JH. Prostaglandin E2 affects proliferation and collagen synthesis by human patellar tendon fibroblasts. Clin J Sport Med. 2004 Jul;14(4):232-6. PubMed PMID: 15273529. Epub 2004/07/27. eng.

57. Khan MH, Li Z, Wang JH. Repeated exposure of tendon to prostaglandin-e2 leads to localized tendon degeneration. Clin J Sport Med. 2005 Jan;15(1):27-33. PubMed PMID: 15654188.

58. Castillo TN, Pouliot MA, Kim HJ, Dragoo JL. Comparison of growth factor and platelet concentration from commercial platelet-rich plasma separation systems. Am J Sports Med. 2011;39(2):266-71.

59. Zimmermann R, Jakubietz R, Jakubietz M, Strasser E, Schlegel A, Wiltfang J, et al. Different preparation methods to obtain platelet components as a source of growth factors for local application. Transfusion. 2001;41(10):1217-24.

60. Italiano JE, Jr., Richardson JL, Patel-Hett S, Battinelli E, Zaslavsky A, Short S, et al. Angiogenesis is regulated by a novel mechanism: pro- and antiangiogenic proteins are organized into separate platelet alpha granules and differentially released. Blood. 2008 Feb 1;111(3):1227-33. PubMed PMID: 17962514. Pubmed Central PMCID: 2214735.

61. Dohan Ehrenfest DM, Andia I, Zumstein MA, Zhang C-Q, Pinto NR, Bielecki T. Classification of platelet concentrates (Platelet-Rich Plasma-PRP, Platelet-Rich Fibrin-PRF) for topical and infiltrative use in orthopedic and sports medicine: current consensus, clinical implications and perspectives. Muscles, ligaments and tendons journal. 2014 Jan-Mar;4(1):3-9. PubMed PMID: PMC4049647.

62. Stolzing A, Jones E, McGonagle D, Scutt A. Age-related changes in human bone marrow-derived mesenchymal stem cells: consequences for cell therapies. Mech Ageing Dev. 2008;129(3):163-73.

63. Liu H-Y, Huang C-F, Lin T-C, Tsai C-Y, Tina Chen S-Y, Liu A, et al. Delayed animal aging through the recovery of stem cell senescence by platelet rich plasma. Biomaterials. 2014;35(37):9767-76.

64. Mastrangelo AN, Haus BM, Vavken P, Palmer MP, Machan JT, Murray MM. Immature animals have higher cellular density in the healing anterior cruciate ligament than adolescent or adult animals. Journal of Orthopaedic Research. 2010;28(8):1100-6.

65. Zhou Z, Akinbiyi T, Xu L, Ramcharan M, Leong DJ, Ros SJ, et al. Tendon-derived stem/progenitor cell aging: defective self-renewal and altered fate. Aging cell. 2010 Oct;9(5):911-5. PubMed PMID: 20569237. Pubmed Central PMCID: 2944918. Epub 2010/06/24. eng.

66. Giraldo CE, López C, Álvarez ME, Samudio IJ, Prades M, Carmona JU. Effects of the breed, sex and age on cellular content and growth factor release from equine pure-platelet rich plasma and pure-platelet rich gel. BMC Veterinary Research. 2013;9(1):1-10.

67. Evanson JR, Guyton MK, Oliver DL, Hire JM, Topolski RL, Zumbrun SD, et al. Gender and age differences in growth factor concentrations from platelet-rich plasma in adults. Mil Med. 2014;179(7):799-805.

68. Kubo K, Kanehisa H, Fukunaga T. Gender differences in the viscoelastic properties of tendon structures. Eur J Appl Physiol. 2003;88(6):520-6.

69. Nyyssönen T, Lüthje P, Kröger H. The Increasing Incidence and Difference in Sex Distribution of Achilles Tendon Rupture in Finland in 1987–1999. Scandinavian Journal of Surgery. 2008 September 1, 2008;97(3):272-5.

70. Guo S, DiPietro LA. Factors Affecting Wound Healing. Journal of Dental Research. 2010 March 1, 2010;89(3):219-29.

71. Mueller MD, Vigne JL, Minchenko A, Lebovic DI, Leitman DC, Taylor RN. Regulation of vascular endothelial growth factor (VEGF) gene transcription by estrogen receptors alpha and beta. Proc Natl Acad Sci U S A. 2000;97(20):10972-7.

72. Denger S, Bahr-Ivacevic T, Brand H, Reid G, Blake J, Seifert M, et al. Transcriptome profiling of estrogen-regulated genes in human primary osteoblasts reveals an osteoblast-specific regulation of the insulin-like growth factor binding protein 4 gene. Mol Endocrinol. 2008;22(2):361-79.

73. Slauterbeck J, Clevenger C, Lundberg W, Burchfield DM. Estrogen level alters the failure load of the rabbit anterior cruciate ligament. J Orthop Res. 1999;17(3):405-8.

74. Gilliver SC, Ashworth JJ, Ashcroft GS. The hormonal regulation of cutaneous wound healing. Clin Dermatol. 2007;25(1):56-62.

75. Yang G, Im H, Wang J. Repetitive mechanical stretching modulates IL-1beta induced COX-2, MMP-1 expression, and PGE2 production in human patellar tendon fibroblasts. Genes and Development. 2005;363:166-72.

76. Rajabi H, Shahin HS, Norouzian M, Mehrabani D, Nazhvani SD. The Healing Effects of Aquatic Activities and Allogenic Injection of Platelet-Rich Plasma (PRP) on Injuries of Achilles Tendon in Experimental Rat. World Journal of Plastic Surgery. 2015;4(1):66-73.

77. Thomopoulos S, Williams GR, Soslowsky LJ. Tendon to bone healing: differences in biomechanical, structural, and compositional properties due to a range of activity levels. J Biomech Eng. 2003;125(1):106-13.

78. Zhang J, Wang JH. Prostaglandin E2 (PGE2) exerts biphasic effects on human tendon stem cells. PloS one. 2014;9(2):e87706.

CHAPTER 12

Infiltrations of PRGF to Treat Ligament and Tendon Injuries in the Hip and Pelvis

AUTHORS

Kraeutler MJ.[1], Garabekyan T.[2], Mei-Dan O.[1]

[1] University of Colorado School of Medicine, Department of Orthopedics, Aurora CO 80045
[2] Southern California Hip Institute, North Hollywood CA 91602

SUMMARY

In recent years, platelet-rich plasma (PRP) has gained popularity within the orthopaedic community as a treatment modality to enhance tissue healing. This chapter aims to concisely present the current indications for PRP injections in the treatment of hip and pelvic pathologies and to describe some novel applications for PRP which have not yet been reported in the literature. With regard to hip and pelvic pathologies, PRP injections are used most commonly as a non-operative intervention, and have been described in the literature to treat osteoarthritis of the hip joint as well as tendinopathy of the hamstrings, adductor longus, and gluteus medius. In contrast, most of the surgical applications of PRP for the hip are novel, with few reported studies in the literature. Because of the increasing awareness of PRP's beneficial effects on musculoskeletal healing and thus the growing number of indications for its use, this review also describes some novel applications for PRP, including osteitis pubis, post-microfracture of the hip, tears of the rectus femoris, and avulsion of the sartorius muscle.

E. Anitua et al. (eds.), *Platelet Rich Plasma in Orthopaedics and Sports Medicine*,
https://doi.org/10.1007/978-3-319-63730-3_12

1. INTRODUCTION

Platelet-rich plasma (PRP) has gained popularity within the last decade among the orthopaedic community as a treatment modality to enhance tissue healing. The term platelet-rich plasma may be applied to any fraction of autologous blood that contains a higher concentration of platelets than baseline[1]. Thus, this term is non-specific and factors such as the concentration of platelets and leukocytes as well as centrifugation methods have differed between studies. DeLong et al[2] developed the PAW classification system to aid in comparing different protocols of PRP preparation. This classification system is based on the absolute number of platelets (P), the method of platelet activation (A), and the presence/absence of white cells (W).

Recently, PRP has been utilized for numerous musculoskeletal indications such as rotator cuff repair[3,4], patellar tendinopathy[5], knee osteoarthritis[6], lateral epicondylitis[7], osteochondral lesions of the talus[8,9], and many other orthopaedic conditions. PRP induces musculoskeletal healing through a number of effects. As a treatment modality for tendon healing, PRP enhances the mobilization of circulation-derived cells[10]. This may include inflammatory cells that secrete cytokines and growth factors as well as fibroblast-like cells that synthesize matrix. Compared to serum, PRP has been shown to significantly increase the deposition of a collagen-rich extracellular matrix[11], with higher collagen I content compared to placebo[12]. Interestingly, PRP-treated tendon tears have actually been shown to contain fewer blood vessels compared to placebo[12], possibly indicating a more physiological healing process. Once PRP enhances the early phase of regeneration, mechanical stimulation is required to promote organized collagen synthesis and remodeling during new tendon development[13].

With muscle strains or contusions, the hematoma that originates contains approximately 94% red blood cells, 4% platelets, and < 1% leukocytes[14]. Compared to whole blood, PRP contains higher concentrations of certain growth factors, in particular platelet-derived growth factor (PDGF) and transforming growth factor-β (TGF-β)[15]. Thus, PRP is theorized to replace the hematoma with a high concentration of platelets and growth factors to promote healing. Furthermore, PRP has been shown to promote angiogenesis through activation of PRP-releasate (PRP-r)[16]. In comparison to tendon and muscle healing, little is known on the mechanisms of PRP in promoting healing of articular cartilage, though this likely involves multiple biological processes including apoptosis, extracellular matrix synthesis, angiogenesis, and inflammation[17]. Because of the increasing awareness of PRP's beneficial effects on musculoskeletal healing and thus the growing number of indications for its use, we present a chapter of the current indications for platelet-rich plasma injections to augment the conservative and surgical treatment of hip and pelvic ligament and tendon pathologies and describe some novel applications for PRP[18]. Although several studies have described the use of PRP for some of these pathologies, other indications for PRP discussed in this chapter have not been published previously. As such, these indications are not yet evidence-based.

2. DECISION-MAKING

After performing an appropriate patient history and physical examination, advanced imaging is typically obtained to better characterize the suspected pathology. With muscle or tendon tears, magnetic resonance imaging (MRI) or ultrasound (US) should be used to determine the exact location and extent of the injury. Depending on the pathology, PRP may be used as a conservative treatment measure or as adjunctive treatment during surgery. When used as a conservative treatment option, PRP may be applicable for tendinopathic changes or partial tendon tears in which the tendon ends are not retracted[1].

The cost of platelet-rich plasma treatment is certainly a factor in the decision-making process. Insurance companies still do not recognize PRP as standard of care, and thus PRP must be paid by patients out of pocket. It has been estimated recently that the cost of PRP is $500 to $1,500 per application[19]. It is important to have an open discussion regarding the cost of PRP injections, given that it may be prohibitively expensive for some patients.

3. PREPARATION AND APPLICATION TECHNIQUES

A sample of whole blood is collected in a sodium citrate tube in order to delay clotting of the blood sample. Once the whole blood sample is collected, centrifugation allows separation of the sample into its component cells and serum. Either one or two centrifugation steps may be used depending on the final product desired. A "soft" spin separates the whole blood sample into three layers: an upper layer consisting mainly of plasma and platelets, a very thin middle layer known as the "buffy coat" that is highly concentrated in WBCs, and a bottom layer consisting mainly of red blood cells (RBCs)[20]. A second, "hard" spin may be used to further concentrate the platelets[20,21]. Following centrifugation, approximately 10% of the initial whole blood volume remains as PRP concentrate[1]. The platelets in the PRP concentrate are activated with calcium chloride and/or autologous or bovine thrombin. These additions are used to initiate the clotting cascade, the release of growth factors from the platelets, and the formation of a fibrin scaffold[21]. Autologous thrombin has been shown to have a lower clot strength compared to bovine thrombin or calcium chloride, with bovine thrombin having the quickest clot initiation time[22]. In an equine model, calcium chloride activation of PRP has been shown to result in greater release of platelet-derived growth factor compared to autologous or bovine thrombin[23]. Calcium chloride also provides the advantage of not using bovine or other non-autologous materials.

Therapeutic doses of PRP require 2.5-5 times the baseline concentration of platelets[24,25], though higher concentrations than this have an inhibitory effect on healing[26]. The white blood cell concentration may also be controlled, with leukocyte-rich PRP (L-PRP) and leukocyte-poor PRP (P-PRP) both being used in the literature. For production of L-PRP, the entire layer of the buffy coat and few RBCs are transferred to an empty sterile tube, while the upper layer and only the superficial buffy coat are transferred for production of P-PRP[20]. Plasma rich in growth factors (PRGF) is a term used to describe a leukocyte-poor PRP which is separated manually (direct visualization using a fine pipette) from the lower fraction of the plasma containing the highest concentration of platelets and growth factors, avoiding the thin WBC layer. PRGF techniques have been shown to produce lower concentrations of growth factors compared to standard PRP kits by 3-4 fold[27] which, according to many studies, may serve as the optimal ratio for tissue healing.

When a tendon or muscle is injured, healing proceeds through three processes: inflammation/degeneration, regeneration, and fibrosis[1]. Although L-PRP has been shown to contain the highest levels of growth factors and cytokines[28], it induces catabolic effects and a significantly greater acute inflammatory response and thus may actually prolong the healing process[28-31]. Thus, the inclusion of white cells defeats the purpose of PRP. On the other hand, P-PRP induces mainly anabolic changes, and while this is generally a beneficial outcome, it could also result in scar tissue formation due to these anabolic effects[28,31]. Still, no randomized or prospective clinical studies have been performed to compare outcomes between leukocyte-rich versus leukocyte-poor PRP.

4. NON-OPERATIVE APPLICATIONS

Platelet-rich plasma injections are used most commonly as an adjunct to conservative treatment. In cases of chronic tendinopathy or osteoarthritis, PRP is typically indicated when first-line treatment (physical therapy, rest) fails. For professional athletes, in-season PRP may be used to reduce pain and improve function as an interim solution until the offseason when the athlete can undergo surgical intervention. This is particularly true for hip labral tears and chronic tendinopathies.

As detailed below, PRP injections have been used to treat tendinopathy of the hamstrings, adductor longus, and gluteus medius. These injections are typically performed under US guidance in the clinic. The number of injections used differs by study, though most reports describe the use of a single PRP injection for a variety of hip pathologies. Prior to injection, patients should fast for a minimum of three hours and should limit water intake to 8 ounces. In addition, patients should avoid the use of non-steroidal anti-inflammatory drugs (NSAIDs) for at least two days prior to and five days following injection, as these medications have been shown to impair platelet function[32].

Hamstring tendinopathy

Chronic tendinopathy or partial tears of the proximal hamstring tendons are common injuries among athletes. These injuries often occur while running, particularly when accelerating. Following severe hamstring injuries, many high level athletes may struggle with sitting on a bike or returning to running. Corticosteroid injections should be avoided as they may result in further tendon weakening and progression to high-grade tearing. PRP injections can be used to facilitate healing when there is partial thickness involvement or tendinosis without retraction. Complete tears, especially if chronic and retracted, are best treated with surgical repair.

A Hamid et al[33] conducted a randomized controlled trial to compare PRP therapy plus a rehabilitation program versus rehabilitation alone in patients with acute hamstring injuries (table 1). Patients in the PRP group were given a single intra-lesional injection of PRP, without addition of an activating agent, under US guidance at an average of 4.6 days following injury. Time to return to play was significantly lower in the PRP group (mean 26.7 days) versus the control group (mean 42.5 days). In addition, the PRP group had significantly lower pain severity scores at all time points up to 7 weeks following intervention.

STUDY	LEVEL OF EVIDENCE	PATHOLOGY	CONTROL GROUP(S)	OUTCOMES MEASURED
A Hamid et al, 2014[33]	II	Acute hamstring injuries	Rehabilitation without PRP	Return to play time, pain severity score, pain interference score
Hamilton et al, 2015[34]	I	Hamstring injuries	Platelet-poor plasma, no injection	Return to play time, reinjury rate
Fader et al, 2015[35]	IV	Chronic proximal hamstring tendinopathy	N/A	VAS pain
Wetzel et al, 2013[36]	III	Proximal hamstring injuries	NSAIDs, physical therapy	VAS, NPRS
Davenport et al, 2015[37]	I	Proximal hamstring tendinopathy	Autologous whole blood	MHHS, Hip Outcome Score-ADL, IHOT-33
Dallaudière et al, 2014[39]	IV	Upper and lower limb tendinopathy	N/A	WOMAC, ultrasound lesion size
Mautner et al, 2013[42]	IV	Chronic tendinopathy	N/A	VAS, assessment of functional pain, overall satisfaction

TABLE 1.CLINICAL STUDIES ON PRP TREATMENT FOR HIP AND PELVIC PATHOLOGIES.
VAS = visual analog scale, NSAIDs = non-steroidal anti-inflammatory drugs, NPRS = Nirschl Phase Rating Scale, MHHS = Modified Harris Hip Score, ADL = activities of daily living, IHOT-33 = International Hip Outcome Tool 33, WOMAC = Western Ontario and McMaster Universities Osteoarthritis Index, OA = osteoarthritis, HA = hyaluronic acid, HHS = Harris Hip Score, AVN = avascular necrosis.

In another randomized controlled trial, Hamilton et al[34] compared PRP, platelet-poor plasma (PPP), and no injection in professional athletes with MRI-positive hamstring injuries. All patients underwent a standardized rehabilitation program. Time to return to sport was found to be significantly lower in the PRP group (mean 21 days) compared with the PPP group (mean 27 days). No significant difference in re-injury rate was noted between the three groups at 2 months or 6 months following intervention.

Fader et al[35] performed a retrospective case series of 18 patients with chronic proximal hamstring tendinopathy. Each patient received a single PRP injection by US guidance. Patients had chronic hamstring pain symptoms for an average of 32.6 months prior to their injection and all patients had attempted other non-surgical treatments such as cortisone injections and physical therapy prior to injection. Based on a visual analog scale (VAS) for pain, patients had an average improvement in pain of 63% at 6 months following PRP injection.

In another study, Wetzel et al[36] performed a retrospective cohort study comparing twelve cases of proximal hamstring injuries treated by a single PRP injection and five patients treated with traditional conservative treatment (TCT) consisting of NSAIDs and physical therapy. Patients in the PRP and TCT groups presented at an average of 9.6 and 7.8 months after injury, respectively. At an average follow-up of 4.5 months, the PRP group demonstrated significantly improved VAS ($p < 0.01$) and Nirschl Phase Rating Scale (NPRS) scores ($p < 0.01$) compared to pre-treatment. At an average follow-up of 2 months, the TCT group did not show the same degree of improvement in VAS ($p = 0.06$) or NPRS scores ($p = 0.06$). However, due to the small sample sizes and differences in follow-up times, it is difficult to discern these outcome differences.

Davenport et al[37] conducted a double-blind, randomized controlled trial comparing a single injection of PRP versus autologous whole blood (WB) for the treatment of proximal hamstring tendinopathy. At follow-up times of 2, 6, and 12 weeks and 6 months, no significant differences were observed between groups with regard to the Modified Harris Hip Score, Hip Outcome Scores for activities of daily living (ADL) and sport-specific function, and International Hip Outcome Tool 33 (IHOT-33). However, compared to baseline, the PRP group demonstrated significant improvements in ADL and IHOT-33 scores, whereas the WB group showed significantly decreased pain with 15-minute sitting at 6 months.

Although conflicting results exist, the majority of published studies have reported successful outcomes of PRP injections for hamstring injuries. The authors use PRP injections for acute hamstring injuries including, in rare cases, complete tears with a small amount of retraction in patients with low activity levels or when patients opt out of surgery.

Adductor tendinopathy/athletic pubalgia

Adductor tendinopathy typically presents with groin pain and is often seen in soccer players due to the frequency of running and cutting movements involved in this sport[38]. Athletic pubalgia is a more general term involving groin pain, often in athletes, with adductor tendinopathy being a frequent concomitant pathology in these patients. Good outcomes have been shown following adductor tenotomy with and without hernioplasty[38], though PRP provides a non-operative treatment option for this pathology.

Adductor longus tendinopathy is a common indication for PRP treatment. Dallaudière et al[39] performed a retrospective case series of 408 consecutive patients treated by a single ultrasound-guided PRP injection for tendinopathy of upper (medial and lateral epicondylar tendons, i.e. golfer's and tennis elbow, respectively) and lower (patellar, Achilles, hamstring, adductor longus, and peroneal tendons) limbs. Patients with hamstring and adductor longus tendinopathy demonstrated significantly improved Western Ontario and McMaster Universities Osteoarthritis Index (WOMAC) scores at 6 weeks and a mean 20.2 months following injection ($p < 0.001$). Ultrasound was also used to assess lesion size at baseline and 6 weeks post-injection, with hamstring and adductor longus tendon lesion size decreasing from an average of 21.2 mm to 2.6 mm during this time ($p < 0.001$).

Interestingly, there is a high incidence of athletic pubalgia symptoms in patients with symptomatic femoroacetabular impingement (FAI)[40]. Hammoud et al[40] showed that 39% of professional athletes presenting with concomitant AP and FAI experienced symptom resolution with surgical treatment of FAI alone. Larson et al[41] demonstrated a return to unrestricted activity in 89% of patients with surgical management of both athletic pubalgia and intra-articular hip pathologies, compared to only 25% in patients undergoing surgical treatment of athletic pubalgia alone.

The authors inject the origin of the adductor longus (AL) tendon for chronic tendinopathy or acute tears (fig. 1). We first exclude the pubic symphysis as the source of the pain (using a lidocaine test) due to its anatomical proximity to the AL. It is also important to conduct full range of motion (ROM) evaluation of the hip joint to exclude concomitant FAI. FAI results in reduced ROM which in turn places increased stress on the AL origin and may result in chronic microtears and tendinopathy. In these cases, PRGF may not be a beneficial long-term solution as the offending mechanism is still present.

When electing to perform PRGF injections for adductor tendinopathy, it is important to have the patient shave the groin area a few days prior to injection for ease of US guidance. These injections can be very painful, though due to the superficial location of the pathology, lidocaine cannot be used. It is recommended that nitric oxide be used as an inhaled anesthetic if possible.

Gluteus medius tendinopathy

The literature is currently lacking in reported outcomes of PRP injection for gluteus medius tendinopathy. However, in a multicenter, retrospective review of 180 patients with chronic tendinopathy[42], 16 patients underwent US-guided PRP injections for gluteus medius tendinopathy with 13 patients demonstrating moderate improvement to complete resolution of symptoms at an average follow-up of 15 months post-injection. However, the PRP injection methodology of this study was non-uniform in that 60% of all patients received one injection, 30% received two, and 10% received three or more injections.

The authors use a series of three injections of PRGF for chronic indications[8] such as gluteus medius or minimus tendinopathy (fig. 2). It is important to

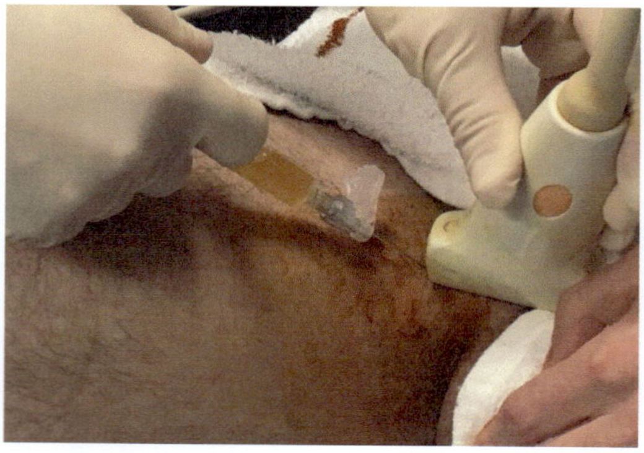

FIG. 1
Ultrasound-guided PRP injection of the adductor longus near its origin on the pubic body.

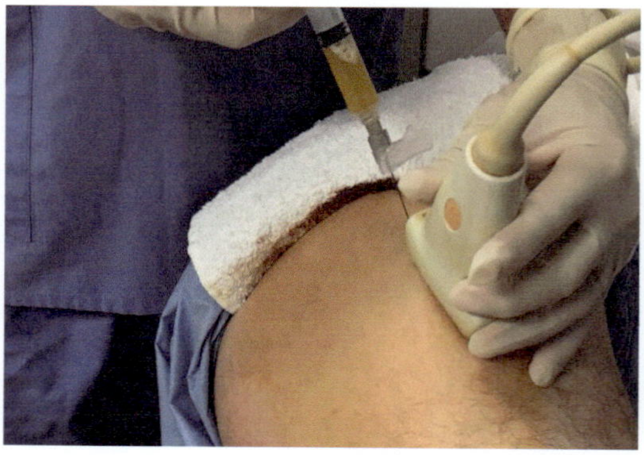

FIG. 2
Ultrasound-guided PRP injection of the gluteus medius near its insertion on the greater trochanter.

conduct a comprehensive physical examination to determine that the reported pain is not referred from the lower back or hip joint. In some cases, a lidocaine test can help to confirm or exclude the gluteus as the primary pathology. It is instrumental to review a high resolution MRI of the region and to determine pre-injection if gluteal bursitis is causing the patient's pain or if tendinopathic changes/tears are present. It is also important to note which tendons are involved, as the minimus tendon is deeper and thus requires proper US guidance during injection. From our experience, the majority of gluteal tendon tears are in the medial/deeper side of the tendon.

As mentioned with hamstring tendinopathy, many practitioners would use steroid injections for greater trochanteric bursitis. However, this is usually a misdiagnosis or a secondary pathology as gluteal tendon tears are often the primary pain source. Although steroid injections can improve pain for a few months, they can also result in atrophy and weakening of the gluteal tendons.

Sartorius avulsion

The sartorius originates on the anterior superior iliac spine (ASIS) apophysis, which begins to ossify between the ages of 13-15 years and fuses with the ilium between the ages of 21-25 years. An ASIS apophyseal avulsion injury occurs most commonly during running with the hip in extension and knee in flexion, or during a kicking motion[43]. Pain and a tearing sensation are the most common symptoms.

Recently, a 16 year old male presented to our clinic with anterolateral left hip pain following a lacrosse injury in which the patient made a cut while sprinting and felt and heard a pop around his hip. MRI showed a proximal sartorius avulsion with a few millimeters of distraction and significant soft tissue and bone edema in the surrounding area (fig. 3). The patient underwent US-guided PRGF injection (fig. 4) and reported complete resolution of symptoms within a week. He returned to full activity with our clearance at five weeks post-injection. A similar technique can be used for other apophyseal avulsion injuries such as that of the hamstrings or rectus femoris.

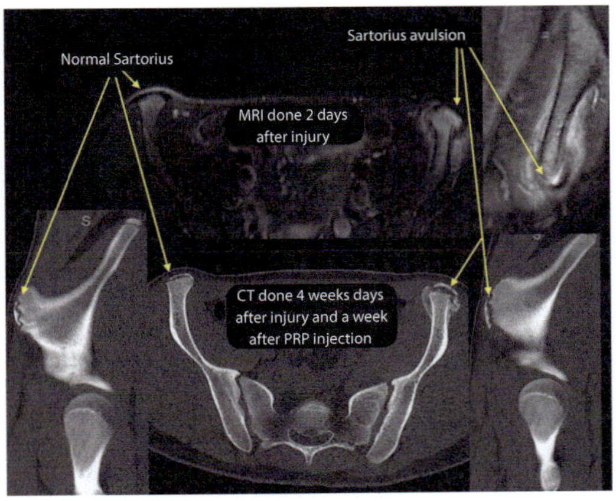

FIG. 3
MRI demonstrating avulsion of the sartorius muscle from its origin on the anterior superior iliac spine (ASIS, top images). CT images comparing a normal sartorius origin on the ASIS (bottom left) and a sartorius avulsion (bottom right).

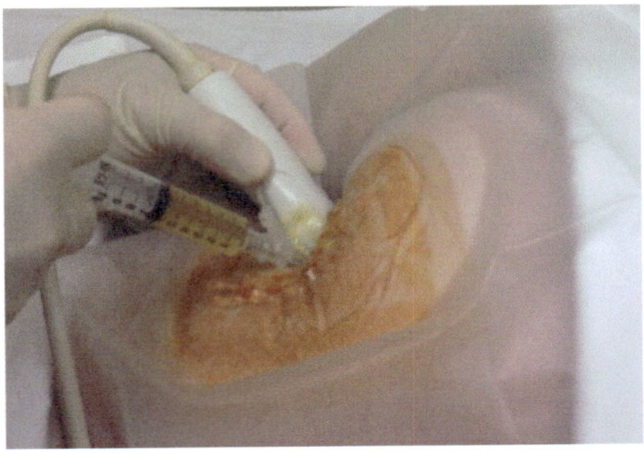

FIG. 4
Ultrasound-guided PRP injection of Hamstrings near its origin on the anterior superior iliac spine.

5.SURGICAL APPLICATIONS

As described above, when used in a non-operative setting, platelet-rich plasma is applied as a liquid injectable. However, in an intraoperative setting, PRP may be injected as a liquid or gel[44], or delivered as a fibrin matrix (platelet-rich fibrin matrix, PRFM)[45]. Most of the surgical applications of PRP for hip and pelvic pathology are novel, with few studies currently in the literature.

Adjuvant therapy for tendon repair

Platelet-rich plasma has been shown to improve healing in patients with acute ruptured Achilles tendons[12,46]. Sánchez et al[46] showed an earlier recovery of range of motion, return to gentle running, and return to training activities in 12 athletes who underwent open suture repair of a complete Achilles tendon rupture with PRP versus standard open suture repair. Alsousou[12] compared biopsy samples of acute ruptured Achilles tendons treated with PRP versus a control group receiving no treatment. The PRP group demonstrated significantly higher collagen I content and a significantly lower modified Bonar score, which indicates improved early tendon healing.

The authors use PRGF injections in patients undergoing surgical repair of the hamstring tendons when the tendon tissue is found to be of low quality and enhancement of the surgical repair is required. Another common indication for PRGF within our practice is in professional athletes for whom there is a need for an expedited recovery and return to play. This is most commonly indicated for the hamstrings, rectus femoris, or a sartorius avulsion.

6. CONCLUSIONS

This chapter describes some of the established as well as novel applications of platelet-rich plasma or plasma rich in growth factors (PRGF) for the treatment of hip and pelvic pathologies. Although the outcomes of many of these applications have not been described in the literature, particularly in high-level studies, from our experience we have found that symptomatic and functional outcomes are successful in the majority of patients. As indications for PRP continue to expand, it will become increasingly important for future studies to state specific methodologies used in the preparation of PRP in order to recognize ideal preparation techniques and the ideal number of PRP injections for each pathology. Leukocyte-poor PRP has the advantages of a reduced inflammatory response and mainly anabolic changes compared to leukocyte-rich PRP, though further, high quality studies are necessary to determine outcome differences between these two PRP preparations.

1. Mei-Dan O, Carmont MR. Novel applications of platelet-rich plasma technology in musculoskeletal medicine and surgery. Operative Techniques in Orthopaedics. 2012;22:56-63.

2. DeLong JM, Russell RP, Mazzocca AD. Platelet-rich plasma: the PAW classification system. Arthroscopy : the journal of arthroscopic & related surgery : official publication of the Arthroscopy Association of North America and the International Arthroscopy Association. 2012;28:998-1009.

3. Castricini R, Longo UG, De Benedetto M, et al. Platelet-rich plasma augmentation for arthroscopic rotator cuff repair: a randomized controlled trial. The American journal of sports medicine. 2011;39:258-65.

4. Mei-Dan O, Carmont MR. Autologous blood products in rotator cuff repair. Medicine and sport science. 2012;57:65-75.

5. Liddle AD, Rodriguez-Merchan EC. Platelet-Rich Plasma in the Treatment of Patellar Tendinopathy: A Systematic Review. The American journal of sports medicine. 2015;43:2583-90.

6. Meheux CJ, McCulloch PC, Lintner DM, Varner KE, Harris JD. Efficacy of Intra-articular Platelet-Rich Plasma Injections in Knee Osteoarthritis: A Systematic Review. Arthroscopy : the journal of arthroscopic & related surgery : official publication of the Arthroscopy Association of North America and the International Arthroscopy Association. 2016;32:495-505.

7. Mishra AK, Skrepnik NV, Edwards SG, et al. Efficacy of platelet-rich plasma for chronic tennis elbow: a double-blind, prospective, multicenter, randomized controlled trial of 230 patients. The American journal of sports medicine. 2014;42:463-71.

8. Mei-Dan O, Carmont MR, Laver L, Mann G, Maffulli N, Nyska M. Platelet-rich plasma or hyaluronate in the management of osteochondral lesions of the talus. The American journal of sports medicine. 2012;40:534-41.

9. Kraeutler MJ, Chahla J, Dean CS, et al. Current Concepts Review Update. Foot & ankle international. 2017;38:331-42.

10. Kajikawa Y, Morihara T, Sakamoto H, et al. Platelet-rich plasma enhances the initial mobilization of circulation-derived cells for tendon healing. Journal of cellular physiology. 2008;215:837-45.

11. Visser LC, Arnoczky SP, Caballero O, Kern A, Ratcliffe A, Gardner KL. Growth factor-rich plasma increases tendon cell proliferation and matrix synthesis on a synthetic scaffold: an in vitro study. Tissue engineering. Part A. 2010;16:1021-9.

12. Alsousou J, Thompson M, Harrison P, Willett K, Franklin S. Effect of platelet-rich plasma on healing tissues in acute ruptured Achilles tendon: a human immunohistochemistry study. Lancet. 2015;385 Suppl 1:S19.

13. Virchenko O, Aspenberg P. How can one platelet injection after tendon injury lead to a stronger tendon after 4 weeks? Interplay between early regeneration and mechanical stimulation. Acta orthopaedica. 2006;77:806-12.

14. Mei-Dan O, Lippi G, Sanchez M, Andia I, Maffulli N. Autologous platelet-rich plasma: a revolution in soft tissue sports injury management? The Physician and sportsmedicine. 2010;38:127-35.

15. Lee JW, Kwon OH, Kim TK, et al. Platelet-rich plasma: quantitative assessment of growth factor levels and comparative analysis of activated and inactivated groups. Archives of plastic surgery. 2013;40:530-5.

16. Kakudo N, Morimoto N, Kushida S, Ogawa T, Kusumoto K. Platelet-rich plasma releasate promotes

angiogenesis in vitro and in vivo. Medical molecular morphology. 2014;47:83-9.

17. Dallari D, Stagni C, Rani N, et al. Ultrasound-Guided Injection of Platelet-Rich Plasma and Hyaluronic Acid, Separately and in Combination, for Hip Osteoarthritis: A Randomized Controlled Study. The American journal of sports medicine. 2016;44:664-71.

18. Kraeutler MJ, Garabekyan T, Mei-Dan O. The use of platelet-rich plasma to augment conservative and surgical treatment of hip and pelvic disorders. Muscles, ligaments and tendons journal. 2016;6:410-19.

19. Samuelson EM, Odum SM, Fleischli JE. The Cost-Effectiveness of Using Platelet-Rich Plasma During Rotator Cuff Repair: A Markov Model Analysis. Arthroscopy : the journal of arthroscopic & related surgery : official publication of the Arthroscopy Association of North America and the International Arthroscopy Association. 2016;32:1237-44.

20. Dhurat R, Sukesh M. Principles and Methods of Preparation of Platelet-Rich Plasma: A Review and Author's Perspective. Journal of cutaneous and aesthetic surgery. 2014;7:189-97.

21. Arnoczky SP, Sheibani-Rad S. The basic science of platelet-rich plasma (PRP): what clinicians need to know. Sports medicine and arthroscopy review. 2013;21:180-5.

22. Ghassab S, Dulin J, Bertone AL. Thromboelastographic Clot Characteristics of Autologous Equine Blood Products After Activation by Autologous Thrombin, Bovine Thrombin, or Calcium Chloride. Veterinary surgery : VS. 2015;44:970-5.

23. Textor JA, Tablin F. Activation of equine platelet-rich plasma: comparison of methods and characterization of equine autologous thrombin. Veterinary surgery : VS. 2012;41:784-94.

24. Graziani F, Ivanovski S, Cei S, Ducci F, Tonetti M, Gabriele M. The in vitro effect of different PRP concentrations on osteoblasts and fibroblasts. Clinical oral implants research. 2006;17:212-9.

25. Weibrich G, Hansen T, Kleis W, Buch R, Hitzler WE. Effect of platelet concentration in platelet-rich plasma on peri-implant bone regeneration. Bone. 2004;34:665-71.

26. Anitua E, Sanchez M, Nurden AT, Nurden P, Orive G, Andia I. New insights into and novel applications for platelet-rich fibrin therapies. Trends in biotechnology. 2006;24:227-34.

27. Weibrich G, Kleis WK, Hitzler WE, Hafner G. Comparison of the platelet concentrate collection system with the plasma-rich-in-growth-factors kit to produce platelet-rich plasma: a technical report. The International journal of oral & maxillofacial implants. 2005;20:118-23.

28. Cavallo C, Filardo G, Mariani E, et al. Comparison of platelet-rich plasma formulations for cartilage healing: an in vitro study. The Journal of bone and joint surgery. American volume. 2014;96:423-9.

29. Dragoo JL, Braun HJ, Durham JL, et al. Comparison of the acute inflammatory response of two commercial platelet-rich plasma systems in healthy rabbit tendons. The American journal of sports medicine. 2012;40:1274-81.

30. McCarrel TM, Minas T, Fortier LA. Optimization of leukocyte concentration in platelet-rich plasma for the treatment of tendinopathy. The Journal of bone and joint surgery. American volume. 2012;94:e143(1-8).

31. Zhou Y, Zhang J, Wu H, Hogan MV, Wang JH. The differential effects of leukocyte-containing and pure platelet-rich plasma (PRP) on tendon stem/progenitor cells - implications of PRP application for the clinical treatment of tendon injuries. Stem cell research & therapy. 2015;6:173.

32. Schippinger G, Pruller F, Divjak M, et al. Autologous Platelet-Rich Plasma Preparations: Influence of Nonsteroidal Anti-inflammatory Drugs on Platelet Function. Orthop J Sports Med. 2015;3:2325967115588896.

33. A Hamid MS, Mohamed Ali MR, Yusof A, George J, Lee LP. Platelet-rich plasma injections for the treatment of hamstring injuries: a randomized controlled trial. The American journal of sports medicine. 2014;42:2410-8.

34. Hamilton B, Tol JL, Almusa E, et al. Platelet-rich plasma does not enhance return to play in hamstring injuries: a randomised controlled trial. British journal of sports medicine. 2015;49:943-50.

35. Fader RR, Mitchell JJ, Traub S, et al. Platelet-rich plasma treatment improves outcomes for chronic proximal hamstring injuries in an athletic population. Muscles, ligaments and tendons journal. 2014;4:461-6.

36. Wetzel RJ, Patel RM, Terry MA. Platelet-rich plasma as an effective treatment for proximal hamstring injuries. Orthopedics. 2013;36:e64-70.

37. Davenport KL, Campos JS, Nguyen J, Saboeiro G, Adler RS, Moley PJ. Ultrasound-Guided Intratendinous Injections With Platelet-Rich Plasma or Autologous Whole Blood for Treatment of Proximal Hamstring Tendinopathy: A Double-Blind Randomized Controlled Trial. Journal of ultrasound in medicine : official journal of the American Institute of Ultrasound in Medicine. 2015;34:1455-63.

38. Mei-Dan O, Lopez V, Carmont MR, et al. Adductor tenotomy as a treatment for groin pain in professional soccer players. Orthopedics. 2013;36:e1189-97.

39. Dallaudiere B, Pesquer L, Meyer P, et al. Intratendinous injection of platelet-rich plasma under US guidance to treat tendinopathy: a long-term pilot study. Journal of vascular and interventional radiology : JVIR. 2014;25:717-23.

40. Hammoud S, Bedi A, Magennis E, Meyers WC, Kelly BT. High incidence of athletic pubalgia symptoms in professional athletes with symptomatic femoroacetabular impingement. Arthroscopy : the journal of arthroscopic & related surgery : official publication of the Arthroscopy Association of North America and the International Arthroscopy Association. 2012;28:1388-95.

41. Larson CM, Pierce BR, Giveans MR. Treatment of athletes with symptomatic intra-articular hip pathology and athletic pubalgia/sports hernia: a case series. Arthroscopy : the journal of arthroscopic & related surgery : official publication of the Arthroscopy Association of North America and the International Arthroscopy Association. 2011;27:768-75.

42. Mautner K, Colberg RE, Malanga G, et al. Outcomes after ultrasound-guided platelet-rich plasma injections for chronic tendinopathy: a multicenter, retrospective review. PM & R : the journal of injury, function, and rehabilitation. 2013;5:169-75.

43. Boyd KT, Peirce NS, Batt ME. Common hip injuries in sport. Sports Med. 1997;24:273-88.

44. Cervellin M, de Girolamo L, Bait C, Denti M, Volpi P. Autologous platelet-rich plasma gel to reduce donor-site morbidity after patellar tendon graft harvesting for anterior cruciate ligament reconstruction: a randomized, controlled clinical study. Knee surgery, sports traumatology, arthroscopy : official journal of the ESSKA. 2012;20:114-20.

45. Rodeo SA, Delos D, Williams RJ, Adler RS, Pearle A, Warren RF. The effect of platelet-rich fibrin matrix on rotator cuff tendon healing: a prospective, randomized clinical study. The American journal of sports medicine. 2012;40:1234-41.

46. Sanchez M, Anitua E, Azofra J, Andia I, Padilla S, Mujika I. Comparison of surgically repaired Achilles tendon tears using platelet-rich fibrin matrices. The American journal of sports medicine. 2007;35:245-51.

CHAPTER 13

A Novel and Versatile Adjuvant Biologic Therapy in the Management of Neuropathies

AUTHORS

Sánchez M.[1], Anitua E.[3,4,5], Delgado D.[2], Garate A.[2], Bilbao AM.[1], Sánchez P.[2], Padilla S.[3,4,5]

[1] Arthroscopic Surgery Unit, Hospital Vithas San José. Vitoria-Gasteiz, Spain.
[2] Advanced Biological Therapy Unit, Hospital Vithas San Jose, Vitoria-Gasteiz, Spain.
[3] BTI-Biotechnology Institute, Vitoria, Spain
[4] Eduardo Anitua Foundation for Biomedical Research. Vitoria-Gasteiz, Spain
[5] University Institute for Regenerative Medicine and Oral Implantology (UIRMI) from the University of Basque Country (UPV/EHU)

SUMMARY

In mammals, axons of injured peripheral nerves (PNI) can and do regenerate, but often the functional recovery is incomplete or suboptimal. In recent years in vivo tissue engineering approaches through molecular intervention and scaffolding are offering promising outcomes. In this sense, evidence is accumulating in both preclinical and clinical settings, indicating that platelet rich plasma (PRP) products, and fibrin scaffold obtained from this technology, hold an important therapeutic potential as a neuroprotective, neurogenic and neuroinflammatory therapeutic modulator system, as well as enhancing the sensory and motor functional nerve muscle unit recovery.

This chapter addresses current molecular and cellular data in intrinsic nerve repair processes and describes a new strategy to harness and enhance these processes by using biochemical and biomechanical cues. In particular, it focuses on autologous fibrin, plasma and platelet-derived growth factors as filler or scaffolds that can synergize with the gold standard therapy and other nerve guidance conduits.

E. Anitua et al. (eds.), *Platelet Rich Plasma in Orthopaedics and Sports Medicine*,
https://doi.org/10.1007/978-3-319-63730-3_13

1. INTRODUCTION

Every year, 350,000 patients are affected by traumatic peripheral nerve injuries, which accounts for $150 billion in annual health care costs[1]. Direct tension-free microsurgical repair and/or the transplantation of a nerve autograft to bridge the gap are the gold standard treatments aimed at enhancing the intrinsic regenerative potential of injured axons[2]. However, such treatments fail to recreate the suitable cellular and molecular microenvironment of peripheral nerve repair[3] in addition to creating, as in the case of autografts, a second iatrogenic injury and morbidity in the donor site[4]. In recent years, biologic strategies to treat peripheral nerve injury (PNI) combined with in vivo tissue engineering approaches through molecular intervention and scaffolding are offering promising outcomes[2,5,6]. Among them, platelet rich plasma (PRP) products hold an important therapeutic potential as a neuroprotective, neurogenic, and neuroinflammatory therapeutic modulator system[5,7-11] and as enhancer of sensory and motor functional nerve-muscle unit recovery[12-14]. PRPs are emerging as an adjuvant biologic in the treatment of peripheral nerve injuries (PNIs) and neuropathies[12-14]. These autologous products are applied either as a filler of nerve conduits or vein-muscle grafts across nerve gaps post trauma by Ultrasound-guided perineural and intraneural infiltrations , or as scaffolds to bridge or wrap the injured nerve stumps[15-18]. Moreover, there are non-traumatic peripheral injuries such as compression, adhesion and fibrosis, (as in the case of carpal tunnel syndrome and fibrotic post-surgical side effects)[19], where this novel approach applied may additionally diminish undesirable consequences such as fibrotic scars and denervated organ atrophy, since this adjuvant therapy can speed up the functional recovery of the nerve-muscle unit[20-24].

Considerable progress has been made in understanding the molecular and cellular events of peripheral nerve regeneration after injury, and this chapter will discuss our current knowledge, and the particular application of plasma rich in growth factors for improving repair and regeneration in PNI.

2. NEUROBIOLOGY OF PERIPHERAL NERVE INJURY AND REPAIR

After injury, approximately 30-40% of sensory neurons die, and these numbers increase as the nerve injury gets closer to the neuron body[25]. Persisting neurons switch their state from a signalling to a growing phenotype through the expression of genes involved in cell survival and axon outgrowth[25,26]. Concomitantly, injured or dying axons signal to Schwann cells (SCs) through their loss of contact, by an as yet poorly understood mechanism, and SCs respond with a radical phenotypic change known as activation or transdifferentiation[27,28]. In addition, supportive stromal cells such as endothelial cells, fibroblasts, and macrophages, will play a key role in the guidance and support of Schwann cell-growing axon regenerative units across first the nerve bridge and then the distal segment to eventually reconnect with their original targets at a rate of about 1mm per day in humans (fig. 1)[25,29].

SCs act as masters and servants in PNI repair, and show a striking chameleonic response to the biological battlefield they are exposed to inside a damaged nerve and are the early detectors of damage (fig. 1). Recent studies have shown that SCs express a variety of Toll-like receptors (TLRs2/3/4) through which SCs recognize these DAMPs, together with resident macrophages also endowed with TLRs, thereby playing a sentinel role to identify nerve injury and hence, activate an inflammatory response known as neuroinflammation[30,31]. In a context-and time-dependent manner, dedifferentiated SCs perform a variety of cell repair tasks from phagocytosing myelin debris to secreting neurotrophic and neurotropic factors (laminin), proliferation and migration, which results in the formation of SC cords and Bungner Bands in the proximal and distal nerve segment, respectively[27,30,32]. Although SCs have the reputation of being the engine of peripheral nerve repair, in the nerve repair complex process they are fuelled by axon growth cones and supportive stromal cells such as macrophages and fibroblasts, the very elements of Wallerian degeneration as a neuroinflammatory process (fig. 1)[27,30,33-35]. The macrophages acting as "jack of all trades" will collaborate with the activated-dedifferentiated SCs in clearing the myelin and other tissue debris. Moreover, these SCs come into direct contact with resident fibroblasts that accumulate in large numbers at the site of injury influencing SC migration and dedifferentiation[27,28,33] (fig. 1). Moreover, emerging evidence suggests that macrophage plasticity contributes to peripheral nerve regeneration via distinct mechanisms: by phagocyitosing myelin debris, synthesizing trophic factors such as VEGF and promoting angiogenesis, producing collagen type VI, modulating the proliferation and migration of SCs, and influencing the resolution of inflammation through the polarization from M1 to M2 phenotype[34-36]. Cattin et al[34] confirmed an idea suggested by Chen et al[37] that blood vessels might provide substrate or signalling for axon growth guidance and SC migration, by showing that macrophages selectively sense hypoxia in the area of nerve bridge and drive angiogenesis via the VEGF-secretion pathway at the nerve bridge (fig. 1). In addition, these SCs come into direct contact with resident fibroblasts that accumulate in large numbers at the site of injury influencing SC migration and dedifferentiation[27,28,33] (fig. 1).

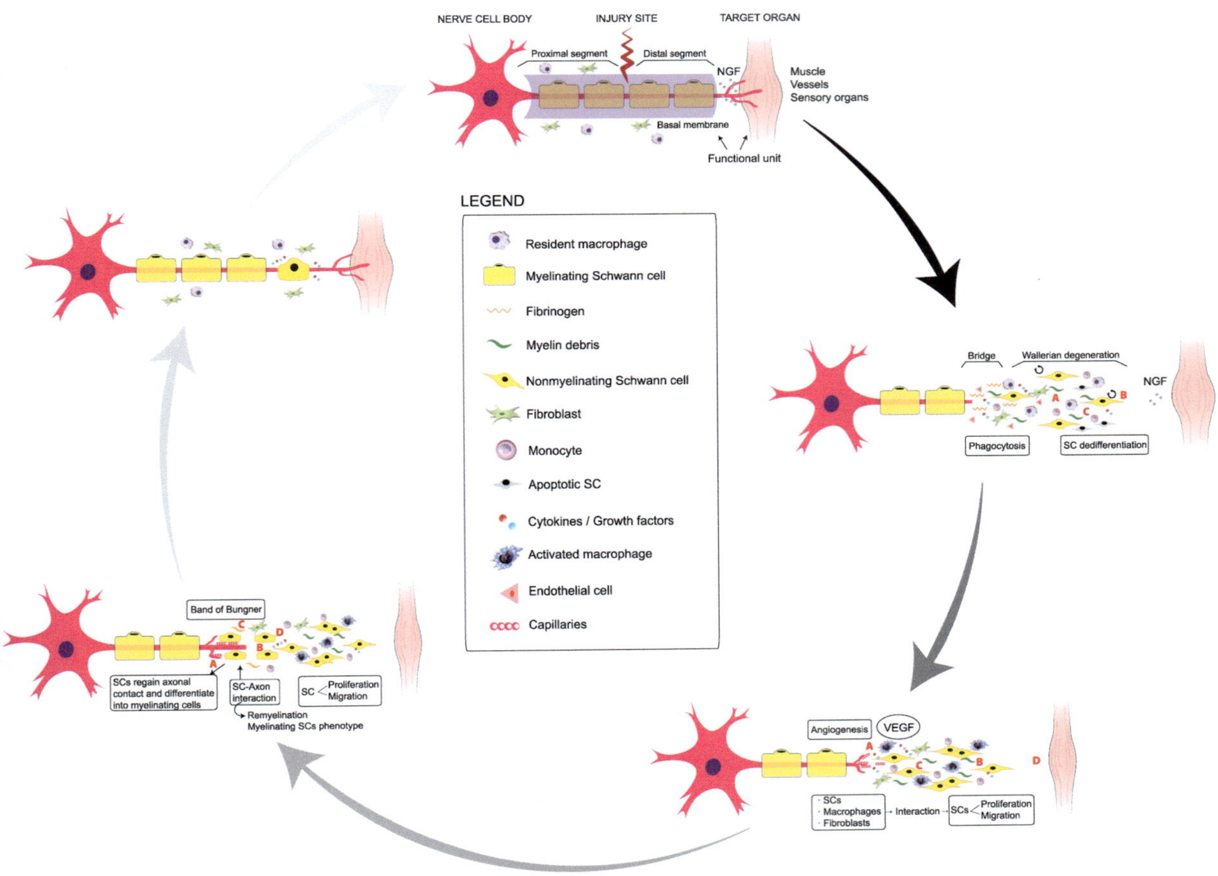

FIG. 1 SPONTANEOUS PERIPHERAL NERVE REGENERATION IS A MULTICELLULAR AND PLEIOTROPIC PROCESS
Schwann cells are the master and servant in peripheral nerve regeneration while macrophages act as "Jack of all trades". The partnership between the transdifferentiated SCs and macrophages induce the latter to synthesize VEGF. In addition to stimulating the proliferation of endothelial cells, and thereby promoting new vessels that guide the axon growth, thereby serving as tracks for migrating and proliferating SCs to from a Band of Bungner, VEGF enhances the survival, migration and proliferation of SCs, all of which contribute to the outgrowth of axons, restoration of basal lamina and facilitation of the formation of Band of Bungner at both nerve stumps. (reprinted with permission from Sanchez, M. et al.[29]

Despite the robust repair capacity to regrow peripheral nervous axons shown in the adult mammal[30,34] and meticulous microsurgical nerve repair techniques there are some limiting factors, including the poor vascularization, the patients age, the chronic denervation of SCs, the endoneurial and perineurial fibrosis, the misguided axonal growth, the vast distance that axon growth cones must cover to reinnervate target organs/tissues, as well as their atrophy, and the rate of regeneration[25,32,38,39]. Therefore, three key events significantly contribute to axonal outgrowth, namely, angiogenesis, axon-SC partnership, and a permissive and inductive microenvironment where as important as the absence of inhibitory molecules is the presence of nerve guidance, and neurotropic and neurotrophic factors.

3. PLASMA RICH PLASMA: AN INJECTABLE SCAFFOLD TO ASSIST IN NERVE REPAIR

Platelet rich plasma (PRPs) are blood-derived biological drug delivery products that have emerged as a novel and versatile formulation to enhance repair and regeneration in the treatment of musculoskeletal conditions including osteoarthritis and chondral pathologies, non-union fractures, acute and chronic tendinopathies, muscle strains, and peripheral nerve injuries and neuropathies[12,40-42].

These varied products consist of a pool of growth factors (GFs), microparticles, and other bioactive

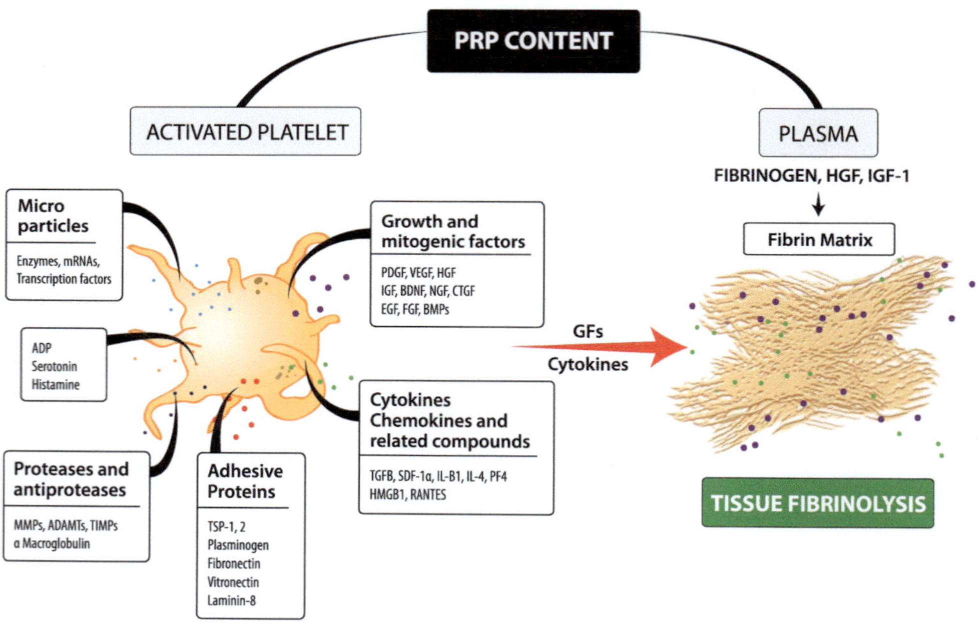

FIG. 2
Illustration of some biological mediators of platelet-rich plasma (PRP) that govern tissue repair by still poorly undestood mechanisms. There are biomolecules and several growth factors which come either from platelet activation and plasma or both. Several of these bioactive mediators and other growth factors or proteins remain trapped through fibrin heparan sulfate-binding domains, in a three-dimensional transient fibrin matrix to be released later by tissue fibrinolysis. ADAMTs: A disintegrin and metalloprotease with thrombospondin motifs; ADP: adenosine diphosphate; BDNF: brain-derived neurotrophic factor; BMPs: bone morphogenetic proteins; CTGF: connective tissue growth factor; EGF: epidermal growth factor; FGF: fibroblast growth factor; GFs: growth factors; HGF: hepatocyte growth factor; HMGB1: high mobility group box 1; IGF: insulin-like growth factor; IL-β1: interleukin-β1; MMPs: matrix metalloproteinases; NGF: nerve growth factor; PDGF: platelet-derived growth factor; PF4: platelet factor 4; RANTES: regulated upon activation, normal T cell expressed and presumably secreted; SDF-1α: stromal cell-derived factor-1α; TGFB: transforming growth factor beta; TIMPs: tissue inhibitors of metalloproteinases; TSP-1: thrombospondin-1; VEGF: vascular en- dothelial growth factor. (reprinted with permission from Sanchez, M. et al.[29]

mediators stemmed from platelet activation and plasma (fig. 2)[29]. Many of these biomolecules are trapped, through fibrin heparan sulfate-binding domains, in a three-dimensional transient fibrin matrix generated from the polymerization of plasmatic fibrinogen, thereby regulating the tissue concentration of GFs, as is the case in biological repair[43].

Once PRP is infiltrated intraneurally as a liquid-to-gel injectable scaffold, or wrapped around the injured nerve gap as a matrix-like viscous and malleable structure, or both,[12] (fig. 3) tissue fibrinolysis breaks the fibrin down, thereby releasing cell signalling molecules such as neurotrophic (NGF, BDGF, IGF-1, PDGF, VEGF, HGF) and neurotropic factors (fibrin, fibronectin, and vitronectin)[9].

Growing in vitro and in vivo evidence suggests that the biomolecules conveyed by PRPs are instrumental agents that modulate early inflammation, stem cell-like myelinating Schwann cell activation, macrophage polarization, as well as the active resolution of inflammation, angiogenesis, and fibrogenesis, thereby acting as key drivers of full nerve functional recovery[27,34,44-46] (Table I and II)[6].

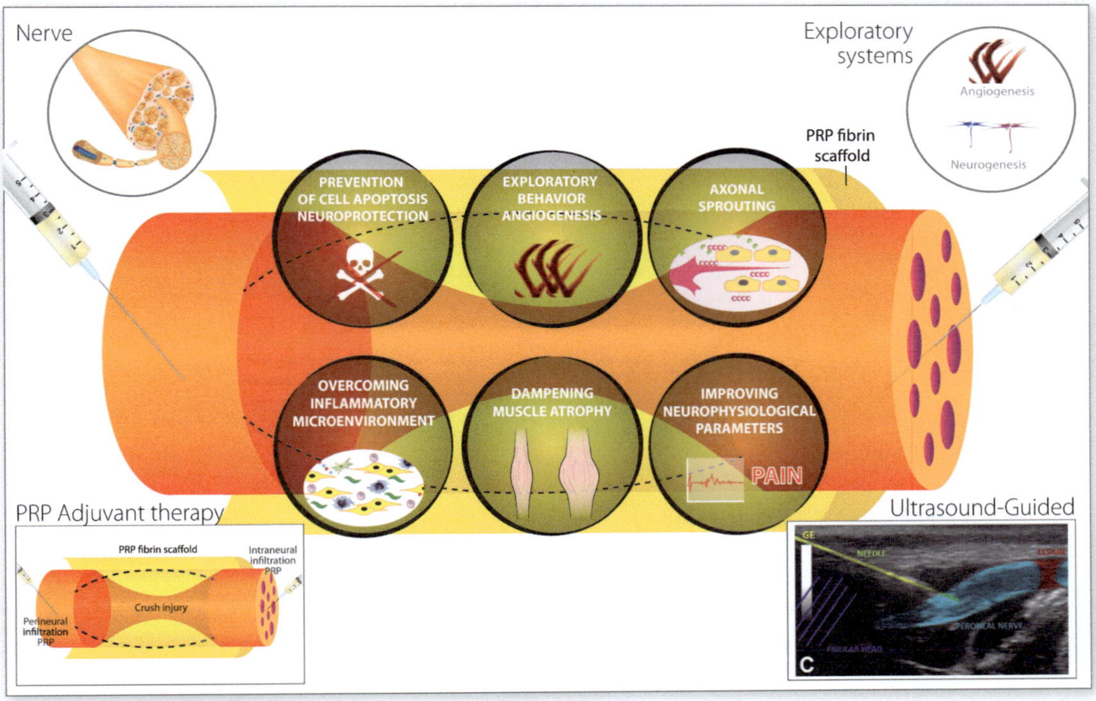

FIG. 3
Six lines of evidence suggest the therapeutic potential use of PRPs on neural tissue repair and regeneration.
These include the prevention of cell apoptosis and neuroprotection, the stimulation of angiogenesis, the modulation of inflammatory microenvironment, the enhancement of axonal outgrowth and nerve guidance, the dampening of both denervated muscle atrophy and scarring that follow peripheral nerve trauma and damage, and the improvement of neurologic parameters in humans. (reprinted with permission from Sanchez, M. et al.[29]

Cell type/Animal model	Intervention	Outcome	Reference
Human bone marrow stem cells	Cells cultured with PRP scaffolds enriched with NGF, BDGF and retinoic acid.	Prevention of cell apoptosis and differentiation in neural phenotype.	Zurita et al. 2010
Bone marrow stromal cells and Wistar rats with intracerebral hemorrhage	Intracerebral administration of cells embedded in PRP scaffold	Increment of cell viability and biological, neurological and functional activity	Vaquero et al. 2013
Sprague-Dawley rats with bilateral cavernous nerve crush	Injection of 200μL of PRP into the corpus cavernosum immediately after crush injury	Preservation of myelinated axons and prevention of cell apotosis	Wu et al. 2012
Albino guinea pigs with facial nerve transection	Injection of 5mL of PRP and perineural microsuture	Improvement in function, increment of neurotrophic factors and preservation of axons and myelin	Cho et al. 2010
Primary cortical and hippocampal neurons from Wistar rat embryos cultured with amyloid-β peptide	Cell incubation with 7% and 10% PRP during 48 hours.	Increment of cell survival in primary neurons	Anitua et al. 2013
Double-transgenic APP/PS1 mice (model of Alzheimer disease)	Intranasal administration of 3μL of PRP, 3 times per week for 4 weeks.	Decrease in brain Aβ deposition, neuroprotection and reduction of inflammation	Anitua et al. 2014
BALB/c mice with hind limb sichemia	Inyection of 6-18μL of PRP into the adductor and quadriceps region 24 hours after surgery	Enhancement of reperfusion and reduction of fibrotic tissue	Anitua et al. 2015
Sprague-Dawley rats with 10-mm sciatic nerve gap	Inside-out vein graft filled with 0.15-2 mL of PRP	Increment of neoangeogenesis, number of myelinated axons and diameter of axons and myelin sheat.	Kim et al. 2014
Schwann cells from sciatic nerves of Sprague-Dawley rats	Cells cultured with different concentrations of PRP	Stimulation of cell proliferation, migration and neurotrophic function in a dose-dependent manner	Zheng et al. 2016
Brain cortex and spinal cord cocul-ters from Sprague-Dawley rats	Coculters incubated with medium containing 5%-10% of PRP durin 14 days	Promotion of axon growth and number	Takeuchi et al. 2012
New Zeland White rabbits with 10 mm sciatic nerve defect	Implantation of poly (lactic-co-glycolic acid) conduit filled with PRP and Schwann cells in the defect	Increment of the number of regenerating nerve fibers, thickness of the myelin sheath, muscle action potential and nerve conduction velocity	Ye et al. 2012
Rabbit and dog with sciatic nerve cut	"Fibrin suture" with coagulated blood plasma previously enriched with fibrinogen	Growth of new fibers across the junction	Young et al. 1940
Isogenic spontaneous hypertensive rats with sciatic nerve gap	Implantation of vein grafts injected with PRP.	Increment of sciatic functional index	Sabongi et al. 2014
Sprague–Dawley rats 15-mm long sciatic nerve defects	Implantation of acellular nerve allografts loaded with PRP in the nerve gap	Improvement of electrophysiology response for amplitude and conduction velocity , diameter, thickness and numbers of regenerating nerve fiber	Zheng et al. 2014
Wistar rats with 1-cm long sciatic nerve defects	Implantation of collagen nerve conduit with Platelet gel	Improvement of functional and structural outcomes	Kaplan et al. 2011
Wistar albino rats with cross-sectioned sciatic-nerve	Implantation of sutured PRP-membrane sutured around sciatic nerve	Improvement of amplitude and frequency spectrum in the electromyographic data	Giannessi et al. 2014
Sprague-Dawley rats with facial nerve transection	PRP added to perineural sutures	Improvement of functional activity and neurotrophic effect	Farrag et al. 2007
Wistar rats with 1 sciatic nerve transection	PRP added to epineural sutures	Increment of myelin thickness and reduction of latency time in electromyography	Sariguney et al. 2008
Latxa sheep with common peroneal nerve crush injury	PRP membrane placed around the nerve lesion and 3 intraneural injection of 3 mL of PRP, one injection every two weeks.	Earlier electrophysiological response, increment of axonal density and reduction of muscle atrophy	Sánchez et al. 2015
C5tBL/6J mice lesioned with 1-methyl-4phenyl-1,2,3,6-tetrahydropirydine (Parkinson's disease model).	Intranasal administration of 3μL of PRP, 3 times per week for 2 weeks.	Increment of neuroprotection, improvement of motor performance and reduction of inflammatory response, nuclear transcription factor-κβ, nitric oxide, cycloxignase-2 and tumor necrosis factor-alpha.	Anitua et al. 2015
New Zeland white rabbits with carpal tunnel syndrome dextrose-induced median nerve injury	Injection of 0.3 mL of PRP into the carpal tunnel	Improvement of electrophysiological parameters and reduction of nerve swelling	Park et al. 2014
Wistar albino rats with sciatic nerve crush injury	Injections of 15μg of IGF-1 or 0.125 mL of Leukocyte rich-PRP into the crush-injured site	Improvement of functional and sensory recovery of animals treated with IGF-1	Emel et al. 2011

TABLE 1 Summary of in vitro and in vivo effects of Platelet-Rich Plasma (reprinted with permission[6])

Type of study	Clinical cases	Intervention	Outcome	Reference
Case Report n=1	Ulnar nerve trauma at the elbow, with neuropathic pain and nerve dysfunction	12-cm-long nerve gap bridged with a collagen tube filled with autologous platelet-rich fibrin during the surgery at 3.25 years post trauma	Sensory and motor recovery across nerve gap and reduction of neuropathic pain.	Kuffler et al. 2011
Case series n=27	Patients under 58 years with 2-16-cm-long nerve gap in their extremities	Nerve gaps bridged with collagen tubes filled with PRP during the surgery at 0.5-3 years post trauma	Functional recovery	Kuffler et al. 2014
Randomized control study n=20	Patients with benign parotid gland tumor presenting facial muscles and nerve deficit	Superficial parotidectomy using PRP gel	Significant improvements in several clinical parameters	Sacala et al. 2014
Double blind, randomized, control clinical trial n=60	Patients with leprosy peripheral neuropathy	One injection of perineural injection of 1mL of PRP in the posterial tibial and ulnar nerves	Significant two-point discrimination test reduction and significant VAS improvement in week 2.	Anjayani et al. 2014
Retrospective analysis n=10	Patients with persistent pudendal neuralgia after neurolysis and transposition	One injection of PRP around the pudendedal nerve after a transgluteal decompression enclosing the nerve in NeuroWrapNerve Protector	Significant pain reduction	Hibner et al. 2012
Case series n=14	Patients with median nerve injury suffering from carpal tunnel syndrome for over 3 months	One US-guided injection of 1-2 mL of PRP into the region around the median nerve at the proximal edge of carpal tunnel	Pain almost disappeared and upper limb function improved at 1 month after treatmen	Malahias et al. 2015
Case Report n=1	Patients with peroneal nerve palsy with drop foot after multiple ligament injuries of the knee	Serial US-guided intraneural and perineural infiltrations of 3-8 mL of PRP.	Significant pain and function recovery with EMG signs of reinnervation for the peroneus longus and the tibialis anterior.	Sánchez et al. 2014
Case Report n=1	6-year-old boy with perinatal cerebral palsy	On intravenous injection of 25 mL of PRP	Clear improvement in cognitive and language spheres.	Alcazar et al. 2015

TABLE 2 Summary of clinical studies of Platelet-Rich Plasma and nerve (reprinted with permission[6])

4. THE SCIENTIFIC RATIONALE BEHIND THE USE OF PRPS TO ASSIST PNI REPAIR

Six lines of evidence suggest the therapeutic potential of PRPs on neural tissue repair and regeneration (table I and II)[6]. These include the prevention of cell apoptosis and neuroprotection, the stimulation of angiogenesis, the modulation of inflammatory microenvironment, the enhancement of axonal outgrowth and nerve guidance, the dampening of both denervated muscle atrophy and scarring that follow peripheral nerve trauma and damage, and the improvement of neurologic parameters in humans (fig. 3)[29].

Neuroprotection and prevention of cell apoptosis

Several GFs present in PRP including, NGF, BDNF, PDGF, VEGF, IGF-1, TGFB alone or in combination have been shown to exert an antiapoptotic and neuroprotective effect on mesenchymal stem cells (MSCs), neurons, SCs, and human neural stem cells[45,47-51]. PRP fibrin scaffolds enriched with NGF, BDGF, and retinoic acid and loaded with bone marrow stromal cells (BMSCs), enhance their survival and differentiation into the neural phenotype[52]. In addition, when this PRP scaffold was transplanted into the brain the viability and biologic activity of allogenic BMSC increased[53]. Moreover, neuroprotective and antifibrotic beneficial effects[22,54] were reported with the injection of PRP into the corpus cavernosum in a bilateral cavernous nerve injury rat model and applying PRP in a facial nerve suture in a guinea pig model. A recent in vitro study on neuronal cultures of mouse model of Alzheimer disease[8], showed that the neurotoxicity induced by aggregated β-amyloid added in primary neuronal cultures was significantly reduced, and the living cell number after the co-treatment with PRP increased. In addition, in the chronic intranasal administration of PRP on Alzheimer´s disease mouse model, this treatment elicits neuroprotection which is likely mediated by the activation of the antiapoptotic PIEK/Akt signalling pathway[55].

Stimulation of angiogenesis

Despite the crucial role that blood vessels play as trackers of the axonal growth cones across the injury site, and the meaningful evidence that PRP promotes angiogenesis in bone, tendon, and muscle[11,56-58] there is still a scarcity of studies assessing angiogenesis in nerve repair. Borselli et al 48 showed in an ischemic limb rodent model with a loss of neuromuscular junction (NMJ) innervation that an injectable scaffold loaded with VEGF and IGF-1 accelerated regeneration of damaged NMJs together with an enhancement of angiogenesis. In a rat model it has been reported that sciatic nerve gaps of 10 mm repaired with vein graft filled with PRP exhibited a more prominent early neoangiogenesis than sciatic nerve gaps treated with nerve autograft alone[17]. In this regard, it should be taken into account that fibrin is a pivotal element within PRP that provides extracellular matrix tissue with a robust and permissive 3-D matrix for angiogenesis[59].

Enhancing axonal outgrowth capacity

The crucial role played by GF within the PRP has been highlighted in a rat brain-spinal cord cocultured system, where the addition of PRP supernatant promoted an increase in the size and number of axons, a positive effect that was significantly suppressed when antibodies against IGF-1 and VEGF were added[23]. As a cellular carrier, two studies in acute nerve injury model in guinea pig and rabbits applied PRP and seeded the acellular carrier with either MSCs or SCs, reporting beneficial effects on axonal counts, myelination and electrophysiological parameters[21,54]. One example of the use of PRP as a filler of acellular nerve allografts (ANA PRP) is the work of Zheng et al[7] which, having previously shown a dose-dependent effect of PRP on the proliferation, migration and, neurotrophic function in rat SCs cutured with PRP, subsequently showed significant improvements in diameter, thickness, and numbers of myelinating axons as well as an enhancement of electrophysiological parameters in sciatic nerve injury repaired with autografts and ANA PRP in a rat model[44]. Using a simple inside-out vein autograft or an inside-out vein autograft filled with PRP to bridge the sciatic nerve gap in a rat model, Kim et al.[17] observed that the number of myelinated axons, the axon diameter and myelin sheath were significantly superior when PRP was used as a filler. These results are in accord with the work of Kaplan et al., who used platelet gels as filler of collagen nerve conduit with improvement in functional and structural outcomes in an injury model of rat sciatic nerve[60]. Using platelet-rich fibrin (PRF) as a filler of silicon nerve guidance[61] or nerve grafts[62] in a rat model, animals treated with PRP improved functional recovery and showed a superior sciatic functional index compared with non-treated animals. However, the researchers did not find morphometric or structural improvements[61,62]. The application of PRP as a suturable membrane to wrap the neurorraphy in an acute injury model of sciatic nerve neurotmesis showed diverse positive effects. Gianessi et al. observed a stronger EMG signal, a significantly larger axonal density, and a lower scar tissue in animals treated with PRP suturable membranes, and remains of PRP membranes were still present after 6 weeks post-surgery[15]. In this sense, two studies reported the positive effects of using PRP as adjuvant in nerve suture. Farrag et al[18] reported that PRP may enhance the myelin thickness and increase the axon counts when injured nerve is sutured and assisted with PRP, whereas Sariguney et al[24] found no positive effects on axonal size in sutured nerves assisted with PRP. However, they showed a better functional outcome associated with improvement in the myelin thickness and the onset latency. In applying PRP as both filler of the injured nerve and as a scaffold to coat the nerve crush on sheep, Sanchez et al.[12] reported an earlier electrophysiological response, a higher axonal density, and lower muscle atrophy in treated animals compared with the saline or spontaneous regeneration groups.

Overcoming the inflammatory microenvironment

Though indirect, two important pieces of evidence in neural tissue support the antiinflammatory effect of PRP. Anitua et al reported that astrocytes cultured with β-amyloid expressed proinflammatory cytokines, but this effect was completely blocked when the culture was supplemented with PRP, an effect mediated by the suppression of the nuclear transcription factor-κB (NF-κB) on astrocytes[55]. In a mouse model of Parkinson´s disease, Anitua et al[10] showed that the neuroinflammatory process, mediated by microglia, was reduced, together with an improvement in motor performance, responses that were associated with a robust reduction in NF-kB activation, nitric oxide, cyclooxygenase, and tumor necrosis factor expression in the brain[10]. In a rabbit model of dextrose-induced median nerve injury, the injection of PRP into the carpal tunnel of rabbits injured 4 weeks before, exerted a significant reduction in nerve swelling compared with the control group[63].

Dampening the denervated target muscle atrophy

Several animal studies have demonstrated that the application of PRP as a filler, a suturable membrane, or both, induce an earlier axonal regeneration and functional recovery[12,15,17,18,22,24,47]. This is the case reported by Sanchez et al[12] on sheep, where nerves repaired with PRP were associated with an earlier electrophysiological recovery and lower muscle atrophy, suggesting that PRP application may dampen the target muscle atrophy. In addition, another recovery burden in nerve repair is scarring, which has been reported to be minimized by the repair of sciatic injured nerve assisted with PRP[15]. Anitua et al[11] showed that intramuscular injection of PRP 24 hours after the induction of limb ischemia in mice, mitigates fibrosis and muscle atrophy. These results are in agreement with the reduction of atrophy in denervated muscle reported when muscle was infiltrated with cells[64], effects suggested to be mediated by the IGF-1[65]. Moreover, TGFB, an important GF within PRP, attenuates the adverse effects of chronically denervated Schwann cells, and reactivated SCs support axon regeneration in vivo[66].

The improvement of neurologic parameters in humans

In the wake of promising results in animal experimentation, PRP has been applied either as filler of nerve conduits across post traumatic nerve gaps[5,67], as a liquid dynamic scaffold infiltrated perineurally[13,16,68], intraneurally, or both (as in the case of a peroneal nerve palsy[20] (and other damaged nerves). Furthermore, it has also been applied as scaffold or fibrin membranes[5,67,69] with beneficial outcomes and better functional recovery. Kuffler applied autologous platelet rich fibrin as a filler of a collagen tube, proceeding to bridge the 12 cm nerve gap 3.25 years after an ulnar nerve trauma, and to recovery of both muscle and sensory function[67]. In a recent series of cases of surgical nerve repair, Kuffler[5] reported functional recovery in patients under 58 years whose nerve gaps of 2-16 cm were treated with collagen tube filled with PRP, after 0.5-3 years of trauma.

In a double-blind, randomized, clinical trial, the application of perineural PRP injections in tibial and ulnar nerves has shown sensory improvement in leprosy peripheral neuropathy[13]. In a retrospective analysis of 10 patients with persistent pudendal neuralgia, who underwent a second trans-gluteal decompression of the pudendal nerve, they injected activated PRP around the coated nerve, reporting a significant reduction in pain[68]. In a case series of fourteen patients with carpal tunnel syndrome, a single ultrasound-guided injection of PRP around the median nerve led to the disappearance of pain in eight patients, and pain alleviation in three patients at three months of follow-up[16]. Another case report, in this case applying sequential proximal and distal ultrasound-guided PRP injections intraneurally and perineurally (fig. 3) in a common peroneal nerve palsy, Sanchez et al reported a significant functional recovery assessed by electromyographic signs of reinnervation for both peroneus longus and tibialis anterior muscles as well as almost full recovery of sensitivity[12]. It has been reported that the intravenous injection of 25cc of concentrated platelet-rich plasma in a 6-year-old-boy with perinatal cerebral palsy is safe, and significantly improved the cognitive and language spheres[70].

5. CONCLUDING REMARKS AND FUTURE DIRECTIONS

The ultimate goal of any peripheral nerve repair strategy is the restoration of nerve-target organ function, while minimizing therapeutic side effects. PRPs are versatile and safe biological products to be harnessed by surgeons and clinicians as an adjuvant therapeutic tool to enhance the robust intrinsic nerve repair processes and overcome post-traumatic and neuropathic inhibitory microenvironment by the combinatorial strategy of delivering neurotrophic and neurotropic factors. They may assist nerve conduit guidances and grafts as a filler, as a liquid in intraneural and perineural ultrasound-guided injections in nerve entrapments and fibrosis, and as a scaffold to bridge or wrap the injured nerve gap.

There are several areas in which the application of PRPs might be modified to improve the functional outcomes in assisting neuropathies and nerve repair techniques. So far, in the majority of studies on animals (Table I) and humans (Table II), PRP has been applied around the nerve, namely, perineurally[13,16,68,69]. We have applied PRP perineurally and intraneurally both in animal and humans (table I and II). We have implemented this combination after having already ascertained, in a sheep model, that intraneural injections of PRP previously stained with methylene blue diffused homogenously across the nerve with no adverse effects[6]. Second, when we treat nerve palsy or neuropathies such as the common peroneal nerve or carpal tunnel syndrome, the only way to accurately place PRP at the site of injury is by ultrasound-guided injections that confirm accuracy by direct visualization of US imaging. Third, we recommend performing a combination of intraneural and perineural injections, several times depending on the clinical evolution of the patient in case of nerve palsy or carpal tunnel syndrome. In the case of assisting surgical repair by PRP as in the case of end-to-end neurorrhaphy, nerve compression, or nerve entrapment, we recommend combining intraneural and perineural infiltrations of liquid PRP with the application of a PRP membrane as scaffold, which wraps the injured area as indicated in figure 3. These modifications affecting the way PRP is currently used might in our opinion produce significant functional benefits.

1. Griffin JW, Hogan MV, Chhabra AB, Deal DN. Peripheral nerve repair and reconstruction. The Journal of bone and joint surgery. American volume. 2013;95:2144-51.

2. Fowler JR, Lavasani M, Huard J, Goitz RJ. Biologic strategies to improve nerve regeneration after peripheral nerve repair. Journal of reconstructive microsurgery. 2015;31:243-8.

3. Faroni A, Mobasseri SA, Kingham PJ, Reid AJ. Peripheral nerve regeneration: experimental strategies and future perspectives. Advanced drug delivery reviews. 2015;82-83:160-7.

4. Belkas JS, Shoichet MS, Midha R. Peripheral nerve regeneration through guidance tubes. Neurol Res. 2004;26:151-60.

5. Kuffler DP. An assessment of current techniques for inducing axon regeneration and neurological recovery following peripheral nerve trauma. Progress in neurobiology. 2014;116:1-12.

6. Sánchez M, Anitua E, Delgado D, et al. Platelet-rich plasma, a source of autologous growth factors and biomimetic scaffold for peripheral nerve regeneration. Expert opinion on biological therapy. 2016:1-16.

7. Zheng C, Zhu Q, Liu X, et al. Effect of platelet-rich plasma (PRP) concentration on proliferation, neurotrophic function and migration of Schwann cells in vitro. Journal of tissue engineering and regenerative medicine. 2016;10:428-36.

8. Anitua E, Pascual C, Perez-Gonzalez R, et al. Intranasal delivery of plasma and platelet growth factors using PRGF-Endoret system enhances neurogenesis in a mouse model of Alzheimer's disease. PloS one. 2013;8:e73118.

9. Anitua E, Prado R, Azkargorta M, et al. High-throughput proteomic characterization of plasma rich in growth factors (PRGF-Endoret)-derived fibrin clot interactome. Journal of tissue engineering and regenerative medicine. 2015;9:E1-E12.

10. Anitua E, Pascual C, Perez-Gonzalez R, Orive G, Carro E. Intranasal PRGF-Endoret enhances neuronal survival and attenuates NF-kappaB-dependent inflammation process in a mouse model of Parkinson's disease. Journal of controlled release : official journal of the Controlled Release Society. 2015;203:170-80.

11. Anitua E, Pelacho B, Prado R, et al. Infiltration of plasma rich in growth factors enhances in vivo angiogenesis and improves reperfusion and tissue remodeling after severe hind limb ischemia. Journal of Controlled Release. 2015;202:31-39.

12. Sanchez M, Anitua E, Delgado D, et al. Ultrasound-guided plasma rich in growth factors injections and scaffolds hasten motor nerve functional recovery in an ovine model of nerve crush injury. Journal of tissue engineering and regenerative medicine. 2015:DOI: 10.1002/term.2079.

13. Anjayani S, Wirohadidjojo YW, Adam AM, Suwandi D, Seweng A, Amiruddin MD. Sensory improvement of leprosy peripheral neuropathy in patients treated with perineural injection of platelet-rich plasma. Int J Dermatol. 2014;53:109-13.

14. Kuffler DP. Platelet-Rich Plasma Promotes Axon Regeneration, Wound Healing, and Pain Reduction: Fact or Fiction. Molecular neurobiology. 2015;52:990-1014.

15. Giannessi E, Coli A, Stornelli MR, et al. An autologously generated platelet-rich plasma suturable membrane may enhance peripheral nerve regeneration after neurorraphy in an acute injury model of sciatic nerve neurotmesis. Journal of reconstructive microsurgery. 2014;30:617-26.

16. Malahias MA, Johnson EO, Babis GC, Nikolaou VS. Single injection of platelet-rich plasma as a novel

treatment of carpal tunnel syndrome. Neural Regen Res. 2015;10:1856-9.

17. Kim JY, Jeon WJ, Kim DH, Kim YH, Youn I, Park JW. An inside-out vein graft filled with platelet-rich plasma for repair of a short sciatic nerve defect in rats. Neural regeneration research. 2014;9:1351.

18. Farrag TY, Lehar M, Verhaegen P, Carson KA, Byrne PJ. Effect of platelet rich plasma and fibrin sealant on facial nerve regeneration in a rat model. The Laryngoscope. 2007;117:157-65.

19. Dodla M, Bellamkond R, Atala A. Peripheral nerve regeneration. Foundations of Regenerative Medicines: Clinical & Therapeutic Applications. 2008:1270-82.

20. Sanchez M, Yoshioka T, Ortega M, Delgado D, Anitua E. Ultrasound-guided platelet-rich plasma injections for the treatment of common peroneal nerve palsy associated with multiple ligament injuries of the knee. Knee surgery, sports traumatology, arthroscopy : official journal of the ESSKA. 2014;22:1084-9.

21. Ye F, Li H, Qiao G, et al. Platelet-rich plasma gel in combination with Schwann cells for repair of sciatic nerve injury. Neural Regen Res. 2012;7:2286-92.

22. Wu CC, Wu YN, Ho HO, Chen KC, Sheu MT, Chiang HS. The neuroprotective effect of platelet-rich plasma on erectile function in bilateral cavernous nerve injury rat model. The journal of sexual medicine. 2012;9:2838-48.

23. Takeuchi M, Kamei N, Shinomiya R, et al. Human platelet-rich plasma promotes axon growth in brain-spinal cord coculture. Neuroreport. 2012;23:712-6.

24. Sariguney Y, Yavuzer R, Elmas C, Yenicesu I, Bolay H, Atabay K. Effect of platelet-rich plasma on peripheral nerve regeneration. Journal of reconstructive microsurgery. 2008;24:159-67.

25. Hall S. The response to injury in the peripheral nervous system. The Journal of bone and joint surgery. British volume. 2005;87:1309-19.

26. Allodi I, Udina E, Navarro X. Specificity of peripheral nerve regeneration: interactions at the axon level. Progress in neurobiology. 2012;98:16-37.

27. Jessen KR, Mirsky R, Lloyd AC. Schwann Cells: Development and Role in Nerve Repair. Cold Spring Harbor perspectives in biology. 2015;7:a020487.

28. Arthur-Farraj PJ, Latouche M, Wilton DK, et al. c-Jun reprograms Schwann cells of injured nerves to generate a repair cell essential for regeneration. Neuron. 2012;75:633-47.

29. Sanchez M, Garate A, Delgado D, Padilla S. Platelet-rich plasma, an adjuvant biological therapy to assist peripheral nerve repair. Neural Regen Res. 2017;12:47-52.

30. Gaudet AD, Popovich PG, Ramer MS. Wallerian degeneration: gaining perspective on inflammatory events after peripheral nerve injury. J Neuroinflammation. 2011;8:110.

31. Martini R, Fischer S, Lopez-Vales R, David S. Interactions between Schwann cells and macrophages in injury and inherited demyelinating disease. Glia. 2008;56:1566-77.

32. Zochodne DW. The challenges and beauty of peripheral nerve regrowth. J Peripher Nerv Syst. 2012;17:1-18.

33. Parrinello S, Napoli I, Ribeiro S, et al. EphB signaling directs peripheral nerve regeneration through Sox2-dependent Schwann cell sorting. Cell. 2010;143:145-55.

34. Cattin AL, Burden JJ, Van Emmenis L, et al. Macrophage-Induced Blood Vessels Guide Schwann Cell-Mediated Regeneration of Peripheral Nerves. Cell. 2015;162:1127-39.

35. Chen P, Piao X, Bonaldo P. Role of macrophages in Wallerian degeneration and axonal regeneration after peripheral nerve injury. Acta Neuropathol. 2015;130:605-18.

36. Mokarram N, Merchant A, Mukhatyar V, Patel G, Bellamkonda RV. Effect of modulating macrophage phenotype on peripheral nerve repair. Biomaterials. 2012;33:8793-801.

37. Chen YY, McDonald D, Cheng C, Magnowski B, Durand J, Zochodne DW. Axon and Schwann cell partnership during nerve regrowth. Journal of neuropathology and experimental neurology. 2005;64:613-22.

38. Scheib J, Hoke A. Advances in peripheral nerve regeneration. Nat Rev Neurol. 2013;9:668-76.

39. Painter MW, Brosius Lutz A, Cheng YC, et al. Diminished Schwann cell repair responses underlie age-associated impaired axonal regeneration. Neuron. 2014;83:331-43.

40. Sanchez M, Anitua E, Orive G, Mujika I, Andia I. Platelet-rich therapies in the treatment of orthopaedic sport injuries. Sports Med. 2009;39:345-54.

41. Anitua E, Alkhraisat MH, Orive G. Perspectives and challenges in regenerative medicine using plasma rich in growth factors. Journal of controlled release : official journal of the Controlled Release Society. 2012;157:29-38.

42. Padilla S, Sanchez M, Orive G, Anitua E. Human-Based Biological and Biomimetic Autologous Therapies for Musculoskeletal Tissue Regeneration. Trends in biotechnology. 2016.

43. Aird WC. Endothelial biomedicine. Cambridge university press; 2007. N.W.Shworak. Heparan sulfate.

44. Zheng C, Zhu Q, Liu X, et al. Improved peripheral nerve regeneration using acellular nerve allografts loaded with platelet-rich plasma. Tissue engineering. Part A. 2014;20:3228-40.

45. Sondell M, Lundborg G, Kanje M. Vascular endothelial growth factor has neurotrophic activity and stimulates axonal outgrowth, enhancing cell survival and Schwann cell proliferation in the peripheral nervous system. The Journal of neuroscience : the official journal of the Society for Neuroscience. 1999;19:5731-40.

46. Jiang H, Qu W, Li Y, Zhong W, Zhang W. Platelet-derived growth factors-BB and fibroblast growth factors-base induced proliferation of Schwann cells in a 3D environment. Neurochem Res. 2013;38:346-55.

47. Emel E, Ergun SS, Kotan D, et al. Effects of insulin-like growth factor-I and platelet-rich plasma on sciatic nerve crush injury in a rat model. Journal of neurosurgery. 2011;114:522-8.

48. Borselli C, Storrie H, Benesch-Lee F, et al. Functional muscle regeneration with combined delivery of angiogenesis and myogenesis factors. Proceedings of the National Academy of Sciences of the United States of America. 2010;107:3287-92.

49. Luo H, Zhang Y, Zhang Z, Jin Y. The protection of MSCs from apoptosis in nerve regeneration by TGFβ1 through reducing inflammation and promoting VEGF-dependent angiogenesis. Biomaterials. 2012;33:4277-87.

50. Lee AC, Yu VM, Lowe JB, 3rd, et al. Controlled release of nerve growth factor enhances sciatic nerve regeneration. Experimental neurology. 2003;184:295-303.

51. Rao SN, Pearse DD. Regulating Axonal Responses to Injury: The Intersection between Signaling Pathways Involved in Axon Myelination and The Inhibition of Axon Regeneration. Front Mol Neurosci. 2016;9:33.

52. Zurita M, Otero L, Aguayo C, et al. Cell therapy for spinal cord repair: optimization of biologic scaffolds for survival and neural differentiation of human bone marrow stromal cells. Cytotherapy. 2010;12:522-37.

53. Vaquero J, Otero L, Bonilla C, et al. Cell therapy with bone marrow stromal cells after intracerebral hemorrhage: impact of platelet-rich plasma scaffolds. Cytotherapy. 2013;15:33-43.

54. Cho HH, Jang S, Lee SC, et al. Effect of neural-induced mesenchymal stem cells and platelet-rich plasma on facial nerve regeneration in an acute nerve injury model. The Laryngoscope. 2010;120:907-13.

55. Anitua E, Pascual C, Antequera D, et al. Plasma rich in growth factors (PRGF-Endoret) reduces neuropathologic hallmarks and improves cognitive functions in an Alzheimer's disease mouse model. Neurobiol Aging. 2014;35:1582-95.

56. Yokota K, Ishida O, Sunagawa T, Suzuki O, Nakamae A, Ochi M. Platelet-rich plasma accelerated surgical angio-genesis in vascular-implanted necrotic bone: an experimental study in rabbits. Acta orthopaedica. 2008;79:106-10.

57. Bosch G, Moleman M, Barneveld A, van Weeren PR, van Schie HT. The effect of platelet-rich plasma on the neovascularization of surgically created equine superficial digital flexor tendon lesions. Scandinavian journal of medicine & science in sports. 2011;21:554-61.

58. Sanchez M, Anitua E, Azofra J, Prado R, Muruzabal F, Andia I. Ligamentization of tendon grafts treated with an endogenous preparation rich in growth factors: gross morphology and histology. Arthroscopy : the journal of arthroscopic & related surgery : official publication of the Arthroscopy Association of North America and the International Arthroscopy Association. 2010;26:470-80.

59. Hall H. Modified fibrin hydrogel matrices: both, 3D-scaffolds and local and controlled release systems to stimulate angiogenesis. Current pharmaceutical design. 2007;13:3597-607.

60. Kaplan S, Piskin A, Ayyildiz M, et al. The effect of melatonin and platelet gel on sciatic nerve repair: an electrophysiological and stereological study. Microsurgery. 2011;31:306-13.

61. Lichtenfels M, Colome L, Sebben AD, Braga-Silva J. Effect of Platelet Rich Plasma and Platelet Rich Fibrin on sciatic nerve regeneration in a rat model. Microsurgery. 2013;33:383-90.

62. Sabongi RG, De Rizzo LALM, Fernandes M, et al. Nerve regeneration: is there an alternative to nervous graft? Journal of reconstructive microsurgery. 2014;30:607-16.

63. Park GY, Kwon DR. Platelet-rich plasma limits the nerve injury caused by 10% dextrose in the rabbit median nerve. Muscle & nerve. 2014;49:56-60.

64. Schaakxs D, Kalbermatten DF, Raffoul W, Wiberg M, Kingham PJ. Regenerative cell injection in denervated muscle reduces atrophy and enhances recovery following nerve repair. Muscle & nerve. 2013;47:691-701.

65. Shavlakadze T, White JD, Davies M, Hoh JF, Grounds MD. Insulin-like growth factor I slows the rate of denervation induced skeletal muscle atrophy. Neuromuscul Disord. 2005;15:139-46.

66. Sulaiman OA, Gordon T. Transforming growth factor-beta and forskolin attenuate the adverse effects of long-term Schwann cell denervation on peripheral nerve regeneration in vivo. Glia. 2002;37:206-18.

67. Kuffler DP, Reyes O, Sosa IJ, Santiago-Figueroa J. Neurological recovery across a 12-cm-long ulnar nerve gap repaired 3.25 years post trauma: case report. Neurosurgery. 2011;69:E1321-6.

68. Hibner M, Castellanos ME, Drachman D, Balducci J. Repeat operation for treatment of persistent pudendal nerve entrapment after pudendal neurolysis. J Minim Invasive Gynecol. 2012;19:325-30.

69. Scala M, Mereu P, Spagnolo F, et al. The use of platelet-rich plasma gel in patients with mixed tumour undergoing superficial parotidectomy: a randomized study. In Vivo. 2014;28:121-4.

70. Alcaraz J, Oliver A, Sanchez JM. Platelet-Rich Plasma in a Patient with Cerebral Palsy. Am J Case Rep. 2015;16:469-72.

CHAPTER 14

PRGF Molecular Intervention: a Bridge from Spontaneity to Muscle Repair

AUTHORS

Sánchez M.[1,2], Anitua E.[3,4,5], Aizpurua B.[1], Delgado D.[2], Sánchez P.[2], Guadilla J.[1], Padilla S.[3,4,5]

[1] Arthroscopic Surgery Unit (UCA). Vitoria-Gasteiz, Spain. Hospital Vithas San Jose, Vitoria-Gasteiz, Spain
[2] Advanced Biological Therapy Unit, Hospital Vithas San Jose, Vitoria-Gasteiz, Spain
[3] Biotechnology Institute (BTI). Vitoria-Gasteiz, Spain
[4] Foundation Eduardo Anitua. Vitoria-Gasteiz, Spain
[5] University Institute for Regenerative Medicine and Oral Implantology (UIRMI) from the University of Basque Country (UPV/EHU)

SUMMARY

Muscle injuries are some of the most common sport injuries, accounting for between 10% and 55% of all such lesions. Although the skeletal muscle is a plastic organ capable of efficiently responding to environmental changes, the appropriate treatment of muscle injuries remains a daunting clinical challenge in sports medicine. There is a great deal of evidence in basic science pointing towards growth factors such as TGFB, HGF or IGF and fibrin matrix as the key players in cellular events required for muscle repair and regeneration process, namely, myogenesis, angiogenesis, and fibrogenesis. An innovative biological approach to the treatment of muscle injuries is the application of Plasma Rich in Growth Factors (PRGF) in intramuscular infiltrations. PRGF delivers growth factors, cytokines and adhesive proteins present in platelets and plasma, as well as other biologically active proteins conveyed by the plasma such as fibrinogen, prothrombin, and fibronectin among others. But the application of this autologous mimetic biomaterial embedded with a pool of growth factors, acting as a smart dynamic scaffold, must be carried out [taking into account a] using a particular biological approach.

E. Anitua et al. (eds.), *Platelet Rich Plasma in Orthopaedics and Sports Medicine*,
https://doi.org/10.1007/978-3-319-63730-3_14

1. INTRODUCTION

Muscle injury is one of the most common traumas in sports irrespective of the level of sport practiced, accounting for 10% to 55% of all such injuries[1] and encompasses contusions, strains, and lacerations. The most common mechanism of skeletal muscle strain in elite sportsmen is the concentric/eccentric muscle movements associated with high levels of explosive force in response to sharp changes in direction and speed. This is the case in sprinting and jumping, where the excessive tensile force generated in response to sharp changes in direction and speed[2] leads to muscle injury causing tears in the blood vessels of the muscle tissue. The severity of these types of injuries is measured by the athlete´s functional inability to train and compete, in addition to the increased risk of recurrent injury. In many cases this functional loss or compromise may last 30–40 days.

In spite of the fact that skeletal muscle may be seen as the paradigm of tissue plasticity which conserves and shares modules of regulatory pathways and transcription factors of embryonic myogenesis and development, to be redeployed for tissue repair after muscle injury[3,4], the appropriate treatment of muscle injuries remains a daunting clinical challenge in sports medicine[1,5,6].

There is a great deal of evidence in basic science pointing towards growth factors such as TGFB, HGF or IGF and fibrin matrix as the key players in cellular events required for muscle repair and regeneration process, namely, myogenesis, angiogenesis, and fibrogenesis[7]. Drawing on the regenerative potential of platelets, thrombin, plasma biomolecules and fibrin matrix[8-10], several systems of producing autologous Platelet Rich Plasma (PRP) derivates have been developed and aimed at triggering and enhancing the natural in vivo tissue morphogenesis and regenerative capacity[11] by targeting "the stem cell zone" microenvironment of damaged and healthy tissue-areas[12].

This novel biological approach could be an important option to treat muscle tears in light of the knowledge and insight gained in both basic science about the role of growth factors and fibrin matrix in muscle tissue repair process[13-18] and in the promising results yielded by this approach in musculoskeletal system pathologies[11,19,20].

2. TISSUE-BASED PHENOMENA IN SKELETAL MUSCLE INJURY AND REPAIR

Although it is tempting to refer almost exclusively to myogenesis as the pivotal parenchymal cell process in muscle repair and regenerations, there is a great deal of evidence showing that muscle repair and functional recovery[21,22] also rely on other stromal cell events such as inflammation involving monocytes and macrophages[23-27], angiogenesis[28], fibrogenesis[2,29], reinnervation[30-32] and physical stress[1,33,34] (figs. 1-2).

Immediately following muscle tear, the massive entry of calcium into the damaged myofiber and subsequent activation of complement and proteases such as calpains, will lead to myofiber necrosis and destructuring of the constituents of ECM[17,32,35,36]. Moreover, the disruption of vessels and acute injury will both generate a haematoma and activate satellite cells (SCs), platelets, endothelial cells (ECs), fibro/adipogenic progenitor (FAPs) and muscle connective tissue (MCT) fibroblasts[37-39]. The haematoma that fills the gap created between the already necrotic and retracted myofiber stumps[2,17,35] will turn into a fibrin clot and will temporarily serve as provisional extracellular matrix (ECM) that will house the development of stromal and parenchymal cell events such as angiogenesis, myogenesis, fibrogenesis and innervation of the new-formed tissue[2,29,40]. Platelets and endothelial cells release cytokines and growth factors that, together with the injured tissue damage-associated molecular patterns (DAMPs)[25,41,42], recruit, attract, and activate neutrophils, resident

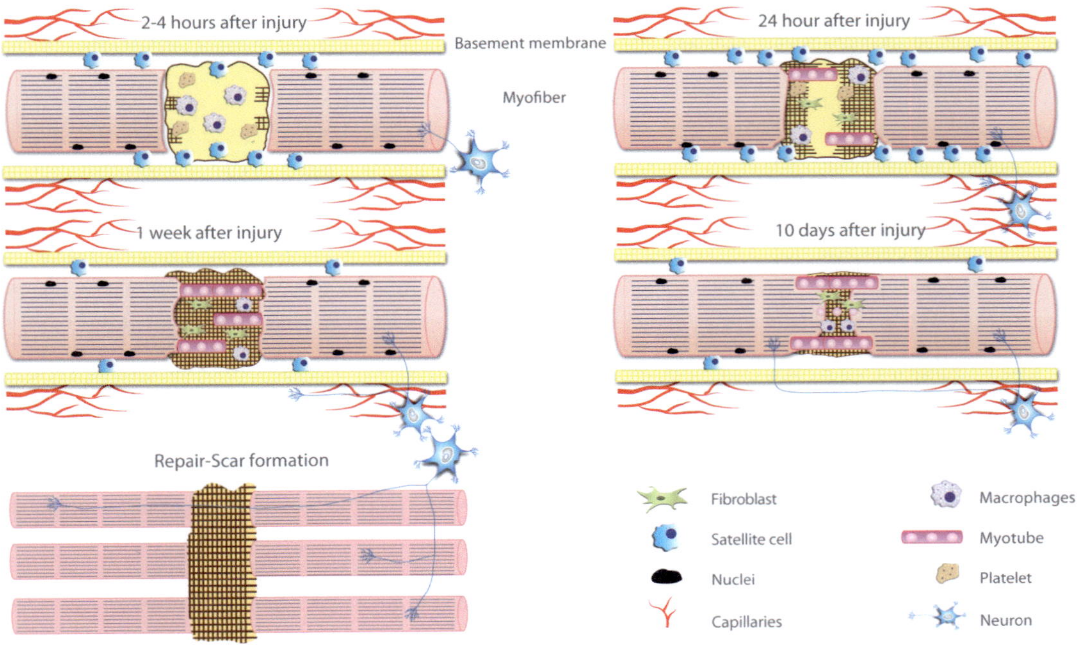

FIG. 1
The most important cell-based phenomena during the repair of muscle injuries. (Reprinted with permission from Sanchez et al[7]).

macrophages, and circulating monocytes to the injured area. Whereas neutrophils appear to play a minor role in the repair process besides exacerbating myofiber damage[24,43,44], monocyte-derived cells are the main players of the innate immune system in muscle repair process, and adopt, in this sterile though necrotic microenvironment, a proinflammatory phenotype M1 (macrophage type 1)[39]. These M1 phagocytose tissue debris, clean the necrotic zone and release growth factors, cytokines and cell adhesion molecules that, together with those coming from the degranulation of activated platelets and through influencing the cell fates and behavior of SCs, monocytes, ECs, pericytes and fibrobasts, will support muscle tissue homeostasis and repair[25,26,38,39,41].

Once they have undergone necrosis myofibers have a poor potential to regenerate themselves given that they are postmitotic cells[40]. However, new muscle tissue can be formed partially from the activation of SCs[32,45,46]. These precursor muscle stem cells[16,17,47] lie sandwiched between sarcolemma and the basal lamina (BL), which is a highly specialized interstitial connective tissue within the ECM. In spite of an impaired basal lamina and the toxic milieu brought about primarily by infiltrated neutrophil, inflammatory macrophages[48], and ECM fragments , satellite cells along with other survivor cells, are activated and migrate to the site of injury within 2h after injury, though some of them undergo self-renewal for replenishing the SC pool[45,49]. Once at the site of injury, SCs proliferate and differentiate into fusion-competent myoblasts which will differentiate and fuse with one another to form myotubes and new myofibers by about 7 days in injured mouse muscle[40,49], or with existing damaged myofiber to repair them[21,32].

Angiogenesis is carried out by the activation of quiescent ECs that in mammalian skeletal muscle show a potential to rapidly proliferate after being activated by angiogenic stimuli coming from the injured area such as DAMPs and growth factors, namely, VEGF and PDGF[28]. The sprouting of small blood vessels takes place in this fibrous callus that now joins the ends of the various broken fibers while the fibrin matrix continues to be infiltrated with macrophages. These new capillaries will later undergo a maturation and stabilization process which involve pericytes, to eventually end up generating a structured network of capillaries[21,50]. Moreover, neovascularization appears to be crucial in functional and structural muscle regeneration, furnishing the new tissue with oxygen and other nutrients as well as with blood-derived cells, at the same time as removing carbon dioxide and other tissue-waste products[2,21].

Fibrogenesis is another key component of toolkit-defense system that (see chapter 3) has evolved to rapidly fix and replace the necrotic areas and the initial formed fibrin clot with new ECM and connective tissue[2,38,39] in order to address the loss of connective tissue, to seal off the injured area, and repair or generate the BL[29,38]. When the aseptic yet hypoxic and necrotic microenvironment lingers over time, or when neovascularization is compromised, the M1 phenotype persists, which leads to a non-resolving fibrogenesis where a myofibroblast profile and fibrogenesis will take over myogenesis thereby generating an excessive and persistent deposition of ECM which results in a fibrotic scar tissue[26,29,36,40,51-53]. For myogenesis, angiogenesis and innervation to develop functionally, the integrity of the BL and the 3D structure provided by the fibrin adhesive protein matrix that support ECM and cell-cell adhesion is of paramount importance[17,54,55]. Repair of the BL is the first key step in reconstruction of the neural canal since BL not only ensures subsequent compartmentalization of the repair phenomena[54], it is also involved in mechanical support, myogenesis, and synaptogenesis. Moreover, the molecular composition of the muscle BL endows it with adhesive and inductive functions for a variety of cell fates during muscle repair[4,36,54].

Innervation is essential for growth and maturation of newly formed myofibres as well as for the re-expression of myosin heavy chains[4,40]. It is important that the newly formed granulation tissue which joins the damaged fibers together does not form a barrier to the axon´s progression from neighboring nerve endings[2,33] nor surround them with fibrotic tissue resulting from an excess collagen synthesis or defective metalloproteinase (MMPs) synthesis[33,51]. This progression of axons leads toward the old synaptic site where the original neuromuscular junction (NMJ) was located or to the basal lamina of new myotubes[17], thereby allowing the restoration of full muscular function, a process which might take months[2].

During the repair process, the existence of a mechanical stimulus causes integrins to laterally bind the edges of muscle cells to the extracellular matrix via laminins, thereby preventing them from retracting and thus contributing to the repair process[33]. Controlled physical stress helps to reorient type I collagen, thereby enhancing the penetration and alignment of myoblasts and stimulating remodeling[1,21,56].

All these biological defense system modules are tightly coordinated through the secretion of growth factors and cytokines primarily but not exclusively released by SCs, macrophages, platelets, ECs , and myofibroblasts[16,38,47,49,57] (fig. 2).

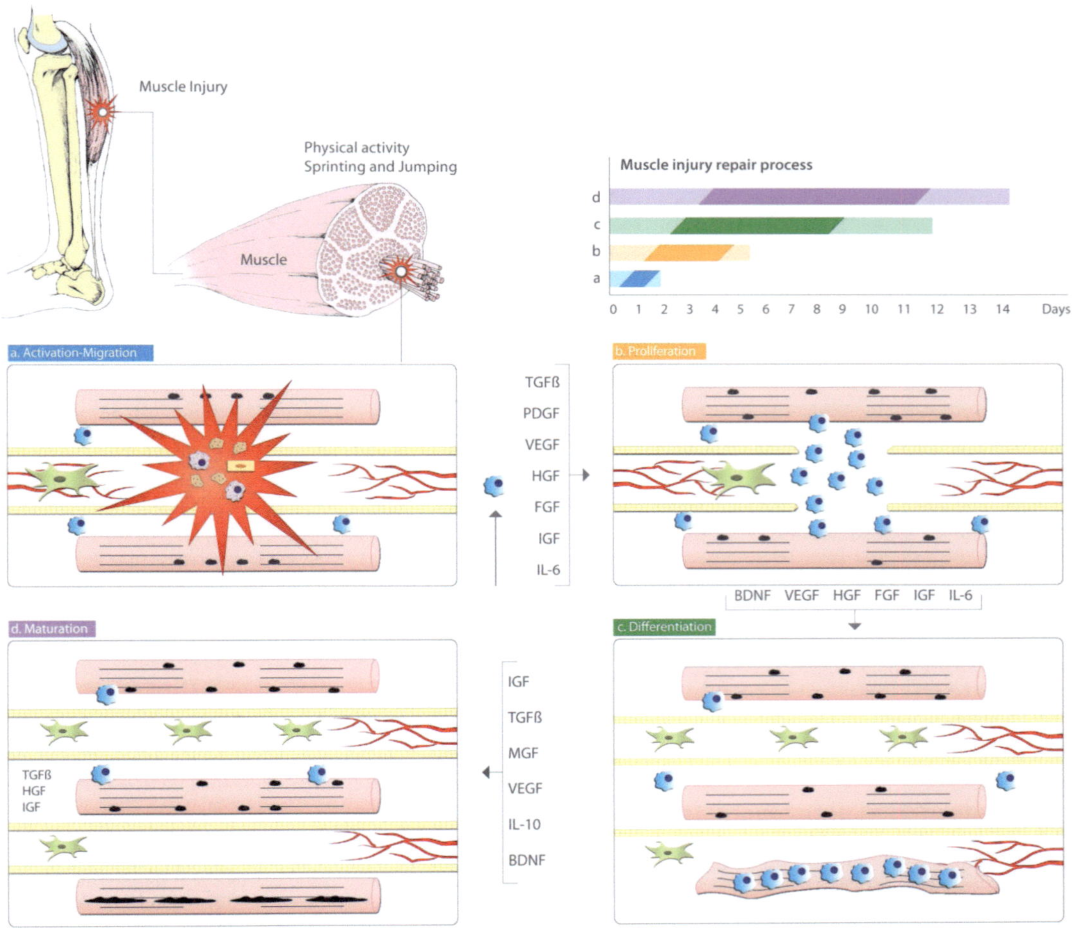

FIG. 2
The key role played by satellite cells (muscle stem cells) in muscle repair under the control of various growth factors. (Reprinted with permission from Sanchez et al[7]).

3. CELLULAR AND MOLECULAR MECHANISMS REGULATING MUSCLE REPAIR AND REGENERATION

Mammalian muscles are made up of tissues with quite different proliferative activity of their cell; cells that have left the cell cycle and do not undergo mitotic division in postnatal life such as neurons or myofibers and quiescent cells such as fibroblasts, SCs, and ECs with low or no level of proliferation. But SCs and ECs can, in response to environmental cues such as mechanical injury through DAMPs[16,17,38,47,50], undergo a boost in mitotic, migratory, and secretory activity. Following muscle injury, a short inflammatory stage ensues (in the first 24-48 hours after injury)[27,49], primarily stemming from the presence of DAMPs that are first recognized by transmembrane toll-like receptors (TLRs) of platelets, ECs, and resident macrophages, and then activated[58]. These activated cells located at the fibrin clot will secrete TNF, IL-6, MCP1 (monocyte chemoattractan protein

1) which along with VEGF[59], attract blood monocytes and more epimysium/perimysium resident macrophages to the damaged area[25,27,32,43]. Simultaneously, at the injured site, the presence of HGF coming from inflammatory macrophages (M1), and activated platelets and ECs, promote cell cycle reentry of quiescent SCs, and FGF, TGFB, IGF1, PDGF and VEGF will stimulate their proliferation and promote the migration of activated SCs and myoblasts to the repair area as well as protect stromal cells and myofibres from an apoptotic fate[13,18,22,40,49]. Moreover, stromal-derived factor 1 (SDF1) released by platelets and fibroblasts, is a mitogenic and motogenic factor for stem and progenitor cells as well as for circulant monocyte and resident macrophages which will migrate to the injury sites and modulate their phenotype in a context sensitive manner[10,22,24,25,60,61]. This SDF1 (known as CXCL12) also plays an important role in angiogenesis by recruiting endothelial progenitor cells (EPCs) from bone marrow through a CXCR4 dependent mechanism[62]. TGFB with pleiotrophic effects will promote SCs proliferation and FAP activation, proliferation and differentiation towards fibroblasts, at the same time inhibiting myoblast differentiation[29,40,63-65]. Moreover, skeletal muscle, like many other musculoskeletal tissues, contain multipotent mesenchymal progenitor cells, termed fibro/adipogenic progenitors (FAPs) and muscle connective tissue (MCT) fibroblasts[37,38,66], and they rapidly enter the cell cycle in response to acute muscle damage, and might be at the origin of fat accumulation and fibrosis in skeletal muscle[66]. The antiapoptotic effect on parenchymal and stromal cells is mainly driven by IGF-I and II, HGF, FGF, VEGF, and it appears to be crucial for myogenesis to be redeployed as in embryo development[4,49] although doing so in a hostile and necrotic tissue-injured microenvironment, and sometimes with impaired or with no basal lamina as an instructive scaffold that in embryonic myogenesis acts as template[27,32].

In the wake of phagocitic activity of M1 and the new microenvironment created within this callus by the secretory activity of M1, fibroblasts, myoblasts, and ECs, a pivotal event in the muscle repair will occur 48-72 hours after injury[25,53], namely, the resolution of inflammation, and macrophages, that exhibit a remarkable ability to reprogram their gene expression profile[25,61,67], will switch from a pro-inflammatory macrophage (M1) to a healing or trophic macrophage profile (M2)[24,25,53] releasing mainly TGF-β and IL-10[25,52]. The fibrin matrix generated as a transient ECM along with other biomolecules of the ECM may retain several growth factors such as FGF, HGF, TGFB, VEGF, BDNF previously released by platelets, macrophages, ECs and newly activated fibroblasts[21,36,68] through the cell surface heparan sulphate binding domains of heparin sulfate proteoglycans (HSPGs)[68,69] to be gradually freed up later 68 thereby controlling morphogen gradients at the repair scenario[70,71]. IGF-I released by myoblasts, endothelial cells and now trophic M2, will stimulate the proliferation and differentiation of myoblasts, promote cell survival[16,36,47,59] and modulate inflammation through the suppression of macropage MIF and transcription factor NF-kB, thereby reducing fibrosis and myonecrosis 14. In addition, the release of platelet factor 4 (PF4) released by platelets prevents monocyte apoptosis, promotes trophic M2[60] and may restore cells to a noninflammatory phenotype. Overall, these stromal and parenchymal events will favour a trophic microenvironment as well as dampen inflammation, and may well contribute to the resolution of inflammation, and thereby shorten the repair process[5].

Quiescent endothelial cells will enter the cell cycle in the presence of microenvironmental stimuli such as DAMPs and VEGF, the latter as a hierarchically superior master switch of the angiogenic cascade[50.] The anatomical proximity among endothelial cells (ECs), pericytes and satellite cells make this area work as a stem cell zone, mainly through the cross-talking through VEGF, HGF, IL-6, and Angiopoietin-1(Ang1)[29] which are, together with PDGF and FGF, pivotal in generating, organizing, and maintaining the microvasculature[21] as well as in the development of myogenesis[28,55]. Moreover, this close association of many quiescent cell types (SCs, ECs and Neural stem cells (NSCs)) with the vasculature allows the modulation of these cell-fate decisions via metabolic cues, circadian rhythms, temperature, mechanical stress as well as providing a feedback with humoral factors and cells from the immune system[12]. Another early event in the stromal cell response to muscle injury is the activation, migration and proliferation of fibroblasts that, in presence of TGFB and PDGF, take on a myofibroblast phenotype[29,38] and are, in cooperation with myofibers, responsible for tissue homeostasis, and synthesis and secretion of ECM components such as collagens, laminins, tenascin C, metalloproteinases (MMPs), tissue inhibitors of metalloproteinases (TIMPs), and TGFB[2,29,36,38] among others. These activated fibroblasts, under the stimulation of TGFB, are highly secretory and synthetic cells[2,29,33,41], and infiltrate the fibrin clot that now joins the ends of the various broken fibers. The mechanical and biochemical features of the newly secreted ECM along with the provisional fibrin matrix play a role as adhesive cell contacts, and serve as reservoir of growth factors such as VEGF, PDGF, TGFB that will be release gradually, thereby modulating macrophages, myofibroblasts, and survival and fate of myotubes[22,29,38,72,73]. After muscle injury, the absence or disruption of innervation is the major cause of poor restoration of tissue, leading to compromised function[32,33]. Reinnervation and the creation of a new neuromuscular junction (NMJ) in the repaired or regenerated fibers, via the basement membrane, may be driven by growth of new axons from adjacent nerves[47]. These events, often absent from in vitro studies, might well be mediated by nerve growth factor (NGF) and IGF-1, both present in the damaged tissue and synthesized by muscle cells and fibroblasts under paracrine influence[47] in addition to biomechanical signaling (Brain-derived neurotrophic factor BDNF, Glial growth factor GGF) and ECM stiffness which modulates the phenotype and fate of several types of cells such as SCs, activated resident fibroblasts (myofibroblasts), ECs, macrophages and Schwann cells[21,73,74].

Regulating the gene expression products (TGF-β1, IGF-1, IL-10, BDGF, VEGF, collagens, fibronectin, tenascin-C) of SCs, activated resident fibroblasts, ECs, macrophages and Schwann cells appears to be essential in the success of muscle repair[1,21,27,29] and mechanical and chemical signals such as mechanogrowth factor (MGF or CTGF) and insulin-like growth factor-1 expressed in autocrine and paracrine manner, and coming from the cell environment, might well complement each other[14,73]. It should also be noted that the presence of tenascin C in the extracellular matrix, the synthesis of which is induced by mechanical stress, is a prerequisite for muscle reinnervation[36,64]. In the clinical setting, early gradual mechanical loading stimulates gene expression of trophic factors and signals such as cyclooxygenase-1 (COX-1), FGFb, hypoxia-inducible factor (1HIF-1), and BDNF influencing maturation and the correct patterning of myotubes, collagens and tenascin-C[32,33]. Both the gradual and controlled mechanical stimulus that induces IGF synthesis by muscle cells (by endocrine and paracrine activity)[32,63] and the paracrine and autocrine synthesis of growth factors such as HGF and TGF-β by fibroblasts during the final remodeling phase, appear to be essential, since both these signals may have a synergistic effect on the activity of the fibroblasts that are remodeling the ECM[36,75] and repaired tissue. Moderate sustained mechanical load modulates the fusion and ensuing alignment of myoblasts into myofibres[21] and may minimize or even avoid the formation of scar tissue by inhibiting the NF-kB of muscle cells[76] among them fibroblasts which can promote fibrotic scar[77]. The aforementioned events, which play a crucial role in balancing tissue remodeling versus fibrotic scar in injured muscle[32,33] imply that what is true for an isolated myofiber is not necessarily true for the entire muscle[22].

4. AN INNOVATIVE BIOLOGICAL APPROACH TO THE TREATMENT OF MUSCLE INJURIES: PLASMA RICH IN GROWTH FACTORS

There is an increasing body of evidence in basic science pointing out that growth factors and fibrin matrix are instrumental in the muscle repair and regeneration process[13,18,20,21,36,40,57,78].

One innovative biological approach is the application of Platelet Rich Plasma (PRP) in intra-muscular infiltrations[5]. Autologous blood-derived products convey growth factors, cytokines, and morphogens contained in the platelets, as well as fibrinogen and other plasmatic proteins in a biologically balanced aggregate, managed and delivered in a pharmacological manner[11] which may account for two special features: the resolution of inflammation and avoidance of fibrosis. In addition to conveying GFs, PRGF provides the damaged tissue with a transient biological fibrin scaffold which stems from the polymerization of fibrinogen, a pleiotropic blood protein that regulates coagulation, inflammation, and tissue regeneration[10,79].

Our group has been designing rigorous and well-defined protocols for the application of different PRGF-based formulations in several acute and chronic-degenerative pathologies, yielding extremely promising clinical and surgical outcomes in oral and maxilofacial surgery[11], in musculoskeletal system pathologies[78,80] as well as in other medical fields[11]. A wealth of preclinical works suggest that PRP early intervention in muscle injury significantly improves several molecular and cellular events involved in muscle regeneration[15,51,81-83]. Although several clinical studies seem to shed light on the effect of PRP on muscle damage repair with promising functional outcomes[5,6,19,20,84-86], it is fair to say that so far the only clinical trials conducted so far have shown no improvement of muscle injuries treated with PRP 87. However, it is worth highlighting that the delayed administration, and the low dosage of GF conveyed by 3 ml of PRP injection in the Reurink clinical trial may well have rendered PRP treatment ineffective[88]. In an elegant study conducted by Dimauro et al[81] on animal model of muscle injury, the authors showed that the early PRP application, namely, immediately after the injury, exerted a multi-directional effect on myogenic regulators and growth factors involved in inflammation and myogenesis.

Two main challenges remain unresolved when it comes to muscle injury treatment: the slow down of the functional recovery and the relapses, both linked to fibrotic scar after the muscle tear. These concerns have prompted some researchers to conduct intense research to customize PRPs using antibodies to neutralize TGFB and myostatin in order to reduce fibrosis and optimize myogenesis[51,82,89]. However, and due both to the dynamic nature of fibroblast-satellite cell interaction and to the pleiotrophism of growth factors, therapeutic interventions aimed at minimizing fibrosis after muscle injury will need to be carefully controlled in order to avoid interfering with the early pro-regenerative crosstalk among FAPs, MCT fibroblasts, and satellite cells[37,38].

5. PRGF PROTOCOL USED IN MUSCLE INJURIES

An optimal treatment for muscle injury repair should convey a mimetic biomaterial embedded with a pool of growth factors acting as a smart scaffold[21] which might sustain a gradual delivery of growth factors as a niche therapy[12] at the dysfunctional and deregulated injured site instead of a bolus delivery modality[18,68,90]. This biomaterial must promote myogenesis, angiogenesis and innervation as well as modulate immune response and fibrogenesis in order to generate a functional muscle repair[18,21,38,39,51].

We propose the following general principles in the application of PRGF as a local molecular intervention to the muscle injury treatment[91].

5.1. The process to produce PRGF

The patients are advised not to eat fatty food in the 6 hours prior to the blood extraction. Thirty-six mL of peripheral venous blood is withdrawn into 9-mL tubes containing 3.8% (wt/vol) sodium citrate. Occasionally, due to the size of the lesion, it may be necessary to extract further amounts of blood. Once the blood is centrifuged (BTI technology, Vitoria, Spain), the upper volume of plasma F1 is collected in a tube. The 2-mL plasma fraction located just above the sedimented white and red blood cells (buffy coat), is collected in another tube but without aspirating the buffy coat. This plasma fraction F2 presents a moderate enrichment in platelets (2-3 fold the platelet count of peripheral blood) with scarce leukocytes.

5.2. Injured area preparation

While the nurse is obtaining the PRGF (centrifugation, separation of fractions F1 and F2), the patient is clinically examined to correctly assess and mark the area of maximum tenderness and /or swelling. After pinpointing the injured site, the area of skin to be infiltrated is prepared and demarcated with disposable cloths as a sterile field and antiseptic solution is applied (fig. 3a). By using an ultrasound longitudinal 8.0-13.0 MHz multi-frequency linear probe which is wrapped with a sterile cover (fig. 3a), the injury and, if applicable, the possible hematoma associated with the muscle tear (seromas, fibrosis and degenerated areas in case of chronic injuries), are located (fig. 3b). We choose the anatomical location of injection based on ultrasound and clinical criteria. The use of local anesthesia must be avoided.

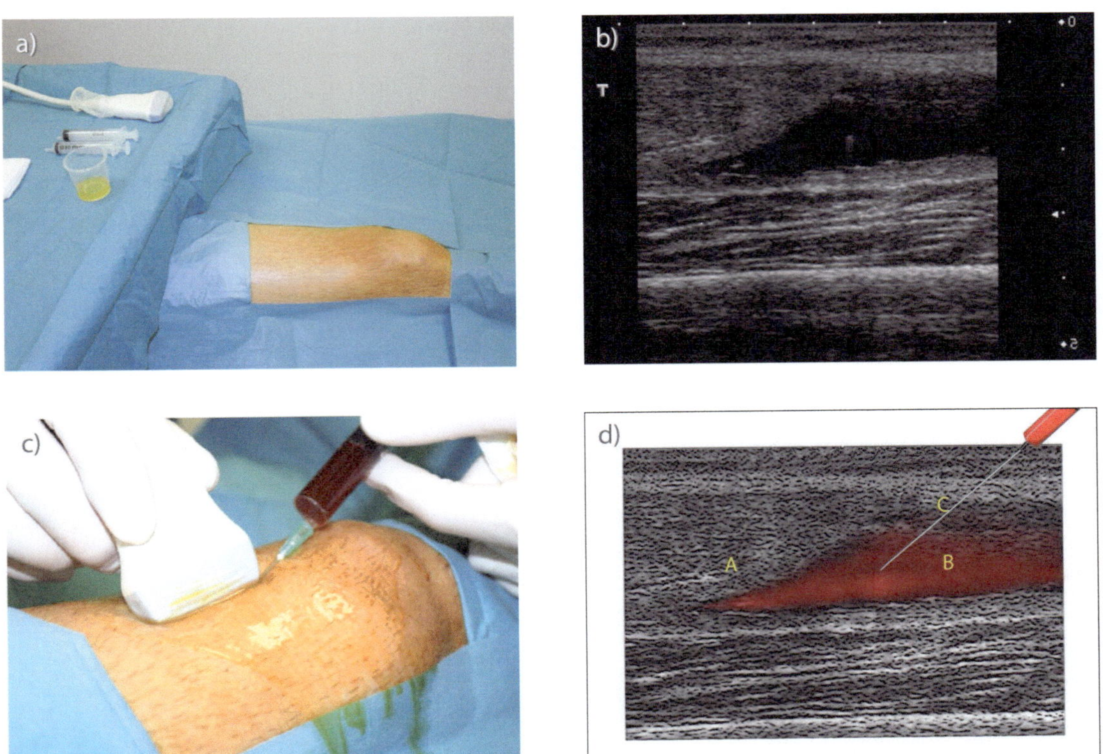

FIG. 3
Preparation of the sterile field (A) required to perform ultrasound control (B) with which we identify the damaged areas, and evacuation of hematoma if exists (C and D). (Reprinted with permission from Sanchez et al[7]).

5.3. Muscle injury site infiltration procedure

Hematoma, seroma, or cysts, if present, are punctured/evacuated using a 18-G needle (figs 3c and d) always under ultrasound guidance (figs 3c and d). Once the hematoma is evacuated, the F2 of PRGF is activated with calcium chloride (10% wt/vol). PRGF-Endoret activated liquid formulation is, in the ensuing 1-3 minutes, injected into the injury site under ultrasound guidance (figs. 4a and b). Although the amount of PRGF infiltrated should be the maximum possible and is usually around 8 mL, this volume could reach 10–12mL depending on the size of the muscle and extent and severity of the damaged area. Once the injury site has been infiltrated, areas adjacent to the site must be systematically infiltrated as well. Therefore, we allocate PRGF infiltration into the peripheral healthy muscle surrounding the injury, including interfascicular and interfibrillar regions (a source of resident macrophages and FAPs), by redirecting the needle in all directions— ventral, lateral, medial, and dorsal, thereby reaching the injury/stump, proximal-stump, distal-fascia, or deep and proximal interfascicular zone (fig. 4b) in order to truly conduct a deregulated area niche therapy[17]. In figure 5, we summarize the most important steps of our procedure. We primarily make use of the F2 fraction, and only when high volumes of PRGF are required, do we draw on the F1 to infiltrate the peripheral areas applying the same activation procedure as with the F2.

PRGF muscle infiltrations are aimed at recruiting, activating and mobilizing satellite cells and resident macrophages[25] which contribute to muscle reparation processes by cell signaling soluble factors[16,17,49,57] besides the already activated ECs, macrophages, and platelets in the injured area. Once the activated PRGF is injected, this liquid-to-gel transition 3D injectable scaffold allows a successful filling of the muscle gaps and defects. With a local and gradual activation ("in vitro" and "in vivo") and a homogeneous distribution through and interaction with the ECM of tissue, it is converted into a matrix-like viscous and malleable structure[11,90]. This fibrin-scaffold formed "in situ" as a provisional extracellular matrix and containing binding sites for cell adhesion as well as proteins such as thrombospondin-1 (TSP-1), alpha-1-antitrypsin fibronectin, acute phase proteins or proteins related to lipid metabolisms[10,90], serves as a highway for mechanical energy to transit from the environment to the cell, thereby bridging cell-to-cell tissue transition, promoting multi-cellular assembly, providing mechanical support and plastic-elastic stiffness which has a drastic impact on fates of diverse cell types such as muscle stem cells[92,93], and endowing tissues with a suitable mechanical and chemical microenvironment for biological restoration. In addition, fibrin matrix, by heparin-binding domains, may sequester growth factors such as PDGF, FGF, HGF, BDNF, and VEGF[18,68,70] and gradually release them later, exerting a synergistic action on tissue repair [18,68]. Finally, ice is applied to the infiltration area for about 10 minutes.

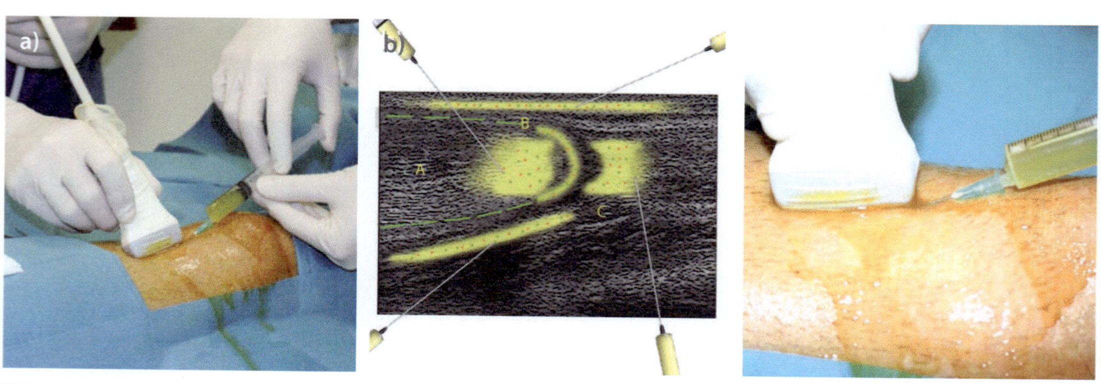

FIG. 4
A)PRGF infiltration at the site injury with correct orientation of the needle, always performed with ultrasound guidance. B)Ultrasound scheme showing the allocation of liquid activated PRGF at the injury site and into surrounding interfascicular and interfibrillar areas. (reprinted with permission from Sanchez et al[7]).

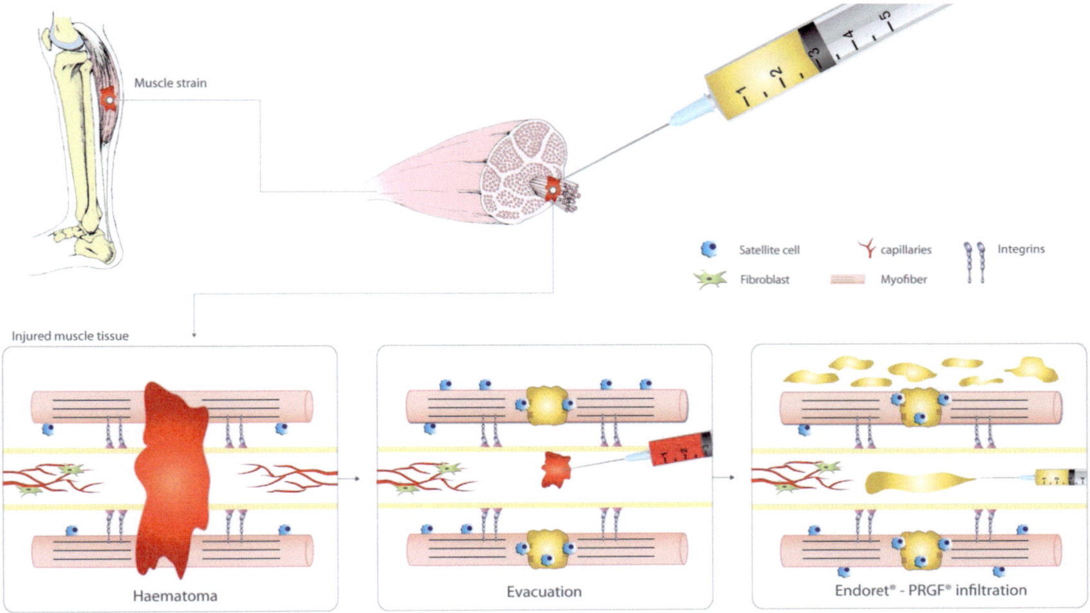

FIG. 5
A summary of the most important phases during percutaneous intramuscular infiltration of liquid activated PRGF. (Reprinted with permission from Sanchez et al[7]).

5.4. Post-infiltration protocol

The patient is advised to apply cold therapy 2-3 times and restrict physical activities during the first 24 hours. Both clinical and ultrasonographic monitoring are performed weekly during patient follow-up in order to evaluate the potential need for more infiltrations. In general, we recommend 2-3 infiltrations, on a weekly basis (relying on the myogenesis and myoblast replication process)[32,35,40]. This decision is based on ultrasound images and pain that the patient presents during the period of treatment, and more than three injections are not normally required. Since muscle tissue is a complex mechano-sensitive tissue, every pharmacological and surgical therapy should be assisted by mechanotherapy. In this respect, and as a clinical application of cell mechanotransduction, a post-infiltration rehabilitation program must be included in a synergistic manner which would play a crucial role in promoting the repair and remodeling of injured tissue. Therefore, since the limb has to be mobilized in an early and progressive manner[2,33,56], physiotherapy and rehabilitation treatment are mandatory. The generated mechanical stimulus achieves a proper recovery of these patients, since it acts in synergistic concert with the biological effects of PRGF[56]. Complications such as seromas, cysts, or muscle fibrosis, have to be approached based on the same principles used in acute ruptures.

1. Järvinen TA, Kääriäinen M, Äärimaa V, Järvinen M, Kalimo H. Skeletal muscle repair after exercise-induced injury. Skeletal Muscle Repair and Regeneration: Springer; 2008:217-42.

2. Jarvinen TA, Jarvinen TL, Kaariainen M, Kalimo H, Jarvinen M. Muscle injuries: biology and treatment. The American journal of sports medicine. 2005;33:745-64.

3. Tajbakhsh S. Skeletal muscle stem cells in developmental versus regenerative myogenesis. Journal of internal medicine. 2009;266:372-89.

4. Gayraud-Morel B, Chretien F, Tajbakhsh S. Skeletal muscle as a paradigm for regenerative biology and medicine. Regenerative medicine. 2009;4:293-319.

5. Sánchez M AE, Andía I. Application of autologous growth factors on skeletal muscle healing. 2nd World Congress on Regenerative Medicine; 2005; Leizpig, Germany.

6. Wright-Carpenter T, Klein P, Schaferhoff P, Appell HJ, Mir LM, Wehling P. Treatment of muscle injuries by local administration of autologous conditioned serum: a pilot study on sportsmen with muscle strains. International journal of sports medicine. 2004;25:588-93.

7. Sanchez M, Anitua E, Delgado D, Sanchez P, Orive G, Padilla S. Muscle repair: platelet-rich plasma derivates as a bridge from spontaneity to intervention. Injury. 2014;45 Suppl 4:S7-14.

8. Brockes JP, Kumar A. Comparative aspects of animal regeneration. Annual review of cell and developmental biology. 2008;24:525-49.

9. Stellos K, Kopf S, Paul A, et al. Platelets in regeneration. Seminars in thrombosis and hemostasis. 2010;36:175-84.

10. Nurden AT. Platelets, inflammation and tissue regeneration. Thrombosis and haemostasis. 2011;105 Suppl 1:S13-33.

11. Anitua E, Sanchez M, Orive G. Potential of endogenous regenerative technology for in situ regenerative medicine. Advanced drug delivery reviews. 2010;62:741-52.

12. Wagers AJ. The stem cell niche in regenerative medicine. Cell stem cell. 2012;10:362-9.

13. Tatsumi R, Anderson JE, Nevoret CJ, Halevy O, Allen RE. HGF/SF is present in normal adult skeletal muscle and is capable of activating satellite cells. Developmental biology. 1998;194:114-28.

14. Pelosi L, Giacinti C, Nardis C, et al. Local expression of IGF-1 accelerates muscle regeneration by rapidly modulating inflammatory cytokines and chemokines. FASEB journal : official publication of the Federation of American Societies for Experimental Biology. 2007;21:1393-402.

15. Li H, Usas A, Poddar M, et al. Platelet-Rich Plasma Promotes the Proliferation of Human Muscle Derived Progenitor Cells and Maintains Their Stemness. PloS one. 2013;8:e64923.

16. Hawke TJ, Garry DJ. Myogenic satellite cells: physiology to molecular biology. J Appl Physiol (1985). 2001;91:534-51.

17. Grounds MD. Towards understanding skeletal muscle regeneration. Pathology, research and practice. 1991;187:1-22.

18. Borselli C, Storrie H, Benesch-Lee F, et al. Functional muscle regeneration with combined delivery of angiogenesis and myogenesis factors. Proceedings of the National Academy of Sciences of the United States of America. 2010;107:3287-92.

19. Wetzel RJ, Patel RM, Terry MA. Platelet-rich plasma as an effective treatment for proximal hamstring injuries. Orthopedics. 2013;36:e64-70.

20. Hammond JW, Hinton RY, Curl LA, Muriel JM, Lovering RM. Use of autologous platelet-rich plasma to treat muscle strain injuries. The American journal of sports medicine. 2009;37:1135-42.

21. Conboy I, Freimer J, Weisenstein L. 5.526 - Tissue Engineering of Muscle Tissue. In: Ducheyne P, ed. Comprehensive Biomaterials. Oxford: Elsevier; 2011:345-59.

22. Cornelison DD. Context matters: in vivo and in vitro influences on muscle satellite cell activity. Journal of cellular biochemistry. 2008;105:663-9.

23. Grounds MD. Phagocytosis of necrotic muscle in muscle isografts is influenced by the strain, age, and sex of host mice. The Journal of pathology. 1987;153:71-82.

24. Saclier M, Cuvellier S, Magnan M, Mounier R, Chazaud B. Monocyte/macrophage interactions with myogenic precursor cells during skeletal muscle regeneration. The FEBS journal. 2013;280:4118-30.

25. Chazaud B, Brigitte M, Yacoub-Youssef H, et al. Dual and beneficial roles of macrophages during skeletal muscle regeneration. Exercise and sport sciences reviews. 2009;37:18-22.

26. Bosurgi L, Manfredi AA, Rovere-Querini P. Macrophages in injured skeletal muscle: a perpetuum mobile causing and limiting fibrosis, prompting or restricting resolution and regeneration. Frontiers in immunology. 2011;2:62.

27. Tidball JG, Villalta SA. Regulatory interactions between muscle and the immune system during muscle regeneration. American journal of physiology. Regulatory, integrative and comparative physiology. 2010;298:R1173-87.

28. Christov C, Chretien F, Abou-Khalil R, et al. Muscle satellite cells and endothelial cells: close neighbors and privileged partners. Molecular biology of the cell. 2007;18:1397-409.

29. Serrano AL, Mann CJ, Vidal B, Ardite E, Perdiguero E, Munoz-Canoves P. Cellular and molecular mechanisms regulating fibrosis in skeletal muscle repair and disease. Current topics in developmental biology. 2011;96:167-201.

30. Rantanen J, Ranne J, Hurme T, Kalimo H. Denervated segments of injured skeletal muscle fibers are reinnervated by newly formed neuromuscular junctions. Journal of neuropathology and experimental neurology. 1995;54:188-94.

31. Slater CR, Schiaffino S. Innervation of regenerating muscle. Skeletal Muscle Repair and Regeneration: Springer; 2008:303-34.

32. Ciciliot S, Schiaffino S. Regeneration of mammalian skeletal muscle. Basic mechanisms and clinical implications. Current pharmaceutical design. 2010;16:906-14.

33. Kaariainen M, Jarvinen T, Jarvinen M, Rantanen J, Kalimo H. Relation between myofibers and connective tissue during muscle injury repair. Scandinavian journal of medicine & science in sports. 2000;10:332-7.

34. Tatsumi R, Liu X, Pulido A, et al. Satellite cell activation in stretched skeletal muscle and the role of nitric oxide and hepatocyte growth factor. American journal of physiology. Cell physiology. 2006;290:C1487-94.

35. Prisk V, Huard J. Muscle injuries and repair: the role of prostaglandins and inflammation. Histology and histopathology. 2003;18:1243-56.

36. Grounds MD. Complexity of extracellular matrix and skeletal muscle regeneration. Skeletal Muscle Repair and Regeneration: Springer; 2008:269-302.

37. Joe AW, Yi L, Natarajan A, et al. Muscle injury activates resident fibro/adipogenic progenitors that facilitate myogenesis. Nature cell biology. 2010;12:153-63.

38. Murphy MM, Lawson JA, Mathew SJ, Hutcheson DA, Kardon G. Satellite cells, connective tissue fibroblasts and their interactions are crucial for muscle regeneration. Development. 2011;138:3625-37.

39. Tidball JG, Dorshkind K, Wehling-Henricks M. Shared signaling systems in myeloid cell-mediated muscle regeneration. Development. 2014;141:1184-96.

40. Grounds MD. Regeneration of Muscle. eLS. Chichester: John Wiley & Sons, Ltd; 2011:10.1002/9780470015902.a0001106.pub2.

41. Duffield JS, Lupher M, Thannickal VJ, Wynn TA. Host responses in tissue repair and fibrosis. Annual review of pathology. 2013;8:241-76.

42. Kharraz Y, Guerra J, Mann CJ, Serrano AL, Munoz-Canoves P. Macrophage plasticity and the role of inflammation in skeletal muscle repair. Mediators of inflammation. 2013;2013:491497.

43. Pizza F. Neutrophils and macrophages in muscle damage and repair. Skeletal Muscle Damage and Repair. 2008;49:57.

44. Stoick-Cooper CL, Moon RT, Weidinger G. Advances in signaling in vertebrate regeneration as a prelude to regenerative medicine. Genes & development. 2007;21:1292-315.

45. Relaix F, Zammit PS. Satellite cells are essential for skeletal muscle regeneration: the cell on the edge returns centre stage. Development. 2012;139:2845-56.

46. Wagers AJ, Conboy IM. Cellular and molecular signatures of muscle regeneration: current concepts and controversies in adult myogenesis. Cell. 2005;122:659-67.

47. Charge SB, Rudnicki MA. Cellular and molecular regulation of muscle regeneration. Physiological reviews. 2004;84:209-38.

48. Tidball JG. Inflammatory processes in muscle injury and repair. American journal of physiology. Regulatory, integrative and comparative physiology. 2005;288:R345-53.

49. Shi X, Garry DJ. Muscle stem cells in development, regeneration, and disease. Genes & development. 2006;20:1692-708.

50. Augustin. HG. Angiogenesis. Endothelial biomedicine: Cambridge University Press; 2007:1444-56.

51. Li H, Hicks JJ, Wang L, et al. Customized platelet-rich plasma with transforming growth factor beta1 neutralization antibody to reduce fibrosis in skeletal muscle. Biomaterials. 2016;87:147-56.

52. Tidball JG, Wehling-Henricks M. Shifts in macrophage cytokine production drive muscle fibrosis. Nature medicine. 2015;21:665-6.

53. Arnold L, Henry A, Poron F, et al. Inflammatory monocytes recruited after skeletal muscle injury switch into antiinflammatory macrophages to support myogenesis. The Journal of experimental medicine. 2007;204:1057-69.

54. Sanes JR. The basement membrane/basal lamina of skeletal muscle. The Journal of biological chemistry. 2003;278:12601-4.

55. Hoying JBaS, K.W. Building blood vessels. Endothelial Biomedicine: Cambridge University Press; 2007:1712-24.

56. Kannus P, Parkkari J, Jarvinen TL, Jarvinen TA, Jarvinen M. Basic science and clinical studies coincide: active treatment approach is needed after a sports injury. Scandinavian journal of medicine & science in sports. 2003;13:150-4.

57. Grounds MD. Muscle regeneration: molecular aspects and therapeutic implications. Current opinion in neurology. 1999;12:535-43.

58. Semple JW, Italiano JE, Jr., Freedman J. Platelets and the immune continuum. Nature reviews. Immunology. 2011;11:264-74.

59. Chazaud B, Sonnet C, Lafuste P, et al. Satellite cells attract monocytes and use macrophages as a support to escape apoptosis and enhance muscle growth. The Journal of cell biology. 2003;163:1133-43.

60. Gleissner CA, Shaked I, Little KM, Ley K. CXC chemokine ligand 4 induces a unique transcriptome in monocyte-derived macrophages. J Immunol. 2010;184:4810-8.

61. Stout RD, Jiang C, Matta B, Tietzel I, Watkins SK, Suttles J. Macrophages sequentially change their functional phenotype in response to changes in microenvironmental influences. J Immunol. 2005;175:342-9.

62. Zheng H, Fu G, Dai T, Huang H. Migration of endothelial progenitor cells mediated by stromal cell-derived factor-1alpha/CXCR4 via PI3K/Akt/eNOS signal transduction pathway. Journal of cardiovascular pharmacology. 2007;50:274-80.

63. Shortreed K, Johnston A, Hawke T. Satellite cells and muscle repair. Skeletal Muscle Damage and Repair. 2008;1:77-88.

64. Sarasa-Renedo A, Chiquet M. Mechanical signals regulating extracellular matrix gene expression in fibroblasts. Scandinavian journal of medicine & science in sports. 2005;15:223-30.

65. Lemos DR, Babaeijandaghi F, Low M, et al. Nilotinib reduces muscle fibrosis in chronic muscle injury by promoting TNF-mediated apoptosis of fibro/adipogenic progenitors. Nature medicine. 2015;21:786-94.

66. Uezumi A, Ito T, Morikawa D, et al. Fibrosis and adipogenesis originate from a common mesenchymal progenitor in skeletal muscle. Journal of cell science. 2011;124:3654-64.

67. Perdiguero E, Sousa-Victor P, Ruiz-Bonilla V, et al. p38/MKP-1-regulated AKT coordinates macrophage transitions and resolution of inflammation during tissue repair. The Journal of cell biology. 2011;195:307-22.

68. Martino MM, Briquez PS, Ranga A, Lutolf MP, Hubbell JA. Heparin-binding domain of fibrin(ogen) binds growth factors and promotes tissue repair when incorporated within a synthetic matrix. Proceedings of the National Academy of Sciences of the United States of America. 2013;110:4563-8.

69. Shefer G, Yablonka-Reuveni Z. The ins and outs of satellite cell myogenesis: the role of the ruling growth factors. Skeletal Muscle Repair and Regeneration: Springer; 2008:107-44.

70. Sarrazin S, Lamanna WC, Esko JD. Heparan sulfate proteoglycans. Cold Spring Harbor perspectives in biology. 2011;3.

71. Bentzinger CF, Wang YX, Rudnicki MA. Building muscle: molecular regulation of myogenesis. Cold Spring Harbor perspectives in biology. 2012;4:doi 10.1101chsperspect.a008342.

72. Sonnet C, Lafuste P, Arnold L, et al. Human macrophages rescue myoblasts and myotubes from apoptosis through a set of adhesion molecular systems. Journal of cell science. 2006;119:2497-507.

73. Janmey PA, Miller RT. Mechanisms of mechanical signaling in development and disease. Journal of cell science. 2011;124:9-18.

74. Hinz B, Mastrangelo D, Iselin CE, Chaponnier C, Gabbiani G. Mechanical tension controls granulation tissue contractile activity and myofibroblast differentiation. The American journal of pathology. 2001;159:1009-20.

75. Kjaer M. Role of extracellular matrix in adaptation of tendon and skeletal muscle to mechanical loading. Physiological reviews. 2004;84:649-98.

76. Brooks SV, Vasilaki A, Larkin LM, McArdle A, Jackson MJ. Repeated bouts of aerobic exercise lead to reductions in skeletal muscle free radical generation and nuclear factor kappaB activation. The Journal of physiology. 2008;586:3979-90.

77. Peterson JM, Bakkar N, Guttridge DC. NF-kappaB signaling in skeletal muscle health and disease. Current topics in developmental biology. 2011;96:85-119.

78. Padilla S, Sánchez M, Orive G, Anitua E. Human-Based Biological and Biomimetic Autologous Therapies for Musculoskeletal Tissue Regeneration. Trends in biotechnology. 2017;35:192-202.

79. Marcus A. Platelets: their role in hemostasis, thrombosis, and inflammation. Inflammation: basic principles and clinical correlates. 1999:77-95.

80. Sanchez M, Anitua E, Orive G, Mujika I, Andia I. Platelet-rich therapies in the treatment of orthopaedic sport injuries. Sports Med. 2009;39:345-54.

81. Dimauro I, Grasso L, Fittipaldi S, et al. Platelet-rich plasma and skeletal muscle healing: a molecular analysis of the early phases of the regeneration process in an experimental animal model. PloS one. 2014;9:e102993.

82. Miroshmychenko O, Chang W, Dragoo JL. The use of platelet-rich and platelet-poor plasma to enhance differentiation of skeletal myoblasts: Implications for the use of autologous blood products for muscle regeneration. AAOS. Stanford Sports Medicine. July 7-10. The Broadmoor, Colorado. 2016.

83. Borrione P, Grasso L, Chierto E, et al. Experimental model for the study of the effects of platelet-rich plasma on the early phases of muscle healing. Blood transfusion = Trasfusione del sangue. 2014;12 Suppl 1:s221-8.

84. Hamid MS, Yusof A, Mohamed Ali MR. Platelet-rich plasma (PRP) for acute muscle injury: a systematic review. PloS one. 2014;9:e90538.

85. Hamid MSA, Ali MRM, Yusof A, George J, Lee LPC. Platelet-rich plasma injections for the treatment of hamstring injuries a randomized controlled trial. The American journal of sports medicine. 2014;42:2410-18.

86. Loo WL, Lee D, Soon M. Plasma rich in growth factors to treat adductor longus tear. Annals of the Academy of Medicine, Singapore. 2009;38:733.

87. Reurink G, Goudswaard GJ, Moen MH, et al. Platelet-rich plasma injections in acute muscle injury. The New England journal of medicine. 2014;370:2546-7.

88. Anitua E, Sanchez M, Padilla S. More on platelet-rich plasma injections in acute muscle injury. The New England journal of medicine. 2014;371:1264.

89. Terada S, Ota S, Kobayashi M, et al. Use of an antifibrotic agent improves the effect of platelet-rich plasma on muscle healing after injury. The Journal of bone and joint surgery. American volume. 2013;95:980-8.

90. Anitua E, Orive G. Endogenous regenerative technology using plasma- and platelet-derived growth factors. Journal of controlled release : official journal of the Controlled Release Society. 2012;157:317-20.

91. Sánchez M, Albillos J, Angulo F, Santisteban J, Andia I. Platelet-rich plasma in muscle and tendon healing. Operative Techniques in Orthopaedics. 2012;22:16-24.

92. Gilbert PM, Havenstrite KL, Magnusson KE, et al. Substrate elasticity regulates skeletal muscle stem cell self-renewal in culture. Science. 2010;329:1078-81.

93. Discher DE, Mooney DJ, Zandstra PW. Growth factors, matrices, and forces combine and control stem cells. Science. 2009;324:1673-7.

CHAPTER 15

Minimally Invasive PRGF Treatment for Low Back Pain and Degenerative Disc Disease

AUTHORS

Kirchner F.[1], Anitua E.[2,3,4]

[1] Barcelona Traumatology Institute, Mataró, Spain
[2] Eduardo Anitua Foundation for Biomedical Research, Vitoria, Spain
[3] BTI-Biothecnology Institute, Vitoria, Spain
[4] University Institute for Regenerative Medicine and Oral Implantology (UIRMI) from the University of Basque Country (UPV/EHU)

SUMMARY

Low back pain is a complex and disabling condition and its treatment is a challenge. Traditional surgery to treat lumbar spine pathology has unwanted and suboptimal results. There is now a primary medical and clinical research motivation to put into practice minimally invasive therapies, particularly in support of regenerative medicine, in the treatment of spinal pain and degenerative diseases. Infiltrations of autologous platelet rich plasma (PRP) have been widely used as an effective technological approach to tissue repair and improvements in numerous clinical conditions. Lately, PRP has been included in therapies in specific spinal structures to treat spinal lumbar pain associated with degenerative disc pathology and arthrosis. In patients with chronic low back pain, plasma rich in growth factors (PRGF) has been shown to be an efficient new procedure to reduce lumbar and joint pain after intradiscal, intra-articular facet and transforaminal epidural infiltration under fluoroscopic guidance-control in the operating theatre setting.

E. Anitua et al. (eds.), *Platelet Rich Plasma in Orthopaedics and Sports Medicine*,
https://doi.org/10.1007/978-3-319-63730-3_15

1. INTRODUCTION

Low back pain (LBP) is a highly frequently occurring musculoskeletal disorder involving the muscles, nerves (Luschka plexus), ligaments (such as posterior longitudinal ligament) and bones of the spine[1], often related to a lumbar Degenerative Disc Disease (DDD) with multifactorial and multidisciplinary effects, that affects a large global population[2]. LBP is ranked among the top ten causes of worldwide morbidity and disability according to the latest Global Burden of Disease Study 2015, representing an elevated cost for the health system in general[2]. LBP is a complex, personal experience encompassing multidimensional phenomena with physiologic, sensory, affective, cognitive, behavioral, and sociocultural affects[3, 4]. Although in most patients low back pain is self-limiting, there is a subset of patients, whose symptoms will reemerge, labeling the condition as non-specific, chronic low back pain lasting longer than 3 months of evolution. The pain is primarily related to mechanical factors which mediate in muscular strain, intervertebral disc degeneration (IVDD), facet-mediated pain, and radiculopathy, though the precise mechanisms remain to be elucidated. Two fundamental spinal structures specialized in both shock-absorbing and load-bearing are intervertebral discs (IVDs) and facet joints (FJs). In response to mechanical stress, inflammatory synovitis, and degenerative arthritis, these structures undergo chronic degenerative process, which leads to chronic low back pain[5]. Aging is another factor that produces elements of spinal degenerative changes which are the predominant cause of back pain and sciatica in adult population[6, 7]. Magnetic Resonance Imaging (MRI) scan is usually employed as a valuable tool to identify anatomical abnormalities and determine structural and functional degenerative changes of the spine[8-11]. MRI findings change over time on IVDs (such as disc herniations and annular tears), vertebral subchondral bone (VSB, for example Modic changes and intravertebral herniated disc called Schmorl´s nodes) and arthrosis, which are generally used to determine structural and functional regeneration of the spine and the relationship of these pathoanatomical structures with LBP[12, 13]. The degree of lumbar disc degenerative changes can be classified by various grading systems based on changes in type of disc degeneration, signal intensity (such as discal degeneration degree-Pfirrmann Classification), and IVD (IVD height (IDH), vertebral body height (VBH), and lumbar disc pathology) or VSB (endplate degeneration degree-Modic Changes, and total endplate damage Score-TEPS) parameters from MRI scans[14, 15].

A remarkable clinical motivation for reducing pain and treating spinal degenerative disease arises from the need to return patients to their daily routines and improve their life quality. The appropriate treatment remains a daunting challenge despite advances in the management of pain, inflammation and degeneration by pharmacological and surgical procedures. Before a conventional and surgical procedure is performed, the patient should be offered an incrementally progressive treatment plan, beginning with a minimally invasive interventional therapy[16-23] for symptomatic disc herniation and degeneration, and lumbar FJ arthrosis.

2. SPINAL ANATOMY AND BIOLOGY: INTERVERTEBRAL DISC AND FACET JOINT

Intervertebral disc (IVD), vertebral subcondral bone (VSB), and facet joints (FJs) are important anatomical elements of a spinal column multivariate system affected by pain and degenerative pathology (vertebral arthrosis or osteoarthritis (OA) of the spine)[24]. Intervertebral disc is composed of distinct anatomical regions including the central gel-like nucleus pulposus (NP), the peripheral fibrous annulus fibrosus (AF), and cartilaginous endplates (CEP) at the cranial and caudal interface of one side of the disc[25-27]. IVDs provide stable support to contiguous spinal vertebrae and permit movement to the vertebral bodies, in that way affecting plasticity of the spine[9]. Disc cells (such as NP, AF and CEP cells) take part in the production and sustaining of disc matrix macromolecules (mainly proteoglycans and collagens) that finally control the biomechanical function of the IVD[26-28]. The normal adult human IVD is mainly avascular and only innervated in the outermost layer of the annulus fibrosus[1, 26]. Nutrients are necessary to support disc cell activity, viability and function. Nutrient diffusion into the disc represents a balance between rate of nutrient supply (capillary density and transport) and rate of cellular demand (disc cell density and metabolic rate)[26, 29]. In addition, metabolic wastes from IVD cells are removed by the reverse route before they accumulate inside the disc[26].

In adults, at the ends of each IVD is located a endplate bilayer of cartilage (CEP) and bone (VSB)[29] that takes apart the vertebral bone from the IVD itself and prevents the vastly hydrated nucleus pulposus from bulging outward to the neighboring vertebrae[30]. In contrast to IVDs, mainly the central endplate of VSB is well innervated as is the adjacent vertebral marrow[30, 31]. It is known that the VSB plays an important role in spinal function, maintaining IVD integrity and disc nutrition supply[24].

At almost every spinal level, lumbar facets or zygapophyseal joints are three-joint complexes with biomechanical capacity as osseous stabilizers of the posterior spinal column facilitating vertebral articulation[32-34]. The three-dimensional (3D) structure is formed by the three articulations between adjacent vertebrae: one anteriorly situated IVD and a pair of small FJs that interact to form a spinal segmental movement complex[32, 35]. At each spinal level, the bilateral FJs are positioned symmetrically relative to the mid-sagittal plane in the posterolateral regions of the vertebral column[33, 35] and are the only true synovial joints between adjacent spinal levels in humans[35]. Facet is a diarthrodial synovial joint with opposing articular cartilage surfaces that provide a low friction environment and a ligamentous capsule that encloses the joint space. Together with the disc, the bilateral FJs transfers loads and guides and constrains motions in the spine as a result of their geometry and mechanical function[33]. Facet joints are anatomically and functionally distinct from the fibrocartilaginous articulation of the IVD[35]. The posterior and medial aspects of lumbar facets resist forward displacement and rotation. At L4-S1segment, angle varies from 30 to 90 degrees, creating more resistance to forward displacement of the superior articular process during flexion and extension but allowing more rotation as the lumbar spine transitions to sacrum[34]. Joint alignment and load distribution are thought to be major factors in the development and progression of FJ OA. Functionally, the three joints in each motion segment are highly interdependent, such that changes in one affect the other two and vice versa[32, 35]. In the majority of individuals, degenerative pathology begins in the disc and is followed by changes in the facet joints affecting the biomechanics of the 3D complex[35]. As a result of biomechanical changes at one level, pathological changes can occur in the motion segment at surrounding spinal levels. In support of the IVD and FJ interdependence concept, FJ OA in the lumbar spine occurs at the levels mainly affected by disc degeneration (L4–S1)[35]. With DDD, the approximation of the vertebral bodies increases the compression on the FJ and changes the relative position of the matching FJ surfaces. The resultant increase in joint compression accelerates wear of the articular facet, producing OA changes[33].

3. PRGF TREATMENT TO REDUCE LOW BACK PAIN

PRP application is a biological and technological approach to tissue repair which has been shown to be an efficient treatment to attenuate and improve several clinical conditions by reducing pain and regenerating tissue[36-40]. Over the past few years, PRP has been used in clinical studies for treatment of vertebral FJ, surrounding ligaments, nerves and IVD to treat pain related to DDD[17-22].

Since the concept of PRGF (PRGF-Endoret) has been developed and characterized[41-45] the application of PRGF-Endoret[40] has been shown to be an efficient treatment to attenuate knee and hip pain of patients with OA and to improve their clinical condition by reducing joint pain[46, 47]. Recently, it has also been reported in an observational retrospective pilot study that fluoroscopy-guided infiltrations of IVDs and vertebral FJs with PRGF-Endoret in patients with chronic LBP resulted in significant radicular and LBP reduction[18].

In light of prior promising results in basic science[48, 49], in preclinical trials, and in osteoarthritic patients whose chronic pain was significantly reduced after PRGF treatment[47, 50-53], results suggest four synergetic effects of PRGF-Endoret on synovial joint diseases, namely, a chondroprotective, anti-inflammatory, cell-phenotype modulation, and joint pain attenuation. These effects make PRGF a strong candidate for treatment of vertebral FJs and IVDD[54].

4. NEW INTRADISCAL PLUS INTRA-ARTICULAR FACET JOINT PRGF TECHNIQUE

In the surgical room of the health centre, low back PRGF protocol (Figure 1A) setup (Kirchner & Anitua, 2016) is performed by a qualified orthopaedic clinical team under international standards from the latest "World medical association declaration of Helsinki" (Brasil, 2013) revised.

Patients are placed in either prone or lateral position depending on patient circumstances. Using sterile technique, intra-articular facet, IVD, and peridural percutaneous PRGF infiltration is performed under X-ray fluoroscopy with a C-arch (BV Libra, Philips, Eindhoven, The Netherlands). Briefly, the percutaneous IVD infiltration approach is used at an oblique angle between 30 and 35 degrees along the lateral margin of the inferior ar-

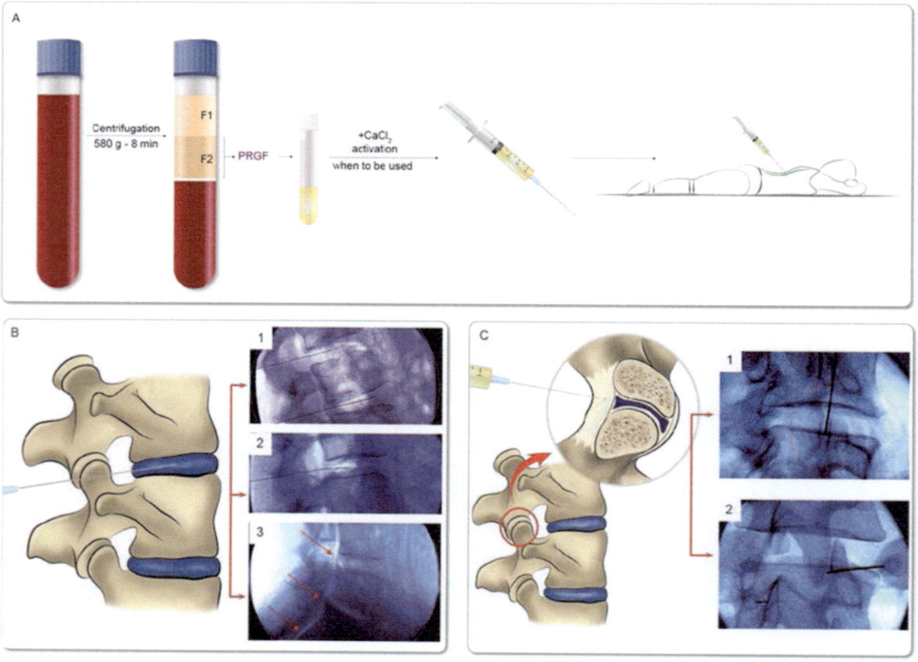

FIG. 1
PRGF preparation and infiltration of disc and lumbar facet joint. (a) Illustrative representation of PRGF obtaining process. Before the percutaneous infiltration, the fraction 2 of PRGF was activated with PRGF activator. (b) Illustration and fluoroscopic-guided lumbar intervertebral disc (insert 1 and 2) images and peridural infiltration (insert 3). (c) Drawing and fluoroscopic-guided lumbar facet joint infiltrations of PRGF showing an intradiscal (insert 1) and intra-articular (insert 2) position of the needle tip (Figure from Kirchner & Anitua, 2016. JCVJS).

ticular process of the vertebrae (Figure 1B, inserts 1 and 2) and through the neuroforamen, while preserving the nerve root. The position of the needle (Quincke needle, 22Ga:178 mm-lenght), which had a manually bent-shaped end, is guided and confirmed under antero-posterior (AP) and lateral fluoroscopic view. Once the needle end is located at the bulging or herniated disc, and checked by infiltrating a little bit of activated PRGF under fluoroscopy, 3 ml of activated PRGF is injected into the NP and the surrounding dehydrated areas while paying careful attention not to allocate more than this PRGF quantity. When the needle is removed from the disc, using the same technical procedure, a peridural infiltration is performed, injecting 1-2 ml of activated PRGF (Figure 1B, insert 3). The spinal FJ infiltration is carried out using the same procedure (Figure 1C, inserts 1 and 2). While the patient lies prone, the joints to be injected are located and marked. After cleaning and draping, the 22-Ga spinal needle is inserted until it contacts the capsule of the joint, and then with careful and refined movements the needle tip enters the joint. Once the needle position is confirmed under fluoroscopy, 1 ml of activated PRGF is injected into each of the zygapophysial or FJs.

5. RESULTS

Intradiscal and facet joint PRGF infiltrations: pain evaluation using VAS outcome

In the retrospective study performed by Kirchner & Anitua 2016[18], the pain assessment was determined using a visual analog scale (VAS) outcome where 0 score denotes "no pain" and a score of 10 denotes "pain as bad as it could be"[3, 55]. The VAS score was evaluated at the first visit before (baseline) and after the procedure at 1, 3, and 6 months. Reduction in VAS score was considered the measure of outcome of interventional therapy with PRGF. The pain reduction after the PRGF-Endoret injections showed a statistically significant drop after the treatment with respect to all the time evaluations. The analysis of the VAS over time showed that at the end point of the study (six months) 91% of patients showed an excellent score (VAS 0-3), 8.1% showed a moderate improvement (VAS 3.1-6.5), and 1.2% were in the inefficient score (VAS 6.6-10) (Figure 2).

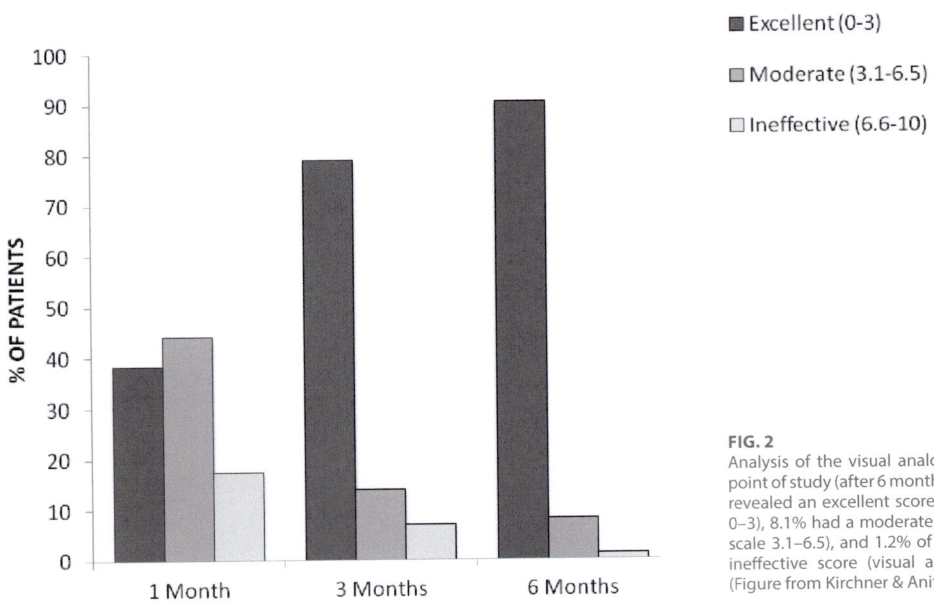

FIG. 2
Analysis of the visual analog scale. At the end point of study (after 6 months), 90.7% of patients revealed an excellent score (visual analog scale 0–3), 8.1% had a moderate score (visual analog scale 3.1–6.5), and 1.2% of patients showed an ineffective score (visual analog scale 6.6–10) (Figure from Kirchner & Anitua, 2016. JCVJS)

Taking into account the limitations and drawbacks addressed at the preliminary study just mentioned[18], and the evidence of other clinical and case reports related to PRP infiltration to treat low back pain[16, 17, 19-22], the authors are confident that infiltrations of IVDs and FJs with PRGF should be considered a valuable therapy in patients with chronic LBP.

Another important point to be considered is the fact that a standardized protocol for PRP infiltration is still not established, and variation of PRP preparation and procedures necessarily results in wide inconsistencies. In addition, the volumes of PRP infiltrations, platelet concentrations, and time differences between injections are still under discussion.

In the treatment of spine pathology PRGF-Endoret therapy, is highly recommended as an additional and specific reinforcing therapy to complete the spinal regenerative process in all patients.

Intradiscal PRGF therapy: Case Report using imaging technique MRI results.

Following an overexertion, a 33 year-old male patient presented to the Traumatology clinic in March 2014 with three months evolution of LBP and symptoms of lumbago and sciatica radiating to the right lower leg and into the foot fingers.

An initial MRI examination in January 2014 revealed decrease of T2-weighted (T2W) discal signal at L5-S1 IVD level indicative of a certain degree

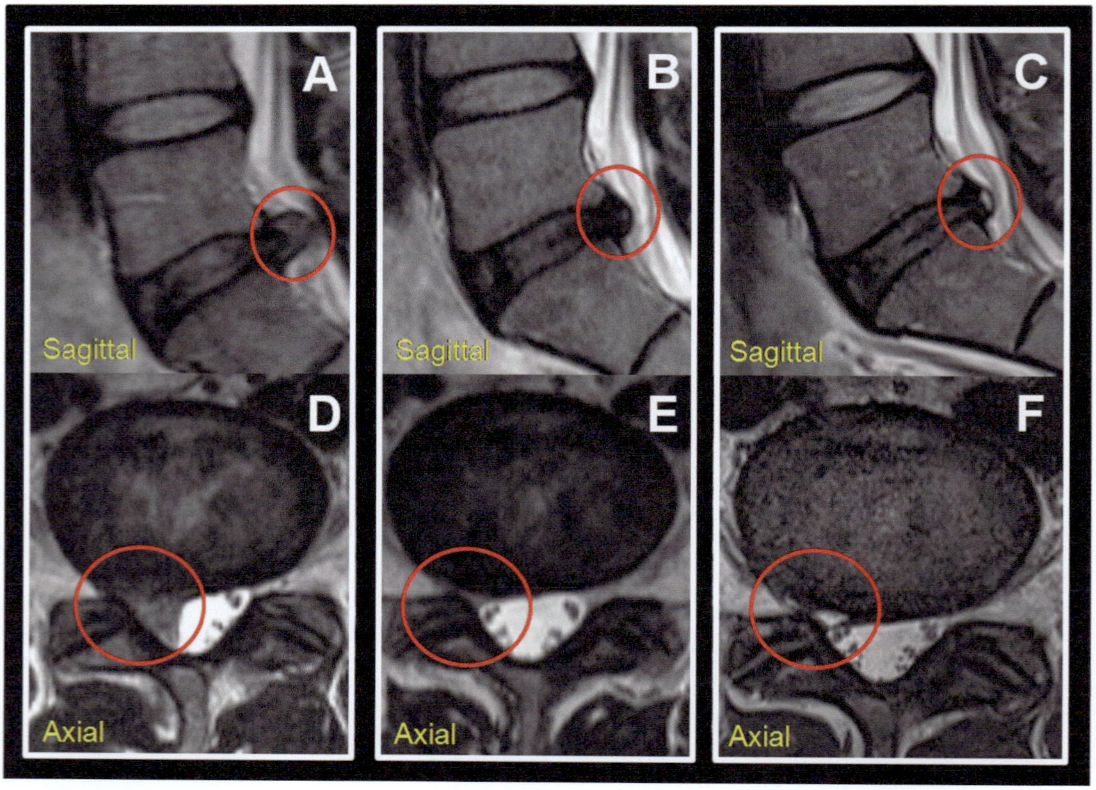

FIG. 3
MRI scan at the lumbar spinal level L5-S1 showing pre and post-PRGF intradiscal treatment T2-weighted (T2W) axial and sagittal section. Red circle delineate extrusion size. (2014) Pre-treatment sagittal (A) and axial (D) MRI scan sections. (2016) Post-treatment MRI sagittal (B) and axial (E) sections. (2017) Final MRI sections at sagittal (C) and axial (F) levels.

of degeneration (Pfirrman degree degeneration grade III), and a significant right-sided postero-paramedial (PP) and preforaminal spinal herniated disc (extrusion) (Figure 3A, 3D) at the L5-S1 IVD space causing compression of thecal sac and right S1 traversing nerve root.

The patient agreed to receive a minimally invasive treatment and underwent three bilateral PRGF applications during his complete therapy. A first, fluoroscopic-guided intradiscal L5-S1, peridural and root percutaneous disc infiltration approach was performed in a surgical suite setting in April 2014. Later, second and third PRGF therapies were completed in an adapted outpatient operating room. The second PRGF infiltration was carried out 20 days after the first PRGF application at L4-L5 and L5-S1 levels. One year after the first PRGF application, the patient received his last PRGF therapy at the same levels as the previous outpatient PRGF infiltrations.

Table 1 reviews the measurements (Figure 4) and findings from MRI scan analysis of the patient before and after PRGF treatment.

A second MRI scan performed approximately two years later (Figure 3B, 3E) revealed a Pfirrmann grade III of degeneration at L5-S1 disc space that was unchanged from the previous posterior lumbar spine MRI examination. The height of L5-S1 disc (Figure 4A) space (IDH) remained decreased compared to the other levels and was slightly variable from the earlier and later lumbar spine MRI

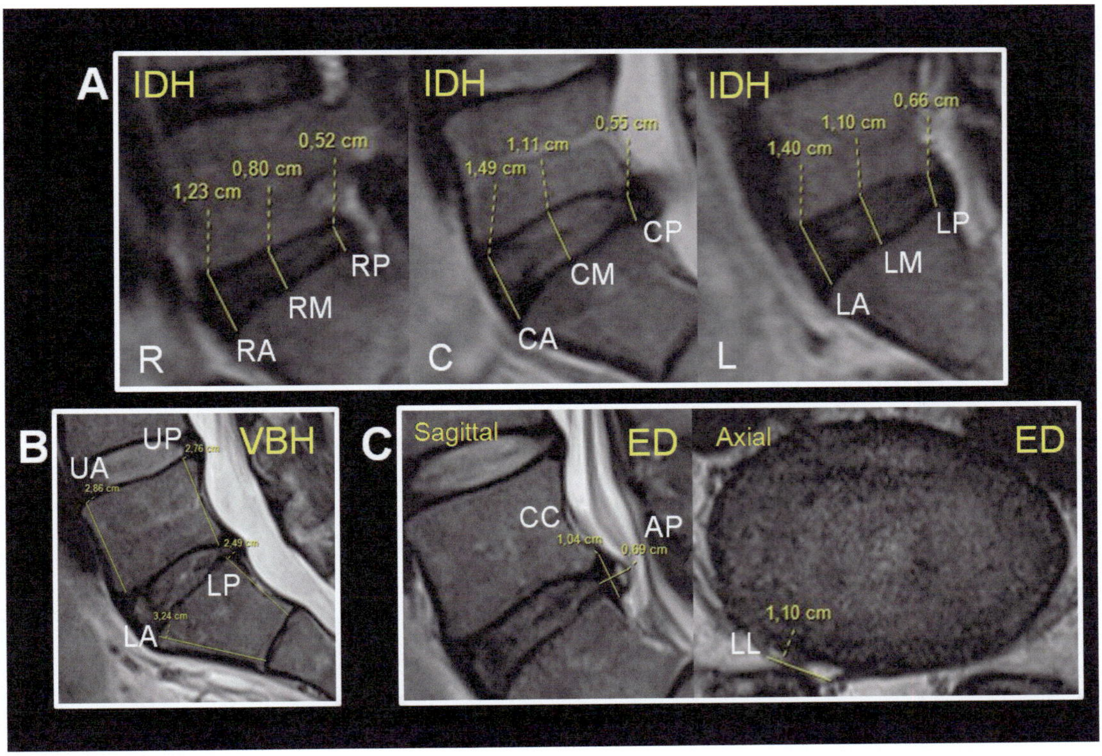

FIG. 4
T2-weighted (T2W) axial and sagittal sections at the lumbar spinal level L5-S1 showing MRI measurements (in mm) using medical imaging remote Workstation AW 4.3 (GE Healthcare). (A) Sagittal measurements of Intervertebral Disc Height (IDH) at Right Anterior (RA), Right Middle (RM), Right Posterior (RP), Centre Anterior (CA), Centre Middle (CM), Centre Posterior (CP), Left Anterior (LP), Left Middle (LM) and Left Posterior (LP) sections; (B) Sagittal measurements of Vertebral Body Height (VBH) at L5-Upper Anterior (UA), L5-Upper Posterior (UP), S1-Lower Anterior (LA), S1-Lower Posterior (LP) sections; and (C) Sagittal and Axial dimension of lumbar disc extrusion diameter at Craneo-caudal (CC), Latero-lateral (LL), and Antero-posterior (AP) sections.

examination. However, an important extrusion resorption (Table 1) was found showing a smaller right-sided PP extrusion diameter (ED) (Figure 4C) at the L5-S1 IVD level evidencing a 42% decrease at latero-lateral (LL) axial section and 22.5% reduction at sagittal AP section without changes at sagittal craneo-caudal (CC) section. No evidence of compression of thecal sac and nerve root on T2W images (T2WI) were observed. Parameters analysed over time for VBH (Figure 4B) showed minimum measurement variation (Table 1). A last, MRI study carried out in January 2017, showed little change with respect to the 2016 MRI report (Table 1, Figure 3C, and 3F). In particular the ED remained diminished and almost the same size as the MRI scans of 2016.

6. DISCUSSION

Kirchner & Anitua[18] showed that a minimally invasive therapy consisting of PRGF-Endoret infiltrations of IVD, FJs and peridural space in patients with chronic LBP resulted in significant pain reduction assessed by VAS outcome. PRGF-Endoret is a treatment without any side effects and no complications were experienced by the patient, so the therapy could be carried out as many times as necessary within the period up to completing the treatment.

At the end of sixth month follow-up period, 91% of patients showed a pain value of 0-3 in the VAS score, which is considered "excellent" in the litera-

MRI parameters: Spine Level L5-S1	Pre-MRI 2014	Post-MRI 2016	Post-MRI 2017
Intervertebral Disc Height (IDH) mm			
Right Anterior (RA)	1.23	1.35	1.42
Right Middle (RM)	0.80	0.95	0.95
Right Posterior (RP)	0.52	0.61	0.52
Centre Anterior (CA)	1.49	1.45	1.51
Centre Middle (CM)	1.11	1.14	1.02
Centre Posterior (CP)	0.55	0.65	0.49
Left Anterior (LP)	1.40	1.19	1.32
Left Middle (LM)	1.10	0.89	0.94
Left Posterior (LP)	0.66	0.66	0.54
Vertebral Body Height (VBH) mm			
L5-Upper Anterior (UA)	2.95	2.91	2.86
L5-Upper Posterior (UP)	2.93	2.72	2.76
S1-Lower Anterior (LA)	3.29	3.20	3.24
S1-Lower Posterior (LP)	2.74	2.47	2.49
Lumbar Disc Pathology	Hernia-Extrusion	Hernia-Extrusion	Hernia-Extrusion
Extrusion diameter (ED) mm			
Craneo-caudal (CC)	1.06	1.06	1.04
Latero-lateral (LL)	1.74	1.01	1.10
Antero-posterior (AP)	1.02	0.79	0.69
Discal Degeneration Degree			
Pfirrmann Classification	Grade III	Grade III	Grade III

TABLE 1
A pre and post-treatment Nuclear Magnetic Resonance (NMR) analysis performed at the L5-S1 discal space and corresponding vertebrae level. According to T2-weighted axial and sagittal sections of the lumbar spine, the networked medical imaging remote Workstation AW 4.3 (GE Healthcare) was used to import, interpret and process DICOM images from MRI scans to categorize and obtain measurements of the following parameters: Intervertebral Disc Height (IDH); Vertebral Body Height (VBH); Lumbar disc pathology; and discal degeneration degree (Pfirrmann Classification).

ture[23]. This result is consistent with the values published by Sanchez et. al.[47] for the treatment of OA of the hip with PRGF infiltration, and comparable to the values reported by Becker and colleagues[56] using epidural perineural injections of autologous conditioned serum (ACS) on patients with lumbar radicular compression, and substantially better than the pain relief shown by infiltrating metylprednisolone in the lumbar FJs[57], triamcinolone in epidural perineural injections[56] or betametasone in periganglionar infiltration[23] in patients with LBP. Nevertheless, the course of treatment reported by Chatuverdi and coauthors[57] reached a peak of 93% of responders at fourth week of treatment and then declined to 62.5% at third month of treatment, an outcome which is not consistent with our results.

The report of Kirchner & Anitua is one of the few in the clinical literatures regarding the use of PRP injections of IVD and FJs as a minimally invasive therapy to treat LBP and IVDD.

Until now, the large number of PRP studies performed on the spine to study pain management and disc pathology have been focused using in vitro (cell cultures) or in vivo (animal model) systems which have produced promising positive results[58-62]. In contrast, so far only two prospective clinical trials have been reported[16, 20, 21] and three papers exist in the literature describing case reports[17, 19, 22] showing positive statistical and clinical improvements based on pain and functional outcomes.

Focusing on clinical studies, at the beginning of 2016, Tuakli-Wosurnu and colleagues reported for the first time pain, function and participant satisfaction outcomes for patients subjected to lumbar intradiscal PRP (Harvest PRP kit, Plymounth, MA, U.S) injection for discogenic LBP[20]. Related to pain outcome, these authors used a Numeric Rating Scale (NRS) to describe pain intensity. After two months follow-up, they reached the maximum mean NRS-pain reduction with statistically significant improvements showing for the participant who received the PRP therapy. Using an approximate comparison of VAS and NRS as two different systems of pain evaluation, higher pain reduction values were registered for Kirchner & Anitua although the maximum mean-VAS score was obtained at six months[18, 20]. However, Levi et. al.[21] using a PRP Harvest Smartprep kit (Harvest, Plymounth, MA, U.S) similar to that used by Tuakli-Wosurnu and coauthors, achieved maximum VAS improvement only in 47% of patients after 6 months with an even lower percentage of patient improvement and VAS score values than Kirchner & Anitua. Levi and colleagues reported as categorical success at least 50% decrease in VAS sore after PRP treatment.

In offering a serviceable comparison, it will be helpful to have three considerations in mind in interpreting the effective differences reported by the above authors: (1) the authors have used two different PRP preparation kits which include a red blood cell-rich and leukocyte PRP preparation (Harvest) and a PRGF formulation without leukocytes (PRGF-Endoret), (2) distinct amounts of PRP volumes to the infiltrated disc were used, and (3) different protocols of PRP total volume infiltration, including the injection of other compounds at the same IVD level, were also performed.

Also notable are the case reports such as Aufiero and colleagues[22], Monfett et. al.[19] and Mascarinas and coauthors[17] which report high VAS and NRS values of pain relieve at different times post- autologous PRP intradiscal procedure.

To date, limited scientific literature exists regarding clinical information on the effect of PRP treatment follow-up and the structural spinal regenerative process. In some cases, a well-known phenomenon for spontaneous regression of herniated lumbar disc material has been documented[63, 64] but the exact mechanism responsible for the regression of herniated IVD is still controversial. Mascarinas and coauthors[17] are the first to have mentioned for a case report of a MRI improvement in disc regeneration after 1 year of intradiscal PRP injection that correlates with improvement in LBP. On the same basis that MRI provides more detailed information about disc herniations, a case report is presented in this chapter showing considerable MRI improvements in IVD resorption after 2 years post PRGF treatment. As biological strategy developed for regeneration of the IVD, PRP may contribute to understanding of the mechanisms underlying the regression of protruded disc herniation. This case description could illustrate the need to achieve results using imaging techniques for lumbar spine such as conventional radiology, MRI or Computerized Tomography-CT[65, 66] in order to correlate improvements of pain and functional outcomes with vertebral related-structure regeneration in the field of spinal regenerative medicine.

Although the relative contribution of various structures in chronic LBP is varied, the pain source is commonly attributed to inflammatory response of FJs and/or IVDD and herniation of cells due to mechanical stress stimuli[57]. FJs and IVDs undergo chronic degenerative process in response to non-physiological mechanical stresses, bringing about collagen and aggrecan cleavage, a decrease of collagen and proteoglycan synthesis, an increase of proteases and cell death which parallels articular cartilage degeneration in OA and whose clinical hallmark is joint pain[35].

There are several potential mechanisms by which PRGF-Endoret infiltrations might either suppress or slow down the progress of IVD and facet degeneration. PRGF- Endoret is an autologous product that conveys a mimetic biomaterial, namely fibrin, which is embedded with a pool of growth factors (fibroblast growth factor (FGF), platelet-derived growth factor (PDGF), insulin-like growth factor-1 (IGF-1), vascular endothelial growth factor (VEGF), transforming growth factor-β (TGF-β), hepatocyte growth factor (HGF), connective tissue growth factor (CTGF), and nerve growth factor (NGF)) stemmed from activated platelets and plasma, and acting as a biological scaffold from which a sustained and a gradual delivery of GFs is released at the dysfunctional and degenerate sites instead of as a bolus delivery modality. Furthermore, a proteomic characterization study of PRGF fibrin matrix[44] reported a significant representation of acute-phase proteins, a strong network of interconnected proteins linked to the nuclear factor kB (NF-kB) pathway. This pathway is in part responsible for the inflammatory response of stressed cells such as chondrocytes, tenocytes, fibroblasts and macrophages. In addition, both, IVD and FJs share many developmental, functional, and biological features with articular cartilage and synovial joints[67].

In vitro, several of the GFs present in PRP such as TGF-β, IGF-1, and CTGF have been shown to exert a powerful effect on extracellular matrix (ECM) synthesis and proliferation in IVD[68, 69]. Furthermore, PDGF and IGF1 have been shown to exert a cell survival action on IVD cells[70]. In addition, through TGF-β or as a PRP whole product, PRP has been shown to promote the synthesis of ECM components such as proteoglycans and collagen in human NP cell cultures[67, 71]. More importantly, PRP administration using biodegradable gelatin hydrogel microspheres into degenerated IVD animal model resulted in a preservation of water and IDH, suppression of the IVD degeneration progression, and a synthesis of proteoclycans 8 weeks after the treatment, highlighting the importance of both delivering GFs in a sustained and gradual manner and the effectiveness for early IVDD intervention[72, 62]. Similar regenerative effects have been reported applying PRP to DDD in animal models[61, 73, 74].

Inflammation is a term that encompasses clinical, physiological, cellular, and molecular phenomena, with pain being the hallmark or the tip of the iceberg underlying pro-inflammatory cytokine release, ECM catabolism, and cell death. Thus, pain and inflammation are flip sides of the same coin, namely, tissue damage. Data coming from animal studies strongly suggest that proinflammatory cytokines such as tumor necrosis factor-α (TNF-α), interleukin-1β (IL-1β), and interleukin-6 (IL-6) are pivotal for the onset and maintenance of pain mainly stemmed from the damaged peripheral tissues[75]. In contrast, anti-inflammatory cytokines such as interleukin-4 (IL-4) and interleukin-10 (IL-10) have analgesic properties[75]. Some components present in PRGF-Endoret (HGF, lipoxin A4 (LXA4), platelet factor 4 (PF4), IGF-1, PDGF, and TGF-β)[48, 76-79] inhibit the NF-kB signaling pathway in several cell lineages including macrophages, chondrocytes, and fibroblasts. NF-kB plays an important role in mediating the gene expression of proinflammatory cytokines such as TNF-α, IL-1β, prostaglandin E2 (PGE2) and cyclooxygenase 1 (COX-1) and cyclooxygenase 2 (COX-2)[80].

As a consequence, it is reasonable to consider that PRGF-Endoret could exert an antiapoptotic, ECM-protective, antiinflammatory and pain reduction effect in a similar manner as in knee and hip synovial joints[52, 53, 81]. In macrophages, the inhibition of the NF-kB might contribute to the polarization from M1 to M2 phenotype, thereby favoring the resolution of inflammation and generating a switch in the ECM from a proinflammatory and algesic milieu to an anti-inflammatory and analgesic context. Furthermore, the in situ generated fibrin matrix would be gradually removed as a result of local activation of the tissue plasminogen activator/plasminogen system. This fibrinolytic remodeling process overlaps with the homing of survival fibrochondrocytes and migratory mesenchymal stem cell (MSCs), which might have been attracted by chemoattractans such as SDF-1, HGF, IGF-1, TGFβ or bFGF sequestered within the fibrin matrix and gradually released during the fibrinolytic-remodelling process[82].

Further case studies and clinical trials using standardized methods are necessary if we are to understand the efficacy of PRGF as a minimally invasive regenerative treatment for spinal pathologies where improvements are reliably measured with respect to pain reduction and recovery of structure and function.

Acknowledgements

We thank Jordi Catala´s radiology team, particularly Adolfo Florensa Suriñach and Laura Lasheras for their collaboration and contribution to the MRI analysis and measurements.

1. Edgar M. The nerve supply of the lumbar intervertebral disc. J Bone Joint Surg Br. 2007;89(9):1135-1139.

2. Vos T, Allen C, Arora M, et al. Global, regional, and national incidence, prevalence, and years lived with disability for 310 diseases and injuries, 1990-2015: a systematic analysis for the Global Burden of Disease Study 2015. Lancet. 2016;388(10053):1545-1602.

3. Mannion AF, Balague F, Pellise F, Cedraschi C. Pain measurement in patients with low back pain. Nat Clin Pr Rheumatol. 2007;3(11):610-618.

4. Hawker GA, Mian S, Kendzerska T, French M. Measures of adult pain: Visual Analog Scale for Pain (VAS Pain), Numeric Rating Scale for Pain (NRS Pain), McGill Pain Questionnaire (MPQ), Short-Form McGill Pain Questionnaire (SF-MPQ), Chronic Pain Grade Scale (CPGS), Short Form-36 Bodily Pain Scale (SF-36 BPS), and Measure of Intermittent and Constant Osteoarthritis Pain (ICOAP). Arthritis Care Res. 2011;63(SUPPL. 11):240-252.

5. Hwang SY, Lee JW, Lee GY, Kang HS. Lumbar facet joint injection: feasibility as an alternative method in high-risk patients. Eur Radiol. 2013;23(11):3153-3160. doi:10.1007/s00330-013-2921-z.

6. Adams MA, Dolan P. Intervertebral disc degeneration: Evidence for two distinct phenotypes. J Anat. 2012;221(6):497-506.

7. de Schepper EI, Damen J, van Meurs JB, et al. The association between lumbar disc degeneration and low back pain: the influence of age, gender, and individual radiographic features. Spine (Phila Pa 1976). 2010;35(5):531-536.

8. Urban JPG, Winlove CP. Pathophysiology of the intervertebral disc and the challeges for MRI. J Magn Reson Imaging. 2007;25(2):419-432.

9. Majumdar S, Link TM, Steinbach LS, Hu S, Kurhanewicz J. Diagnostic Tools and Imaging Methods in Intervertebral Disk Degeneration. Orthop Clin North Am. 2011;42(4):501-511.

10. Brayda-Bruno M, Tibiletti M, Ito K, et al. Advances in the diagnosis of degenerated lumbar discs and their possible clinical application. Eur Spine J. 2014;23(SUPPL. 3):S315-S323

11. Farshad-Amacker NA, Farshad M, Winklehner A, Andreisek G. MR imaging of degenerative disc disease. Eur J Radiol. 2015;84(9):1768-1776.

12. Wassenaar M, Van Rijn RM, Van Tulder MW, et al. Magnetic resonance imaging for diagnosing lumbar spinal pathology in adult patients with low back pain or sciatica: A diagnostic systematic review. Eur Spine J. 2012;21(2):220-227.

13. Panagopoulos J, Hush J, Steffens D, Hancock MJ. Do MRI Findings Change Over a Period of Up to One Year in Patients With Low Back Pain and/or Sciatica? A Systematic Review. Spine (Phila Pa 1976). 2016. doi:10.1097/brs.0000000000001790.

14. Fardon DF, Williams AL, Dohring EJ, Murtagh FR, Gabriel Rothman SL, Sze GK. Lumbar disc nomenclature: Version 2.0 Recommendations of the combined task forces of the North American Spine Society, the American Society of Spine Radiology and the American Society of Neuroradiology. Spine J. 2014;14(11):2525-2545.

15. Rajasekaran S, Venkatadass K, Naresh Babu J, Ganesh K, Shetty AP. Pharmacological enhancement of disc diffusion and differentiation of healthy, ageing and degenerated discs: Results from in-vivo serial post-contrast MRI studies in 365 human lumbar discs. Eur Spine J. 2008;17(5):626-643.

16. Basso M, Cavagnaro L, Zanirato A, et al. What is the clinical evidence on regenerative medicine in intervertebral disc degeneration? Musculoskelet Surg. 2017. doi:10.1007/s12306-017-0462-3.

17. Mascarinas A, Harrison J, Boachie-Adjei K, Lutz G. Regenerative Treatments for Spinal Conditions. Phys Med Rehabil Clin N Am. 2016;27(4):1003-1017.

18. Kirchner F, Anitua E. Intradiscal and intra-articular facet infiltrations with plasma rich in growth factors reduce pain in patients with chronic low back pain. J Craniovertebral Junction Spine. 2016;7(4):250-256.

19. Monfett M, Harrison J, Boachie-Adjei K, Lutz G. Intradiscal platelet-rich plasma (PRP) injections for discogenic low back pain: an update. Int Orthop. 2016;40(6):1321-13288.

20. Tuakli-Wosornu YA, Terry A, Boachie-Adjei K, et al. Lumbar Intradiskal Platelet-Rich Plasma (PRP) Injections: A Prospective, Double-Blind, Randomized Controlled Study. PM R. 2016;8(1):1-10.

21. Levi D, Horn S, Tyszko S, Levin J, Hecht-Leavitt C, Walko E. Intradiscal Platelet-Rich Plasma Injection for Chronic Discogenic Low Back Pain: Preliminary Results from a Prospective Trial. Pain Med. 2016;17(6):1010-1022.

22. Aufiero D, Vincent H, Sampson S, Bodor M. Regenerative Injection Treatment in the Spine: Review and Case Series with Platelet Rich Plasma. J stem cell Res Rev reports. 2015;2(1):1-9.

23. Oder B, Loewe M, Reisegger M, Lang W, Ilias W, Thurnher SA. CT-guided ozone/steroid therapy for the treatment of degenerative spinal disease—effect of age, gender, disc pathology and multi-segmental changes. Neuroradiology. 2008;50(9):777-785.

24. Nguyen C, Poiraudeau S, Rannou F. Vertebral subchondral bone. Osteoporos Int. 2012;23(8 SUPPL):857-860.

25. Moore RJ. The vertebral end-plate : what do we know ? Eur Spine J. 2000;9(2):92-96.

26. Grunhagen T, Shirazi-Adl A, Fairbank JCT, Urban JPG. Intervertebral Disk Nutrition: A Review of Factors Influencing Concentrations of Nutrients and Metabolites. Orthop Clin North Am. 2011;42(4):465-477.

27. Pattappa G, Li Z, Peroglio M, Wismer N, Alini M, Grad S. Diversity of intervertebral disc cells: Phenotype and function. J Anat. 2012;221(6):480-496.

28. Chan WCW, Au TYK, Tam V, Cheah KSE, Chan D. Coming together is a beginning: The making of an intervertebral disc. Birth Defects Res Part C - Embryo Today Rev. 2014;102(1):83-100.

29. Lotz JC, Fields AJ, Liebenberg EC. The role of the vertebral end plate in low back pain. Glob spine J. 2013;3(3):153-164.

30. Moore RJ. The vertebral endplate: Disc degeneration, disc regeneration. Eur Spine J. 2006;15(SUPPL. 3):333-337.

31. Wang Y, Videman T, Battié MC. ISSLS Prize Winner. Lumbar vertebral endplate lesions: associations with disc degeneration and back pain history. Spine (Phila Pa 1976). 2012;37(17):1490-1496.

32. Varlotta GP, Lefkowitz TR, Schweitzer M, et al. The lumbar facet joint: A review of current knowledge: Part 1: Anatomy, biomechanics, and grading. Skeletal Radiol. 2011;40(1):13-23.

33. Jaumard N V, Welch WC, Winkelstein BA. Spinal facet joint biomechanics and mechanotransduction in normal, injury and degenerative conditions. J Biomech Eng. 2011;133(7):1-31.

34. Alonso F, Kirkpatrick CM, Jeong W, et al. Lumbar Facet Tropism: A Comprehensive Review. World Neurosurg. 2017. doi:10.1016/j.wneu.2017.02.114.

35. Gellhorn AC, Katz JN, Suri P. Osteoarthritis of the spine: the facet joints. Nat Rev Rheumatol. 2013;9(4):216-224.

36. Cugat R, Cuscó X, Seijas R, et al. Biologic enhancement of cartilage repair: The role of platelet-rich plasma and other commercially available growth factors. Arthrosc J Arthrosc Relat Surg. 2015;31(4):777-783.

37. Wu PI-K, Diaz R, Borg-Stein J. Platelet-Rich Plasma. Phys Med Rehabil Clin N Am. 2016;27(4):825-853.

38. Filardo G, Kon E, Roffi A, Di Matteo B, Merli ML, Marcacci M. Platelet-rich plasma: why intra-articular? A systematic review of preclinical studies and clinical evidence on PRP for joint degeneration. Knee Surgery, Sport Traumatol Arthrosc. 2015;23(9):2459-2474.

39. Sánchez M, Delgado D, Sánchez P, et al. Platelet rich plasma and knee surgery. Biomed Res Int. 2014;2014:890630. doi:10.1155/2014/890630.

40. Anitua E, Sánchez M, Orive G. Potential of endogenous regenerative technology for in situ regenerative medicine. Adv Drug Deliv Rev. 2010;62(7-8):741-752.

41. Anitua E. Plasma rich in growth factors: preliminary results of use in the preparation of future sites for implants. Int J Oral Maxillofac Implants. 1999;14(4):529-535.

42. Anitua E, Andia I, Ardanza B, Nurden P, Nurden AT. Autologous platelets as a source of proteins for healing and tissue regeneration. Thromb Haemost. 2004;91(1):4-15.

43. Anitua E, Sanchez M, Nurden AT, et al. Autologous fibrin matrices: a potential source of biological mediators that modulate tendon cell activities. J Biomed Mater Res A. 2006;77(2):285-293.

44. Anitua E, Prado R, Azkargorta M, et al. High-throughput proteomic characterization of plasma rich in growth factors (PRGF-Endoret)-derived fibrin clot interactome. J Tissue Eng Regen Med. 2015;9(11):E1-E12.

45. Anitua E, Pascual C, Pérez-Gonzalez R, Orive G, Carro E. Intranasal PRGF-Endoret enhances neuronal survival and attenuates NF-κB-dependent inflammation process in a mouse model of Parkinson's disease. J Control Release. 2015;203:170-180.

46. Anitua E, Sánchez M, Aguirre JJ, Prado R, Padilla S, Orive G. Efficacy and safety of plasma rich in growth factors intra-articular infiltrations in the treatment of knee osteoarthritis. Arthroscopy. 2014;30(8):1006-1017.

47. Sanchez M, Guadilla J, Fiz N, Andia I. Ultrasound-guided platelet-rich plasma injections for the treatment of osteoarthritis of the hip. Rheumatol. 2012;51(1):144-150.

48. Bendinelli P, Matteucci E, Dogliotti G, et al. Molecular basis of anti-inflammatory action of platelet-rich plasma on human chondrocytes: mechanisms of NF-kappaB inhibition via HGF. J Cell Physiol. 2010;225(3):757-766.

49. Anitua E, Sanchez M, De la Fuente M, Zalduendo MM, Orive G. Plasma rich in growth factors (PRGF-Endoret) stimulates tendon and synovial fibroblasts migration and improves the biological properties of hyaluronic acid. Knee Surg Sports Traumatol Arthrosc. 2012;20(9):1657-1665.

50. Sanchez M, Anitua E, Azofra J, Aguirre JJ, Andia I. Intra-articular injection of an autologous preparation rich in growth factors for the treatment of knee OA: a retrospective cohort study. Clin Exp Rheumatol. 2008;26(5):910-913.

51. Wang-Saegusa A, Cugat R, Ares O, Seijas R, Cusco X, Garcia-Balletbo M. Infiltration of plasma rich in growth factors for osteoarthritis of the knee short-term effects on function and quality of life. Arch Orthop Trauma Surg. 2011;131(3):311-317.

52. Sanchez M, Fiz N, Azofra J, et al. A randomized clinical trial evaluating plasma rich in growth factors (PRGF-Endoret) versus hyaluronic acid in the short-term treatment of symptomatic knee osteoarthritis. Arthroscopy. 2012;28(8):1070-1078.

53. Vaquerizo V, Plasencia MÁ, Arribas I, et al. Comparison of intra-articular injections of plasma rich in growth factors (PRGF-Endoret) versus Durolane hyaluronic acid in the treatment of patients with symptomatic osteoarthritis: a randomized controlled trial. Arthroscopy. 2013;29(10):1635-1643.

54. Wang SZ, Rui YF, Tan Q, Wang C. Enhancing intervertebral disc repair and regeneration through biology: platelet-rich plasma as an alternative strategy. Arthritis Res Ther. 2013;15(5):220-228

55. DeLoach LJ, Higgins MS, Caplan AB, Stiff JL. The visual analog scale in the immediate postoperative period: intrasubject variability and correlation with a numeric scale. Anesth Analg. 1998;86(1):102-106.

56. Becker C, Heidersdorf S, Drewlo S, de Rodriguez SZ, Kramer J, Willburger RE. Efficacy of epidural perineural injections with autologous conditioned serum for lumbar radicular compression: an investigator-initiated, prospective, double-blind, reference-controlled study. Spine (Phila Pa 1976). 2007;32(17):1803-1808.

57. Chaturvedi A, Chaturvedi S, Sivasankar R. Image-guided lumbar facet joint infiltration in non-radicular low back pain. Indian J Radiol Imaging. 2009;19(1):29-34.

58. Formica M, Cavagnaro L, Formica C, Mastrogiacomo M, Basso M, Di Martino A. What is the preclinical evidence on platelet rich plasma and intervertebral disc degeneration? Eur Spine J. 2015;24(11):2377-2386.

59. Pirvu TN, Schroeder JE, Peroglio M, et al. Platelet-rich plasma induces annulus fibrosus cell proliferation and matrix production. Eur Spine J. 2014;23(4):745-753.

60. Masuda K, Lotz JC. New challenges for intervertebral disc treatment using regenerative medicine. Tissue Eng Part B Rev. 2010;16(1):147-158.

61. Obata S, Akeda K, Imanishi T, et al. Effect of autologous platelet-rich plasma-releasate on intervertebral disc degeneration in the rabbit anular puncture model: a preclinical study. Arthritis Res Ther. 2012;14(6):R241-R251.

62. Nagae M, Ikeda T, Mikami Y, et al. Intervertebral disc regeneration using platelet-rich plasma and biodegradable gelatin hydrogel microspheres. Tissue Eng. 2007;13(1):147-158.

63. Guinto FC, Hashim H, Stumer M. CT demonstration of disk regression after conservative therapy. Am J Neuroradiol. 1984;5(5):632-633.

64. Hakan T, Gurcan S. Spontaneous Regression of Herniated Lumbar Disc with New Disc Protrusion in the Adjacent Level. Case Rep Orthop. 2016;2016:1538072.

65. Maus T. Imaging the Back Pain Patient. Phys Med Rehabil Clin N Am. 2010;21(4):725-766.

66. Rivers WE, Rimmalapudi V, Heit JJ. Progress in Advanced Imaging Techniques for the Lumbar Spine. Curr Phys Med Rehabil Reports. 2016;4(2):87-98.

67. Chen W-H, Lo W-C, Lee J-J, et al. Tissue-engineered intervertebral disc and chondrogenesis using human nucleus pulposus regulated through TGF-beta1 in platelet-rich plasma. J Cell Physiol. 2006;209(3):744-754.

68. Gruber HE, Fisher Jr. EC, Desai B, Stasky AA, Hoelscher G, Hanley Jr. EN. Human intervertebral disc cells from the annulus: three-dimensional culture in agarose or alginate and responsiveness to TGF-beta1. Exp Cell Res. 1997;235(1):13-21.

69. Pratsinis H, Kletsas D. PDGF, bFGF and IGF-I stimulate the proliferation of intervertebral disc cells in vitro via the activation of the ERK and Akt signaling pathways. Eur Spine J. 2007;16(11):1858-1866.

70. Gruber HE, Norton HJ, Hanley Jr. EN. Anti-apoptotic effects of IGF-1 and PDGF on human intervertebral disc cells in vitro. Spine (Phila Pa 1976). 2000;25(17):2153-2157.

71. Akeda K, An HS, Pichika R, et al. Platelet-rich plasma (PRP) stimulates the extracellular matrix metabolism of porcine nucleus pulposus and anulus fibrosus cells cultured in alginate beads. Spine (Phila Pa 1976). 2006;31(9):959-966.

72. Sawamura K, Ikeda T, Nagae M, et al. Characterization of In Vivo Effects of Platelet-Rich Plasma and Biodegradable Gelatin Hydrogel Microspheres on Degenerated Intervertebral Discs. Tissue Eng Part A. 2009;15(12):3719-3727.

73. Masuda K, An HS. Prevention of disc degeneration with growth factors. Eur Spine J. 2006;15(Suppl. 3):422-432.

74. Masuda K. Biological repair of the degenerated intervertebral disc by the injection of growth factors. Eur Spine J. 2008;17 Suppl 4(Suppl 4):441-451.

75. Uceyler N, Schafers M, Sommer C. Mode of action of cytokines on nociceptive neurons. Exp Brain Res. 2009;196(1):67-78.

76. El-Sharkawy H, Kantarci A, Deady J, et al. Platelet-rich plasma: growth factors and pro- and anti-inflammatory properties. J Periodontol. 2007;78(4):661-669.

77. Montaseri A, Busch F, Mobasheri A, et al. IGF-1 and PDGF-bb suppress IL-1beta-induced cartilage degradation through down-regulation of NF-kappaB signaling: involvement of Src/PI-3K/AKT pathway. PLoS One. 2011;6(12):e28663.

78. Coudriet GM, He J, Trucco M, Mars WM, Piganelli JD. Hepatocyte growth factor modulates interleukin-6 production in bone marrow derived macrophages: implications for inflammatory mediated diseases. PLoS One. 2010;5(11):e15384.

79. van Buul GM, Koevoet WL, Kops N, et al. Platelet-rich plasma releasate inhibits inflammatory processes in osteoarthritic chondrocytes. Am J Sport Med. 2011;39(11):2362-2370.

80. Bonizzi G, Karin M. The two NF-kappaB activation pathways and their role in innate and adaptive immunity. Trends Immunol. 2004;25(6):280-288.

81. Anitua E, Sánchez M, Orive G, Padilla S. A biological therapy to osteoarthritis treatment using platelet-rich plasma. Expert Opin Biol Ther. 2013;13(8):1161-1172.

82. Ratajczak MZ, Majka M, Kucia M, et al. Expression of functional CXCR4 by muscle satellite cells and secretion of SDF-1 by muscle-derived fibroblasts is associated with the presence of both muscle progenitors in bone marrow and hematopoietic stem/progenitor cells in muscles. Stem Cells. 2003;21(3):363-371.

CHAPTER 16

Education and Standardization of Orthobiologics: Past, Present & Future

AUTHORS

Sampson S.[1,2], Vincent H.[3], Ambach M.[1,2]

[1] David Geffen School of Medicine at UCLA, Los Angeles, CA;
[2] The Orthohealing Center, Los Angeles, CA
[3] UC Davis Medical Center, Department of Physical Medicine and Rehabilitation, Sacramento, CA

SUMMARY

Since the beginning of Orthobiologics, the field has continued to evolve and grow, creating a preliminary framework for clinical application in musculoskeletal injuries. With increasing demand from an aging population, and numerous physicians incorporating the techniques into their existing practice, Orthobiologics have started to develop into almost a subspecialty of their own. However, the boom of Orthobiologics has not been matched with an equal surge in high level of evidence studies, leaving much of the field under researched. To date, four generations of Orthobiologics have been identified: Hyaluronic acid (HA), Platelet rich plasma (PRP), Bone marrow concentrate (BMC), and Adipose derived mesenchymal stem cells (aMSC). Although research is limited throughout the field as a whole, larger randomized trials are emerging for the earlier generations showing therapeutic efficacy for tendinopathies and joint osteoarthritis. As the field of Orthobiologics continues to rise, early investigators in the field have a responsibility to strive for cohesiveness and standardization in an attempt to provide the highest level of safety and therapeutic efficacy for patients. In order to satisfy this responsibility and progress in the field of Orthobiologics, it is important to establish a common definition of current Orthobiologic options, improve access to continuing education, and facilitate research collaboration throughout the global medical community.

E. Anitua et al. (eds.), *Platelet Rich Plasma in Orthopaedics and Sports Medicine*,
https://doi.org/10.1007/978-3-319-63730-3_16

1. INTRODUCTION

Over the past 10 years, the field of Orthobiologics has grown rapidly and started to establish a foundation as a potentially safe and efficacious alternative for a variety of musculoskeletal injuries, including osteoarthritis and chronic tendinopathies. With life expectancy on the rise, and an aging population of baby boomers, the demand for viable minimally invasive options is at an all time high. The increased demand has led to scores of physicians attempting to integrate regenerative options into their practices. However, as the exponential growth of Orthobiologics continues to skyrocket, coordinated research efforts haven't been able to match the same trajectory, resulting in a paucity of high level of evidence studies. As the volume of physicians utilizing Orthobiologics continues to rise, the burden is bestowed to early investigators in the field to strive for cohesiveness and standardization in an attempt to provide the highest level of safety and therapeutic efficacy for patients. In order to satisfy this responsibility and progress in the field of Orthobiologics, it is important to establish a common definition of current Orthobiologic options, improve access to continuing education, and facilitate research collaboration throughout the global medical community.

Orthobiologic treatments, as they pertain to the musculoskeletal field, are defined as any treatment modality that utilizes cellular components within the body's native cells, and redirects their use towards damaged or diseased tissues[1,2]. They are often concentrated versions of the body's natural occurring fluids, such as blood, bone marrow, or adipose tissue. Most commonly, they are utilized as an injectable treatment for joints, tendons, or ligaments. Most Orthobiologic injections are performed under image guidance, with either musculoskeletal ultrasound (fig. 1) or fluoroscopic guidance[3]. However, arthroscopy may also be utilized to provide high definition color visualization for accurate cellular deployment. Since the birth of the term Orthobiologics, the field has continued to expand underneath this umbrella term, however the core of Orthobiologic treatments can be classified by 4 generations: hyaluronic acid (HA), platelet rich plasma (PRP), bone marrow concentrate (BMC) and adipose derived mesenchymal stem cells (aMSC) or lipoaspirate.

2. HYALURONIC ACID

The first generation of Orthobiologics is considered to be hyaluronic acid (HA), which has been used as an intra articular injectable in the treatment of Osteoarthritis since the late 1990s. Hyaluronic acid is a naturally occurring protein in the body with viscoelastic properties which help to decrease frictional forces within synovial joints[4]. During joint degradation with Osteoarthritis, the natural concentration of HA within synovial fluid decreases and HA distribution shifts toward lower molecular weight variants, which leads to increased wear and tear on the joint[5]. In addition, intraarticular low molecular weight HA has also been associated with increased pain with OA[6]. The goal of intraarticular HA administration has been to restore the native HA concentration to its nonpathological concentration. However, many other theorized therapeutic mechanisms of HA have been postulated including shock absorp-

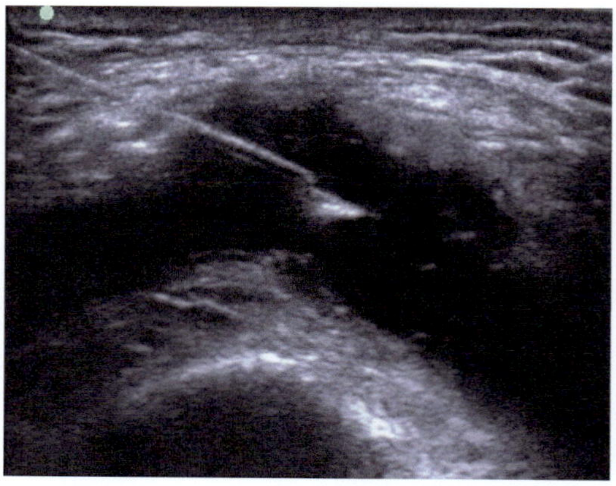

FIG. 1
Right suprapatellar bursae injection under ultrasound guidance.

tion, joint lubrication, anti-inflammatory effects, chrondroprotection, proteoglycan synthesis, and cartilage matrix alterations[5,7]. Although many intrinsic mechanisms have been shown, much of the chrondroprotective and anti-inflammatory mechanisms are correlated with HA binding to cluster of differentiation[44] (CD 44)[8], which inhibits the pro-inflammatory effects of interleukin-1beta, resulting in down regulation of many MMPs associated with cartilage degradation[9].

Although HA is native to intraarticular synovial fluid, the available injectable versions do not currently exist in autologous form, and specific formulations can differ depending on manufacturer and production technique. Some evidence suggests larger molecular weight HA to provide greater anti-inflammatory effects, proteoglycan synthesis, joint lubrication and viscoelastic maintenance compared to lower molecular weight HA counterparts[5]. In addition, avian-derived HA has shown a less favorable safety profile with increased risk for localized intraarticular pseudo septic reactions when compared to HA derived from biological fermentation[10].

The efficacy of intra-articular HA for the treatment of painful symptoms associated with osteoarthritis has been demonstrated in many clinical trials[7], while also providing a superior safety profile when compared to continuous NSAID use for pain control[11-13]. It has also been shown to lengthen the time from diagnosis of OA to time of knee arthroplasty in Medicare (generally senior) patients[14]. Recent OARSI guidelines for the treatment of osteoarthritis suggest "good" level of evidence for the treatment of OA with intraarticular hyaluronic acid[15]. However, previous metaanalyses have illustrated between-study heterogeneity in the efficacy of HA for osteoarthritis, with lower quality studies revealing more efficacious results[16,17], which provides further support for the necessity of high level of evidence studies in the field.

3. PLATELET RICH PLASMA

The second generation of Orthobiologics, platelet rich plasma, was the first autologous Orthobiologic. Although platelet rich plasma (PRP) didn't appear in the sports medicine literature until approximately 2006, it was first used by Ferrari et al in 1987 following open heart surgery[18], and has been used in many other medical fields including ENT, maxillofacial surgery, ophthalmology, urology, dentistry, cosmetic and neurosurgery and wound healing for quite some time. Theoretically, the potent concentration of platelets are injected into soft tissue, tendons, or intraarticularly to stimulate an inflammatory response, as they are comprised of an undifferentiated cocktail of anti-inflammatory, pro-inflammatory, anabolic, and catabolic mediators, in an attempt to elicit the body's natural healing response. The alpha granules within platelets act as the primary storage center for an array of growth factors including transforming growth factor beta (TGFbeta), vascular endothelial growth factor (VEGF), platelet-derived growth factor (PDGF), and epithelial growth factor (EGF) which are thought to be one of the main reasons for its regenerative potential[19,20]. Newer theories on the mechanism of PRP suggest that intraarticular application may potentially alter the entire joint environment through its effects on the signaling cascade, creating a more advantageous inflammatory environment for healing[21]. Changes in the cellular milieu may potentially exert therapeutic benefits by acting on localized joint tissue cells such as synoviocytes or meniscal cells, promoting chemoattraction of the body's native healing cells to damaged tissue[22,23], or through direct analgesic effect[24]. Although research continues to investigate such theories, the specific mechanism of action for PRP's clinical benefits is unknown. However, the etiology of its therapeutic effects are likely multifactorial and potentially variable across different tissue types.

To date, most of the literature on PRP consists of small case series with mixed results and an underwhelming volume of high-level evidence studies. However, as of late, larger randomized controlled trials have demonstrated superior efficacy in areas such as chronic tendinopathies[25,26] and knee osteoarthritis[27]. Research has also been published suggesting therapeutic benefits of combining PRP with other Orthobiologic treatments such as HA[28] or MSCs[29,30], as well as utilizing multiple Orthobiologics in a specific sequence as a treatment protocol for Osteoarthritis[31]. Furthermore, protocols have been established for post-PRP recovery and rehabilitative exercises establishing a preliminary framework for doctors and therapists to provide optimal treatment for return to sport[32].

Platelet rich plasma is derived from a patient's venous blood. Blood is drawn from a patient's vein, processed in a centrifuge, and a cellular concentrate, including the buffy coat, which contains the highest concentration of platelets[20], is extracted and used as an injectable treatment (fig. 2). Many researchers have started to emphasize that not all PRP is created equally. Currently, there are multiple cellular processing techniques for extracting PRP. Some practitioners utilize standardized PRP processing kits, which widely differ by manufacturer in regard to cellular composition and delivery methods. While other practitioners perform more individualized techniques, utilizing single and double spin centrifugation cycles and more precise laboratory procedures [32].

As of late, more clinicians are utilizing point of care cellular cytometry to analyze blood products and establish more cellular standardization of injectable PRP (fig. 3). In an attempt to facilitate uniform PRP classification, researchers have established the PLRA PRP classification, which classifies PRP based on the concentration of platelets, leukocyte, red blood cells, and activation technique[33]. Routine classification usage will lead to more customized PRP formulations to maximize therapeutic efficacy for specific musculoskeletal disorders and aide with interpretation of clinical trials. Initial research suggests that leukocyte poor- PRP may have stronger efficacy with intraarticular application[34,35]. As research continues to expand in the area of PRP, the newest generations of Orthobiologics are also beginning to establish a therapeutic framework.

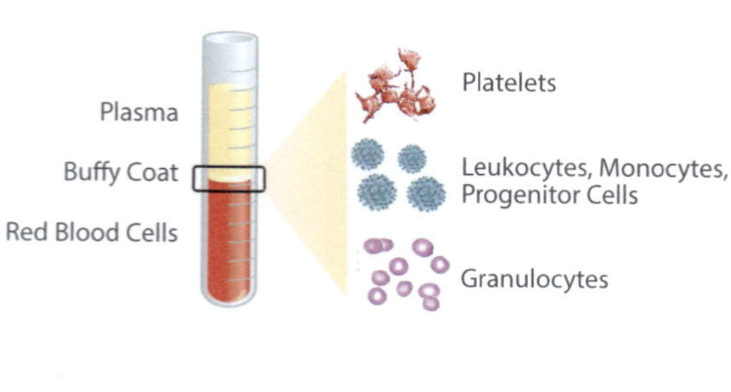

FIG. 2
After venous blood in processed in a centrifuge, it is separated into three layers: Plasma, Buffy coat, and Red blood cells. The buffy coat layer contains the Platelets, which store a variety of potent growth factors, thought to be a primary mechanism of PRP. (Photo courtesy of Ted Sand PhD)

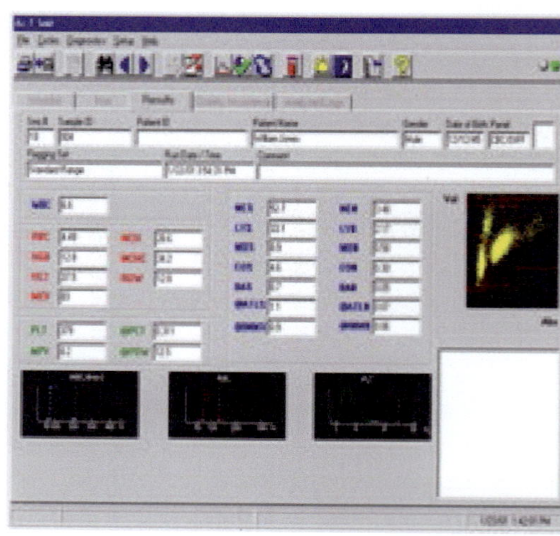

FIG. 3
This is a Cell cytometry analysis of venous blood using the Beckman Coulter ACT 5 DIFF CTL PLUS. This sample is an example of pre-centrifugation data, noted by the normal concentration of platelets. The cytometry data is used to classify PRP based on the PLRA PRP classification system.

4. BONE MARROW CONCENTRATE

Bone Marrow Concentrate (BMC) is considered the 3rd generation of Orthobiologic treatment. It has a potent mixture of mesenchymal stem cells (MSCs), hematopoietic cells, platelets, and cytokines noted for possessing anti-inflammatory, immunomodulatory, and chondrogenic properties, which act as the foundation for its regenerative potential[36]. Although the exact mechanism is unknown, it is hypothesized that the bone marrow concentrate milieu either induces differentiation and proliferation of resident stem cells, or possesses innate chondrogenic potential[36]. Bone Marrow is most commonly aspirated from the posterior iliac crest, utilizing ultrasound or fluoroscopic guidance. The bone marrow aspirate undergoes cellular processing via similar centrifugation mechanisms as platelet rich plasma. Physicians currently have multiple options for marrow concentration, either via standardized manufacturer kits or individualized laboratory techniques, very similar to the PRP options. Similar to PRP, the wide variability with bone marrow aspiration and concentration amongst physicians has added to the ambiguity with standardized treatments and research efforts. As one of the newer generations of Orthobiologics, BMC has a paucity of high-level studies or randomized trials. Although much of the early research has been mixed, some preliminary studies have demonstrated significant patient safety and efficacy with joint Osteoarthritis[31,36-39]. Select practitioners have started to utilize cell cytometry with BMC procedures, similar to the PLRA PRP classification, however no standardized classification exists currently.

5. ADIPOSE DERIVED MESENCHYMAL STEM CELLS (AMSCS)

As the field of Orthobiologics continues to develop, research efforts continue to refine our scientific understanding, opening possibilities for future generations of Orthobiologics. Recent literature has suggested a perivascular origin of MSCs, in the form of pericytes[40], which has led to exploration of other autologous sources of mesenchymal stem cells, including the most recent fourth generation of orthobiologics: Lipoaspirate/Adipose Derived Mesenchymal Stem Cells (or now termed "Medicinal Signaling Cells.)". Compared with BMC, processed lipoaspirate/adipose-derived MSCs (aMSCs) has advantages, in that it is procured in much larger quantities, and with less invasive techniques under local anesthesia and vacuum-assisted lipectomy. Similar to BMC, processed lipoaspirate has exhibited differentiation into chondro¬genic, osteogenic, adipogenic, myogenic, and neurogenic lineages in the presence of lineage-specific induction factors[41,42]. Although, some research has illustrated that aMSCs actually possess larger numbers of MSCs[40], data is mixed as to whether aMSCs have equivalent osteogenic potential as BMC[43,44]. In addition, aMSCs have been shown to be a more potent immunomodulator compared to bone marrow-derived MSCs, albeit the clinical benefit of such difference has yet to be determined[45]. Preliminary research suggests that aMSCs exhibit an anti-inflammatory effect on chrondrocytes and synoviocytes in patients with Osteoarthritis[46]. In addition, one study examined the combination of BMC with aMSC, although an additive effect was not detected[38].

6. FUTURE GENERATIONS

An emerging allogeneic Orthobiologic option, amniotic tissue, has also been shown to be a source of MSCs[47,48]. However, it does not possess the same resident cell volume as BMC and aMSCs[40]. Few human trials exist for human amniotic membrane applications, but small case studies have shown efficacy for elbow tendinopathy[49] and plantar fasciitis[50], while preliminary animal studies have suggested potentially positive applications for tendon injuries[51] and Osteoarthritis[52]. To date, this source of MSCs is the most under researched and one of the newest on the horizon.

7. FUTURE DIRECTIONS

The field of Orthobiologics is faced with the burden of balancing immense growth and diversification with a firm scientific foundation. And, as the separation widens, the lack of standardization and uniformity amongst practitioners is becoming significantly more apparent. All the more, the field as a whole continues to expand at a paramount rate, risking dilution of the core principles of Orthobiologics, if not matched by coordinated research efforts and continuing education. Currently, there are many national organizations and medical societies that have started to integrate orthobiologics, most noticeably AAOSM, Isokinetics, ICRS, as well as many other spine and orthopedic societies. In addition, educational conferences and workshops are beginning to form, teaching practitioners about emerging treatment options, cellular processing, and injection techniques. However, at the moment, the educational environment for Orthobiologics is disjointed, making it difficult for clinicians to not only stay up to date with emerging research, but also gain the hands-on skills needed to safely execute the treatments in their practices.

Rather than providing small breakout sessions as part of a larger broad-spectrum orthopaedic conference, the most comprehensive events in the field of Orthobiologics provide physicians and surgeons with a one-stop-shop for all things Orthobiologics. Most noticeably, The Orthobiologic Institute (TOBI) has established itself as the premier annual event, focusing solely on PRP, BMC, Lipoaspirate, and emerging areas of Orthobiologics. Starting with its first annual symposium just 8 years ago, and a small group of 25 physicians, the annual meeting has swelled to over 500 attendees, representing more than 30 countries, encompassing physicians and surgeons from a myriad of synergistic specialties. The TOBI annual symposium not only provides the most up to date research, but also offers world-class hands-on training at one of the largest cadaver labs in the world, taught by leaders in the field.

In the future, conferences and national organizations that provide continuing education in the field of Orthobiologics may potentially collaborate to form a board certification or certificate of competency for such specialties. Although most physicians are learning Orthobiologic principles after residency training through conferences and workshops, it is likely that the younger generation of physicians will start to gain earlier exposure to Orthobiologics in certain medical specialties such as Physical Medicine and Rehabilitation, Pain Management, Sports Medicine, or Orthopaedic Surgery. In addition, numerous non-accredited fellowship opportunities have started to form as of late, providing new residency graduates with more specialty training underneath an Orthobiologic mentor.

Because of the extensive treatment diversity across the industry, future research efforts for Orthobiologics will incorporate international data registry software to monitor patient outcomes, track patient safety, and analyze cellular compositions for biologic formulations. Recently, a not for profit foundation, the Regenerative Orthobiologics Registry, was started by the coauthors of this chapter to provide a framework for collecting patient data to elevate the field as a whole and improve the safety and quality of Orthobiologic treatments. Larger amounts of PRP, BMC, and Lipoaspirate data will allow for improved efficacy and standardization of treatments, with higher power research studies and more treatment specificity. It is also possible that predictive analytics and integrating Precision Medicine, a medical model that proposes customization of healthcare to each individual, may help guide research efforts and formulate treatment protocols in the future.

As a whole, the field of Orthobiologics is far from where it started. Although, even with some two decades worth of expansion and scientific discovery, the four distinct generations of Orthobiologics lack a true definition as to what they are, and how they should be used. As of now, we can confidently state that hyaluronic acid, platelet rich plasma, bone marrow concentrate, and adipose tissue have established a place for themselves in the future of Orthobiologics. However, investigation into their therapeutic applications, optimal cellular compositions, and treatment protocols lag behind their widespread use. With more commercial biologic options rapidly surfacing, it behooves the industry to establish a proper framework for preexisting biologic options, before moving onto to newer injectables. As the current state of Orthobiologics would have it, the burden lies with the physician to increase their education through annual conferences, such as The Orthobiologic Institute (TOBI), and pursue more collaborative research efforts. Although we cannot predict where the field will be in another 10 years time, by establishing more opportunities for physician education and coordinated research, we can help increase Orthobiologic's credibility and insure its longevity as a minimally invasive tool to combat musculoskeletal disease.

1. Malanga G, Abdelshahed D, Jayaram P. Orthobiologic Interventions Using Ultrasound Guidance. Physical medicine and rehabilitation clinics of North America. 2016;27:717-31.

2. Sampson S VH, Aufiero D. Orthobiologics: A new generation of orthopaedics. Orthopreneur. 2014.

3. Islam A. Ultrasound: a new tool for precisely locating posterior iliac crests to obtain adequate bone marrow trephine biopsy specimen. Journal of clinical pathology. 2013;66:718-20.

4. Miller LE, Block JE. US-Approved Intra-Articular Hyaluronic Acid Injections are Safe and Effective in Patients with Knee Osteoarthritis: Systematic Review and Meta-Analysis of Randomized, Saline-Controlled Trials. Clinical medicine insights. Arthritis and musculoskeletal disorders. 2013;6:57-63.

5. Altman RD, Manjoo A, Fierlinger A, Niazi F, Nicholls M. The mechanism of action for hyaluronic acid treatment in the osteoarthritic knee: a systematic review. BMC Musculoskelet Disord. 2015;16:321.

6. Band PA, Heeter J, Wisniewski HG, et al. Hyaluronan molecular weight distribution is associated with the risk of knee osteoarthritis progression. Osteoarthritis and cartilage / OARS, Osteoarthritis Research Society. 2015;23:70-6.

7. Moreland LW. Intra-articular hyaluronan (hyaluronic acid) and hylans for the treatment of osteoarthritis: mechanisms of action. Arthritis research & therapy. 2003;5:54-67.

8. Karna E, Miltyk W, Surazynski A, Palka JA. Protective effect of hyaluronic acid on interleukin-1-induced deregulation of beta1-integrin and insulin-like growth factor-I receptor signaling and collagen biosynthesis in cultured human chondrocytes. Mol Cell Biochem. 2008;308:57-64.

9. Waddell DD, Kolomytkin OV, Dunn S, Marino AA. Hyaluronan suppresses IL-1beta-induced metalloproteinase activity from synovial tissue. Clinical orthopaedics and related research. 2007;465:241-8.

10. Goldberg VM, Coutts RD. Pseudoseptic reactions to hylan viscosupplementation: diagnosis and treatment. Clinical orthopaedics and related research. 2004:130-7.

11. Bannuru RR, Vaysbrot EE, Sullivan MC, McAlindon TE. Relative efficacy of hyaluronic acid in comparison with NSAIDs for knee osteoarthritis: a systematic review and meta-analysis. Seminars in arthritis and rheumatism. 2014;43:593-9.

12. Bannuru RR, Natov NS, Dasi UR, Schmid CH, McAlindon TE. Therapeutic trajectory following intra-articular hyaluronic acid injection in knee osteoarthritis--meta-analysis. Osteoarthritis and cartilage / OARS, Osteoarthritis Research Society. 2011;19:611-9.

13. Colen S, van den Bekerom MP, Mulier M, Haverkamp D. Hyaluronic acid in the treatment of knee osteoarthritis: a systematic review and meta-analysis with emphasis on the efficacy of different products. BioDrugs : clinical immunotherapeutics, biopharmaceuticals and gene therapy. 2012;26:257-68.

14. Ong KL, Anderson AF, Niazi F, Fierlinger AL, Kurtz SM, Altman RD. Hyaluronic Acid Injections in Medicare Knee Osteoarthritis Patients Are Associated With Longer Time to Knee Arthroplasty. The Journal of arthroplasty. 2016;31:1667-73.

15. McAlindon TE, Bannuru RR, Sullivan MC, et al. OARSI guidelines for the non-surgical management of knee osteoarthritis. Osteoarthritis and cartilage / OARS, Osteoarthritis Research Society. 2014;22:363-88.

16. Wang CT, Lin J, Chang CJ, Lin YT, Hou SM. Therapeutic effects of hyaluronic acid on osteoarthritis of the knee. A meta-analysis of randomized controlled trials. The Journal of bone and joint surgery. American volume. 2004;86-a:538-45.

17. Lo GH, LaValley M, McAlindon T, Felson DT. Intra-articular hyaluronic acid in treatment of knee osteoarthritis: a meta-analysis. JAMA : the journal of the American Medical Association. 2003;290:3115-21.

18. Ferrari M, Zia S, Valbonesi M, et al. A new technique for hemodilution, preparation of autologous platelet-rich plasma and intraoperative blood salvage in cardiac surgery. The International journal of artificial organs. 1987;10:47-50.

19. Alsousou J, Thompson M, Hulley P, Noble A, Willett K. The biology of platelet-rich plasma and its application in trauma and orthopaedic surgery: a review of the literature. The Journal of bone and joint surgery. British volume. 2009;91:987-96.

20. Sampson S, Gerhardt M, Mandelbaum B. Platelet rich plasma injection grafts for musculoskeletal injuries: a review. Current reviews in musculoskeletal medicine. 2008;1:165-74.

21. Filardo G, Kon E, Roffi A, Di Matteo B, Merli ML, Marcacci M. Platelet-rich plasma: why intra-articular? A systematic review of preclinical studies and clinical evidence on PRP for joint degeneration. Knee surgery, sports traumatology, arthroscopy : official journal of the ESSKA. 2015;23:2459-74.

22. Kruger JP, Hondke S, Endres M, Pruss A, Siclari A, Kaps C. Human platelet-rich plasma stimulates migration and chondrogenic differentiation of human subchondral progenitor cells. Journal of orthopaedic research : official publication of the Orthopaedic Research Society. 2012;30:845-52.

23. Kruger JP, Ketzmar AK, Endres M, Pruss A, Siclari A, Kaps C. Human platelet-rich plasma induces chondrogenic differentiation of subchondral progenitor cells in polyglycolic acid-hyaluronan scaffolds. Journal of biomedical materials research. Part B, Applied biomaterials. 2014;102:681-92.

24. Lee HR, Park KM, Joung YK, Park KD, Do SH. Platelet-rich plasma loaded hydrogel scaffold enhances chondrogenic differentiation and maturation with up-regulation of CB1 and CB2. Journal of controlled release : official journal of the Controlled Release Society. 2012;159:332-7.

25. Mishra AK, Skrepnik NV, Edwards SG, et al. Efficacy of platelet-rich plasma for chronic tennis elbow: a double-blind, prospective, multicenter, randomized controlled trial of 230 patients. The American journal of sports medicine. 2014;42:463-71.

26. Rha DW, Park GY, Kim YK, Kim MT, Lee SC. Comparison of the therapeutic effects of ultrasound-guided platelet-rich plasma injection and dry needling in rotator cuff disease: a randomized controlled trial. Clinical rehabilitation. 2013;27:113-22.

27. Patel S, Dhillon MS, Aggarwal S, Marwaha N, Jain A. Treatment with platelet-rich plasma is more effective than placebo for knee osteoarthritis: a prospective, double-blind, randomized trial. The American journal of sports medicine. 2013;41:356-64.

28. Lana JF, Weglein A, Sampson SE, et al. Randomized controlled trial comparing hyaluronic acid, platelet-rich plasma and the combination of both in the treatment of mild and moderate osteoarthritis of the knee. Journal of stem cells & regenerative medicine. 2016;12:69-78.

29. Koh YG, Kwon OR, Kim YS, Choi YJ. Comparative outcomes of open-wedge high tibial osteotomy with platelet-rich plasma alone or in combination with mesenchymal stem cell treatment: a prospective study. Arthroscopy : the journal of arthroscopic & related surgery : official publication of the Arthroscopy Association of North America and the International Arthroscopy Association. 2014;30:1453-60.

30. Pak J, Lee JH, Kartolo WA, Lee SH. Cartilage Regeneration in Human with Adipose Tissue-Derived Stem Cells: Current Status in Clinical Implications. BioMed research international. 2016;2016:4702674.

31. Sampson S, Smith J, Vincent H, Aufiero D, Zall M, Botto-van-Bemden A. Intra-articular bone marrow concentrate injection protocol: short-term efficacy in osteoarthritis. Regenerative medicine. 2016;11:511-20.

32. Maffulli N. Platelet Rich Plasma in Musculoskeletal Practice. 2016.

33. Mautner K, Malanga GA, Smith J, et al. A call for a standard classification system for future biologic research: the rationale for new PRP nomenclature. PM & R : the journal of injury, function, and rehabilitation. 2015;7:S53-9.

34. Braun HJ, Kim HJ, Chu CR, Dragoo JL. The effect of platelet-rich plasma formulations and blood products on human synoviocytes: implications for intra-articular injury and therapy. The American journal of sports medicine. 2014;42:1204-10.

35. Riboh JC, Saltzman BM, Yanke AB, Fortier L, Cole BJ. Effect of Leukocyte Concentration on the Efficacy of Platelet-Rich Plasma in the Treatment of Knee Osteoarthritis. The American journal of sports medicine. 2016;44:792-800.

36. Sampson S, Botto-van Bemden A, Aufiero D. Autologous bone marrow concentrate: review and application of a novel intra-articular orthobiologic for cartilage disease. The Physician and sportsmedicine. 2013;41:7-18.

37. Shapiro SA, Kazmerchak SE, Heckman MG, Zubair AC, O'Connor MI. A Prospective, Single-Blind, Placebo-Controlled Trial of Bone Marrow Aspirate Concentrate for Knee Osteoarthritis. The American journal of sports medicine. 2017;45:82-90.

38. Centeno C, Pitts J, Al-Sayegh H, Freeman M. Efficacy of autologous bone marrow concentrate for knee osteoarthritis with and without adipose graft. BioMed research international. 2014;2014:370621.

39. Centeno CJ, Freeman MD. Percutaneous injection of autologous, culture-expanded mesenchymal stem cells into carpometacarpal hand joints: a case series with an untreated comparison group. Wiener medizinische Wochenschrift (1946). 2014;164:83-7.

40. Murphy MB, Moncivais K, Caplan AI. Mesenchymal stem cells: environmentally responsive therapeutics for regenerative medicine. Experimental & molecular medicine. 2013;45:e54.

41. Zuk PA, Zhu M, Mizuno H, et al. Multilineage cells from human adipose tissue: implications for cell-based therapies. Tissue engineering. 2001;7:211-28.

42. Rodriguez AM, Elabd C, Amri EZ, Ailhaud G, Dani C. The human adipose tissue is a source of multipotent stem cells. Biochimie. 2005;87:125-8.

43. Park SH, Sim WY, Min BH, Yang SS, Khademhosseini A, Kaplan DL. Chip-based comparison of the osteogenesis of human bone marrow- and adipose tissue-derived mesenchymal stem cells under mechanical stimulation. PloS one. 2012;7:e46689.

44. Hung BP, Hutton DL, Kozielski KL, et al. Platelet-Derived Growth Factor BB Enhances Osteogenesis of Adipose-Derived But Not Bone Marrow-Derived Mesenchymal Stromal/Stem Cells. Stem cells. 2015;33:2773-84.

45. Melief SM, Zwaginga JJ, Fibbe WE, Roelofs H. Adipose tissue-derived multipotent stromal cells have a higher immunomodulatory capacity than their bone marrow-derived counterparts. Stem cells translational medicine. 2013;2:455-63.

46. Manferdini C, Maumus M, Gabusi E, et al. Adipose-derived mesenchymal stem cells exert antiinflammatory effects on chondrocytes and synoviocytes from osteoarthritis patients through prostaglandin E2. Arthritis and rheumatism. 2013;65:1271-81.

47. Si YL, Zhao YL, Hao HJ, Fu XB, Han WD. MSCs: Biological characteristics, clinical applications and their outstanding concerns. Ageing research reviews. 2011;10:93-103.

48. Diaz-Prado S, Muinos-Lopez E, Hermida-Gomez T, et al. Human amniotic membrane as an alternative source of stem cells for regenerative medicine. Differentiation; research in biological diversity. 2011;81:162-71.

49. Aufiero D, Sampson S, Onishi K, Bemden V. Treatment of Medial and Lateral Elbow Tendinosis with an Injectable Amniotic Membrane Allograft–A Retrospective Case Series. J Pain Relief. 2016;5:2167-0846.10002.

50. Zelen CM, Poka A, Andrews J. Prospective, randomized, blinded, comparative study of injectable micronized dehydrated amniotic/chorionic membrane allograft for plantar fasciitis--a feasibility study. Foot & ankle international. 2013;34:1332-9.

51. He Q, Li Q, Chen B, Wang Z. Repair of flexor tendon defects of rabbit with tissue engineering method. Chinese journal of traumatology = Zhonghua chuang shang za zhi. 2002;5:200-8.

52. Willett NJ, Thote T, Lin AS, et al. Intra-articular injection of micronized dehydrated human amnion/chorion membrane attenuates osteoarthritis development. Arthritis research & therapy. 2014;16:R47.

MIX
Papier aus verantwortungsvollen Quellen
Paper from responsible sources
FSC® C105338

If you have any concerns about our products,
you can contact us on
ProductSafety@springernature.com

In case Publisher is established outside the EU,
the EU authorized representative is:
Springer Nature Customer Service Center GmbH
Europaplatz 3, 69115 Heidelberg, Germany

Printed by Libri Plureos GmbH
in Hamburg, Germany